PRAISE FOR KIMBERLY SNYDER AND THE *BEAUTY DETOX* SERIES

"The Beauty Detox Power *teaches you how to get to the root of weight issues and let go of blocks to create sustained success in many areas of your life. Kimberly's philosophy reveals that the mental, emotional and spiritual aspects of you, your diet and health are one."*

—Deepak Chopra

"*Kimberly's philosophies about nutrition have really helped me maintain a healthy lifestyle while managing a very busy life. Her program isn't focused on just losing weight; it's more about a complete mind, body and health experience. I start every day with a Glowing Green Smoothie and so does my whole family!"*

—Reese Witherspoon

"*Kimberly Snyder's* The Beauty Detox Solution *intelligently highlights the importance of incorporating large amounts of greens and plant foods in our diets. She also provides the reader with innovative ways to maximize their consumption."*

—Dr. Mehmet Oz

"*I don't like to diet, I like to eat right, and that's what Kim's philosophy is all about. Her food program has had such an impact not only on my body but my health in general. She's brilliant."*

—Drew Barrymore

"*I love Kimberly's holistic approach to health and beauty from the inside out. I start almost every single day with her GGS because it keeps me nourished and energized."*

—Kerry Washington

"*Kimberly's outlook on nutrition stresses lifestyle changes, not fad diets, which was a big awakening for me. I have never felt better since I've been on her program!"*

—Hilary Duff

"*Kimberly Snyder changed my life! She is totally amazing!"*

—Amanda Seyfried

THE BEAUTY DETOX POWER

Nourish Your Mind and Body for Weight Loss and Discover True Joy

KIMBERLY SNYDER, C.N.

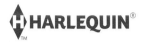

THE BEAUTY **DETOX** POWER

ISBN-13: 978-0-373-89318-8

Photo paired with True Power definition (page vii), Chapter 3 opener photo (page 21), silhouette photo (page 25), Chapter 11 opener photo (page 135), Vishuddha opener photo (page 171), Ajna opener photo (page 177), Sahasrara opener photo (page 184), women seated photo (page 197), yoga photo (page 217), gorilla photo (page 257), Cedric photo (page 262), giraffe photo (page 321) and back cover photo by John Pisani.

Photo of Kuan Yin on page 349 by Kimberly Snyder.

All other photography, including cover shot, by Ylva Erevall.

The health advice presented in this book is intended only as an informative resource guide to help you make informed decisions; it is not meant to replace the advice of a physician or to serve as a guide to self-treatment. Always seek competent medical help for any health condition or if there is any question about the appropriateness of a procedure or health recommendation.

Library of Congress Cataloging-in-Publication Data
Snyder, Kimberly.
  The beauty detox power : nourish your mind and body for weight loss and discover true joy/ Kimberly Snyder, C.N.
     pages cm
  Includes bibliographical references and index.
  ISBN 978-0-373-89318-8 (paperback)
1. Detoxification (Health) 2. Nutrition. 3. Mind and body. 4. Reducing diets—Recipes. 5. Self-care, Health. I. Title.
  RA784.5.S656 2014
  613.2—dc23
          2014033764

www.Harlequin.com

Printed in U.S.A.

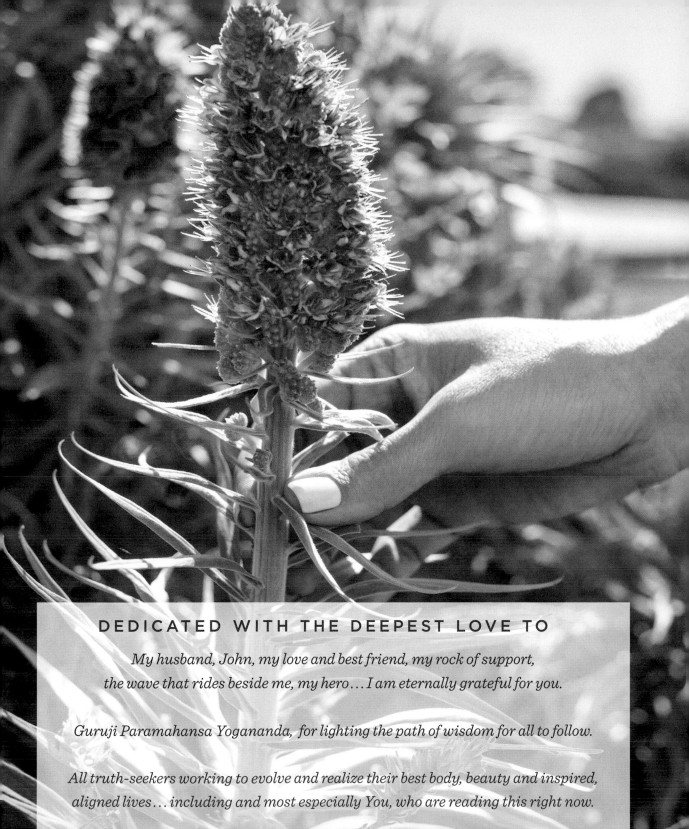

DEDICATED WITH THE DEEPEST LOVE TO

*My husband, John, my love and best friend, my rock of support,
the wave that rides beside me, my hero… I am eternally grateful for you.*

Guruji Paramahansa Yogananda, for lighting the path of wisdom for all to follow.

*All truth-seekers working to evolve and realize their best body, beauty and inspired,
aligned lives… including and most especially You, who are reading this right now.*

You realize that all along there was

something tremendous within you,

and you did not know it.

—Paramahansa Yogananda

True Power

Arises from the alignment between
your thoughts, core beliefs, words and actions.

Comes from within, not from controlling or trying
to grasp at anything outside of you or ego-based.

Allows you to become extraordinarily powerful
and able to shape the body and life you want.

Enables you to surpass perceived limitations.

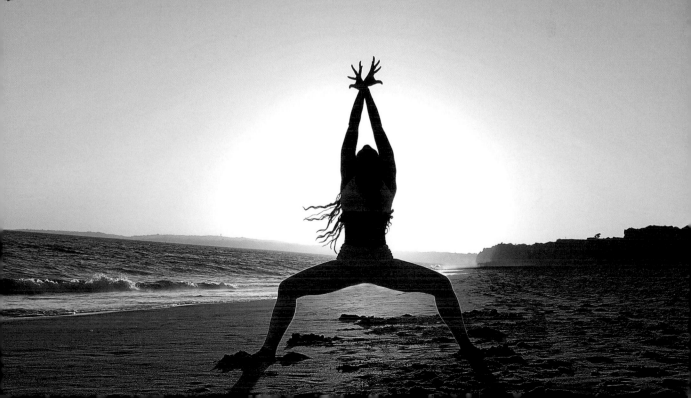

Contents

Introduction

Dearest Friend,

It would have been much easier for me to write another straight food and diet book. Easier because many expected that and easier because what I ended up writing for this book was much more challenging. But easier didn't feel right to me. I wrote this book because there was a burning drive inside me pushing me to do so.

Weight, health and beauty are problematic areas in most of our lives. You don't have to peer too hard to see societal evidence of this: countless diets, weight-loss products and infomercials; the increasing rate of eating disorders, especially among our younger sisters; and even extreme surgical measures, such as liposuction and gastric bypass surgery. This is not even to point out the alarming number of largely lifestyle-induced diseases.

Until now we've been conditioned to think of food as the primary factor in our weight and health. But there's a big truth that is largely unacknowledged in our modern world. You are a whole being made of interconnected aspects. For instance, you may have heard the gut referred to as the "second brain" given how closely the two interact, but you may not realize that repeated emotions and thoughts, both conscious and subconscious, affect the workings of your gut and digestion and can cause you to hold on to excess weight.

In fact, your mind can help you create the body you want, or it can sabotage your efforts to attain your ideal weight and even your beauty. My observations of clients, readers, friends and people all around me (not to mention myself), as well as thorough research, ultimately became the core teaching of this book: There is much more to weight loss, health and beauty beyond food.

I'm not just talking about the well-known phenomenon of emotional eating. Rather, how all parts of your being—your mental, emotional, spiritual and physical aspects—are interconnected and work together to shape your physical body in a rather shocking way. The exciting news is that when you understand how this works, you can actually influence the process with the internal power you already possess.

True power is when you connect to the wholeness that is you, and there is synergy between the mental, physical, emotional and spiritual aspects of your being, and complete alignment between your thoughts (such as "I am healthy and look great," or "I am fat"), core beliefs (such as "Losing weight and keeping it off is hard" or "At a certain age it gets even more difficult to lose weight"), words (that you say to others and about yourself) and actions (such as what you choose to eat). When this happens, you embrace the ability to surpass any limitations you may have put on yourself in the past. You become in touch with your pure, creative power, and you can create anything you want, whether it be improved health, beauty, even the body shape you desire.

Sustained weight loss, optimal health and beauty are not as simple as calories in, working out just like this, and outputting into a particular body shape. We're not robots. I think deep down you've always known that, even as you kept trying new diets. You might be able to list the weight you want to achieve or describe the way you want your body to look. But you may not be aware of the deep, underlying thoughts, beliefs, words and actions that are disconnected from what really serves you and that create enormous struggle, preventing what you want to achieve. Some estimate that your body shape is determined by about 70-80% diet, and 20-30% by exercise.[1] But *The Beauty Detox Power* pulls a third factor into the mix. It's time to turn your mind back on. Your thoughts are essential to your success.

When you have unity between the parts of your being as a whole, which is part of what true power is about, not only will you learn how to sustain weight loss without struggle and force, but you will

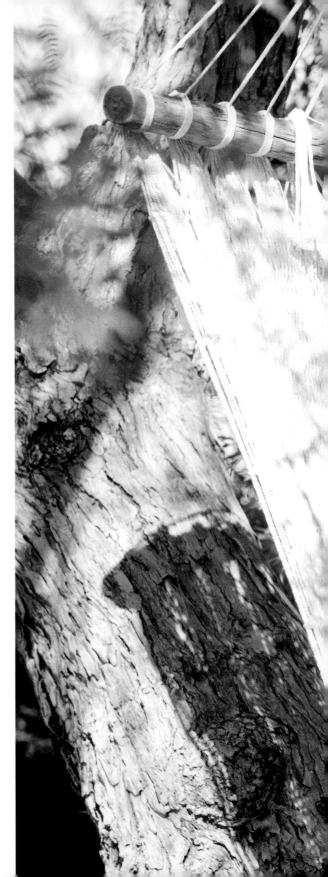

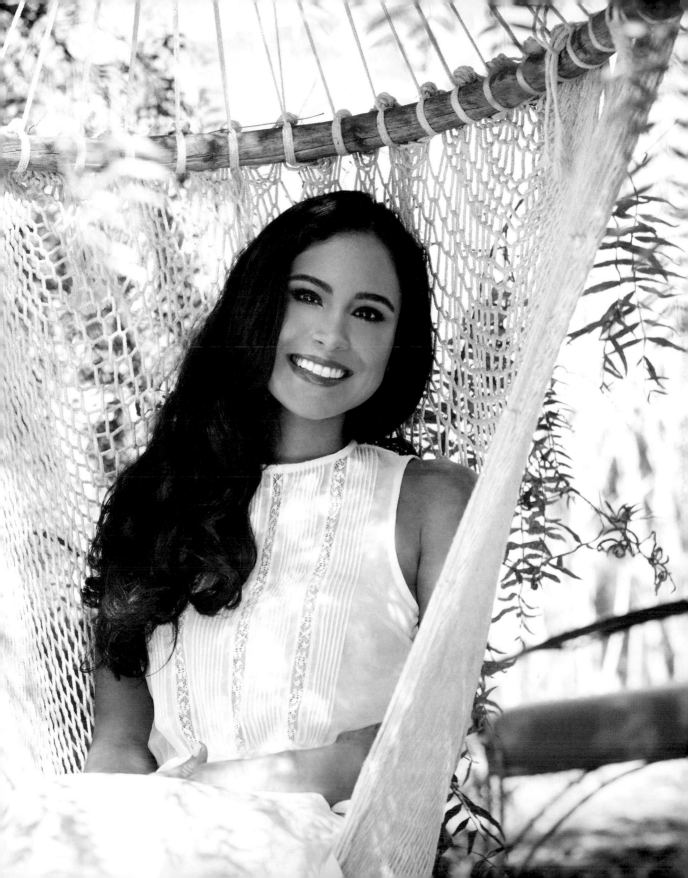

also discover true joy. Joy is largely missing from a vast majority of people's lives. You can buy distractions and temporary pleasures, but you can't buy authentic joy. It can come only from within, and when it does, life keeps getting better and better.

Food is, of course, an essential and important tool in the journey to health, but it's only the first step. This book will explain all the "mysteries" that so many readers and followers on my social media channels are constantly asking me about, such as "How do you stay toned without working out except for yoga?" and "How do you keep your weight down so easily?" and "How are you always so happy?" You'll learn how to create all of this as well as what you specifically want in your own life.

The first time the idea of this book surged out of me—it was clearly not my doing—was during the editing of *The Beauty Detox Foods*. I was swamped with work, but I paused to write the outline for this book because I felt an extremely powerful inner force pushing me to do so. Over a year later, when I was approached to write another book, I wrote an outline without hesitation. Then I remembered the first outline I had written a year earlier, which I had totally forgotten about. I searched for it on my computer and when I pulled it up on my computer screen and compared it to the second outline, I was stunned to discover that the outlines were virtually identical. There was no way I could ignore such clear intuition. This was what I had to write.

This book came straight from my heart. You will find many more personal stories about me and Beauty Detox Transformation stories from individuals I have observed and worked with (with their names changed for privacy) here than in the other *Beauty Detox* books, because I think that is the best way to teach this information. You'll see a lot of quotes from and references to the great yoga guru Paramahansa Yogananda throughout this book, as he has had a tremendous influence on my philosophy. The first time I went to Rishikesh, India, I wandered into a bookshop and was immediately drawn to one of Yogananda's books, *Scientific Healing Affirmations*. As I opened it up and started to read it, I felt a fire of energy surge up my spine, and it was very clear to me that he was going to be my teacher.

In 1920 Yogananda founded the Self-Realization Fellowship, and in the years since, this organization has shared Kriya yoga techniques, based on meditation, with hundreds of thousands of people, including Mahatma Gandhi. Steve Jobs, cofounder and former CEO of Apple Inc., was so inspired by Yogananda throughout his life that he arranged for each of the hundreds of guests at his memorial service to receive a copy of Yogananda's *Autobiography of a Yogi* as his last gift.

Please keep an open heart and mind as you read these pages, because some of this information may be completely new to you. Even the notion that there is more to how you look and feel beyond food may be shocking . . . but I promise you that if you remain receptive, you will benefit immensely from this knowledge.

I organized this book into sections called Power Alignment Shifts, and these sections into chapters. Each of these interrelated sections will help you realize your highest power. Starting with Power Alignment Shift 2, the chapters include a summary of the tips discussed, as well as Power Affirmations to say aloud or silently to yourself to help you start changing your creative thought patterns. And just as this book illustrates how interconnected our mind and body are, the teachings within its covers are all interconnected. You will get far more out of this book if you work through it in its entirety at your own pace, pausing and rereading sections as necessary.

I know it's easy to skip to those parts that interest you most, but I want you to feel and look your best and experience your best life, and that's possible only if you understand all this information. So please set aside a little time to read the entire book thoroughly. You will be very happy that you did!

Thank you for being along with me for this journey. I believe that if you are reading this right now, you were meant to have access to this information. I am deeply honored and grateful to offer this book to you, and it is my sincere intention that it will truly benefit and support you in reaching your highest potential.

Now it's time to start claiming your power and creating your best body, beauty and life. Turn the page and off we go. . . .

With immense gratitude and love,

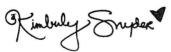

Discover Your True Power

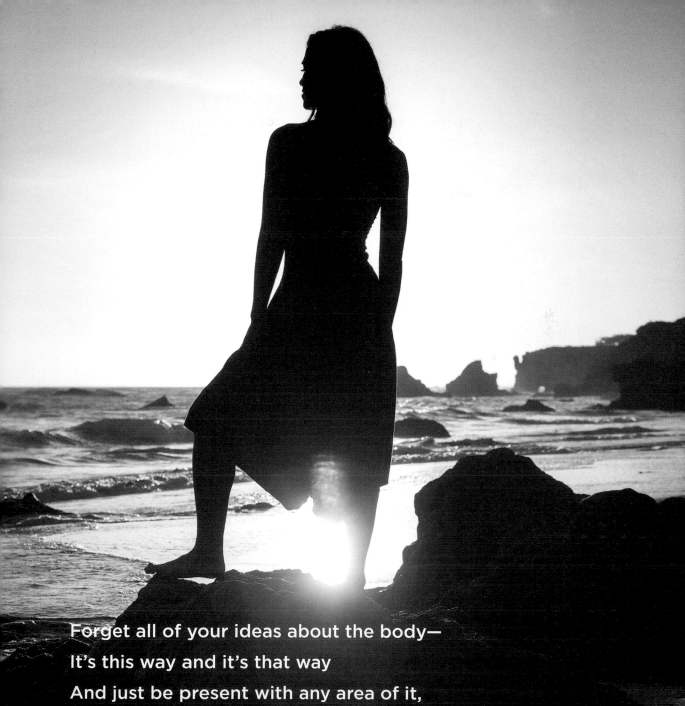

Forget all of your ideas about the body—
It's this way and it's that way
And just be present with any area of it,
this present body
as permeated with limitless space.
Drenched in freedom.

—*The Radiance Sutras*, translated by Lorin Roche[1]

Our journey begins with an important reeducation of food and diet. This will reshape the way you view and think about what you eat, how you view your body, and how you think about weight. Stay open and receptive, as this reeducation process is the true foundation of the entire Beauty Detox program. It is vital to understand these teachings in order to make the positive, deep and lasting changes that you want and deserve to have in your body and in your life.

If you love your body and nourish it from a place of love, instead of just plotting and planning how to make it skinnier, your body will respond with an increased amount of vitality, energy and health . . . and you'll actually realize far superior—and sustainable—results with your weight and beauty.

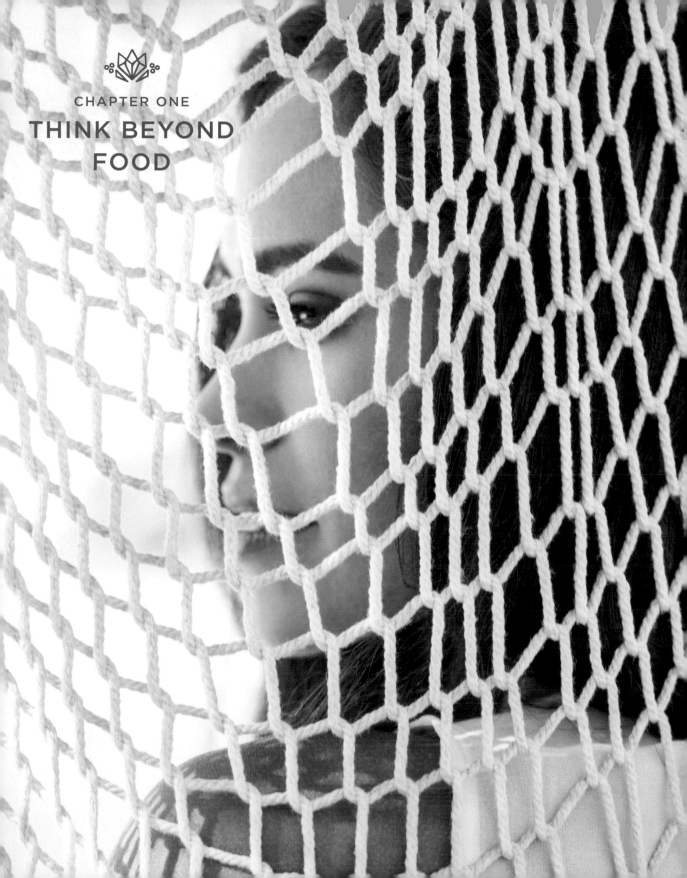

When I started learning about food and diet years ago, one of my teachers told me something I'll never forget. He said, "Food is just the first step to health. It's the beginning of the path." As a student on the road to becoming a nutritionist, I couldn't believe that he would say such a thing. My thoughts went from disbelief (*What the heck is he talking about?*) to a shade of pity (*How sad that he doesn't understand how powerful food is!*) and then became maybe a bit condescending (*Well, he doesn't really know much, does he?*).

At that point, I was passionately focused on my belief that one's diet is the most important part of one's lifestyle with the biggest impact on weight, health and overall well-being. I was inspired and fascinated by the specific properties of foods. It amazed me to learn that antioxidants can neutralize aging free radicals, that there are compounds in certain foods, herbs and spices that can optimize organ functioning and the quality of your blood while simultaneously increasing outer beauty. And I was equally intrigued to discover how certain foods are congestive to the body and can contribute to diseases and aging. I simply wasn't open to the idea that there could be something more important to a person's health than food and diet, and I stubbornly believed that I knew better than my own teacher.

It took me years to integrate his profound words from that day into my own work. I now realize he was teaching me that physical matter is only the beginning. It is easy to start on the path to wellness by changing your diet, since food is visible to the eye and gives you something tangible to focus on. But my teacher was right. There are so many factors beyond food that contribute to our health, weight and, yes, even our beauty. I just couldn't see it at the time.

The Real Defining Factor in Health and Weight Loss

When I think of my reaction to my teacher's words that day, it allows me to reflect on how much I myself have grown as a teacher. After all, we are all lifetime students. And while, of course, I still appreciate the powers of natural foods, I now embrace the fact that there is more that we can do to change and to improve our health and beauty, to transform the shape of our body, and to realize our inner joy, to boot! I have expanded my focus to how true healing actually comes from within. Specific foods can be very supportive to your body in healing itself. *But ultimately change originates and sustains from you and your power.* It's initially daunting, but an exciting and incredibly empowering revelation.

As I examined more and more health information devoted to the minutiae of certain nutrients and more studies attributing "miraculous" healing properties to specific tinctures and powders, I could feel my passion dragging me the other way. I was so sick of hearing about the next super food that also happened to be a "natural" fat burner. Over time, it became clear to me that what's on your plate, which can be precisely quantified and qualified, described in terms of dimensions and measurements, is only one factor contributing to your health and your weight. After observing and working with hundreds of people and spending thousands of hours with them, I understand that weight loss is a result not only of the foods you eat but also of what is going on with you as a whole person.

If you are skeptically wrinkling your nose at this concept, remember that I, too, once firmly believed that food was the be-all and end-all when it came to losing weight. But the nonnegotiable fact remains that we are *not* one-dimensional beings whose health and weight can easily be manipulated by adhering to a numerical formula. Otherwise, we could have all stopped the diet game with the advent of Weight Watchers and everyone would now have the exact figure they desire.

It's obviously true that what one eats can either facilitate or impede weight loss, but more and more I see rarely discussed emotional, mental and spiritual imbalances as underlying root factors in sustained weight loss. By *spiritual* I mean the degree to which you have a conscious connection to the interrelated parts of you that comprise your whole being, as well as a connection to all of life and the universe, however you personally define it.

This is why I've always felt that the word *nutritionist* doesn't adequately describe what I do. I always work with the whole person and approach his or her life holistically, while

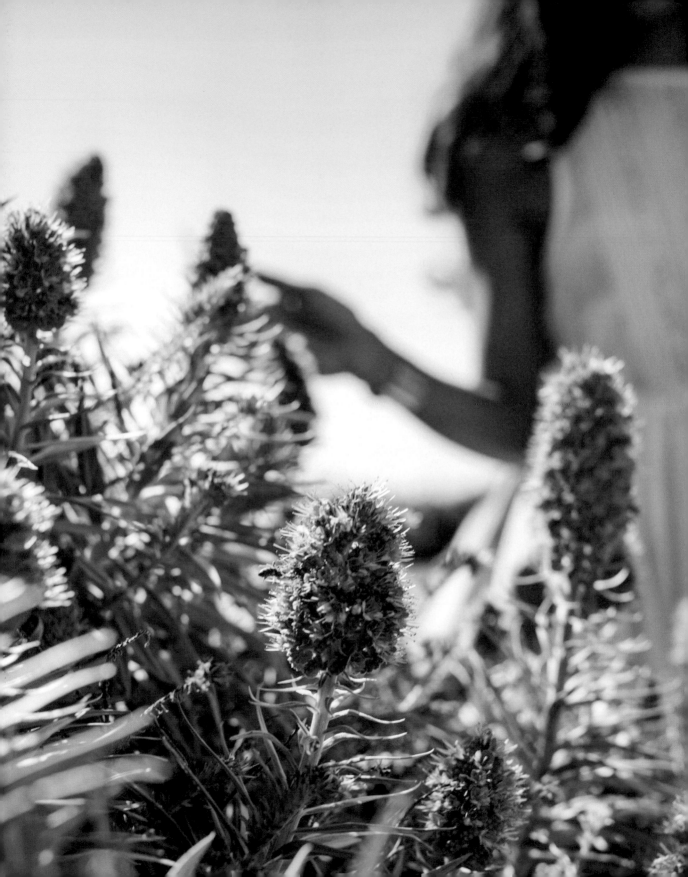

a nutritionist in the standard sense relies on only dietary and food protocols. I prefer the simple term *teacher*. I teach my clients not only about diet but also about the various aspects of balancing and nourishing themselves as whole people, such as becoming mindful of their self-talk, grasping the roots of their underlying beliefs and discerning the ways in which their actions may be contradictory to their goals or intentions. I help them to reconnect to their spiritual side through such methods as meditation, yoga and spending more time in nature.

The core of my teachings is the same whether I'm working with someone on a significant weight-loss goal, those stubborn last five pounds or a general health goal. It goes far beyond the concept of emotional eating. Certainly, consuming more calories than your body needs will often cause you to gain weight, but what I'm referring to here is the way your thought patterns actually shape the visible, physical structure of your body. This happens on a deep, subconscious level. In *Quantum Healing,* Deepak Chopra discusses how some obese people have been known to gain weight on diets containing only the minimal number of calories needed to sustain basal metabolism. He writes, "The reason for this is that the brain can actually alter the metabolism in such a way that the calories are stored as fat instead of being burned up as fuel."[1]

The Interconnectivity of Mind and Body

There are many ways in which our thoughts and emotions affect our bodies. Have you ever been under an extreme amount of stress and ended up gaining weight? Though my weight does not fluctuate by a large amount, I have definitely put on a few extra pounds when there was a big change happening in my life. When I first came to Los Angeles for extended periods to work with clients, the demands on my time and attention by multiple people and the long hours were definitely stressful, and I put on some weight. I could tell because my skinny jeans became even more uncomfortable, and it was around then that I stopped wearing pants with no stretch, which were constant reminders to me of my weight.

The connection between stress, which originates in your mind as a perception of a given situation, and its body-altering outcomes, such as high blood pressure, strokes and heart attacks, has been well researched and widely accepted. Is it so hard to believe that your mind can affect your weight, too?

Dr. Zofia Zukowska, chair of the department of physiology and biophysics at Georgetown University Medical Center, has led numerous studies that reveal that the body reacts to stress by packing on the pounds not due to overeating, but due to the nervous system's response. She says, "[S]tress induces obesity by way of the nerves that go to the fat tissue in that particular region of the body.... Neuropeptide Y stimulates blood vessel formation, which feeds tissue growth, and maybe that gives you increased fat deposits around the waist."[2] In other words, your emotions affect your nervous system, and your body can respond by holding on to fatty elements to help protect your delicate nervous system.[3]

Kathryn's Story

Kathryn was a client of mine who worked in high-end retail. Like many sales jobs, hers was high stress, with constant new goals to hit. Kathryn was also holding on to a lot of anger toward her mother, who had been very cold and critical of Kathryn when she was a child and had never given Kathryn the type of love she wanted. Even as an adult, Kathryn had fought constantly with her mother, who accused her of not behaving "correctly" at family gatherings or of saying the wrong things. She was simply longing for love and validation from her mother, but she was also investing a great deal of energy into holding on to this resentment. At some point in nearly every conversation, she mentioned her "crazy mother," and she often employed destructive tactics, such as not allowing her mother to see her granddaughter for extended periods of time.

When Kathryn came to see me about losing weight, she'd been about thirty pounds heavier than she wanted to be for as long as she could remember. This was uncomfortable on her five-foot-two-inch frame. But even as I glanced between her consultation forms and her facial expressions, I could feel the tense, angry energy that was emanating from her. "So how much weight can I lose in two weeks?" she demanded and then revealed that she wanted to lose weight for a destination wedding she was attending.

The rage toward her mother that she held inside was present in other areas of her life. In the interactions I witnessed, she was snappy and critical of her husband and ceaselessly negative. She complained about everything from restaurants and the weather to driving conditions and her daughter's teachers. She was simply resentful of life in general. And, unsurprisingly, she had battled a lifetime of constipation.

I changed Kathryn's diet, and she started drinking my Glowing Green Smoothie (page 255), a cornerstone of the Beauty Detox dietary program. Previously, she had been following a low-carb, high-protein type of diet, so there had been a lot of fiberless food in her diet that had deposited acidic by-products in her digestive tract. Sure enough, the addition of more fiber to her diet marked the beginning of Kathryn's awakening. I believe it helped to dislodge some stuck energies, and since energy transcends all forms, physical entities like fiber can sometimes be the impetus to create emotional or mental shifts.

Kathryn felt very emotional during the process of shifting her diet. She cried and felt sad and experienced periods of emotional roller coasters characterized by extreme anger ... but she also had glimmers of real peace. It was not what she had expected to happen. After all, she had come to me simply wanting to lose weight. But we discussed what she was feeling extensively, and the more she was able to verbalize "stuck" resentments that she'd held inside her for so long, the more aware she became of their presence in her daily life. Awareness creates space around negative thoughts, a way to acknowledge them so that you can start the process of letting go. It doesn't change what's taken place, but it does create a new understanding that you don't have to keep reacting in the same ways.

It was a long process, but over time Kathryn was able to release a lot of the anger that she had inside. Not coincidentally, her bowel movements also became regular and substantial (nothing less than a thrilling improvement for her health and beauty). The combination of emotional release work and dietary changes allowed Kathryn to shed thirty-three pounds of excess weight and keep it off. Now she is much more present, quicker to smile and far more joyful ... and she also doesn't mention her mother in every conversation anymore!

How Your Emotions Affect Your Vitality

There is a great deal of scientific evidence to support the link between mind and body. In his book *The Second Brain,* Michael D. Gershon, MD, states that there are over a hundred million nerve cells in the small intestine. We have more nerve cells in our gut than in our spine. Gershon notes that the gut is the only organ that contains an intrinsic nervous system, one that is able to "mediate reflexes in the complete absence of input from the brain or spinal chord." He says, "The ugly gut is more intellectual than the heart and may have a greater capacity for 'feeling.'"[4] In other words, your gut (really your digestive tract) is sensitive to what is going on with you emotionally and mentally, not just physically.

We all know that our emotions can affect our stomach. Have you ever felt butterflies in your stomach when you were nervous about something, or even vomited as a result of a bad case of nerves? Emotional thought patterns, such as anxious thoughts or thoughts fueled by low self-esteem, directly impact the nervous system and especially the nerves in the gut. This can impair the gut's vital function, namely, digestion. And impaired digestion may lead to the inefficient release of toxins and waste, making weight loss more difficult.

Researchers have discovered that the neurotransmitter imipramine, which is produced in an abnormal way in people who are depressed, is found not only on brain cells but also on skin cells.[5] Why does the skin produce a "mental" molecule? This phenomenon suggests that feelings, such as depression, affect our entire body, including our skin and its appearance. Insulin, which is a hormone linked to the pancreas, is now known to be produced by the brain, and the stomach is said to produce brain chemicals, such as CCK.[6]

Research conducted at Stanford University reviewed studies on the acute consequences of emotion suppression and found that both expressing and suppressing negative emotions, such as anger, anxiety and tension, can lead to cardiovascular and other issues.[7] The University of Wisconsin and Princeton University collaborated on a study that found that the brain activity related to negative emotions suppresses the body's immune response and thus its ability to fight disease. The study's leader, Richard Davidson, says that emotions play an important role in regulating systems in the body that influence health.[8]

Your mind has a profound effect on your physical body. What you think and how you feel impact your weight and how you look, as well as your overall vitality.

I know that this may seem new to you and different from other ways you've thought about your weight and shaping your body, but it is in our very nature to be a completely whole, interconnected being. Embracing this truth is the foundation for full immersion in the Beauty Detox program, and it is the key to your best body and most joyful life.

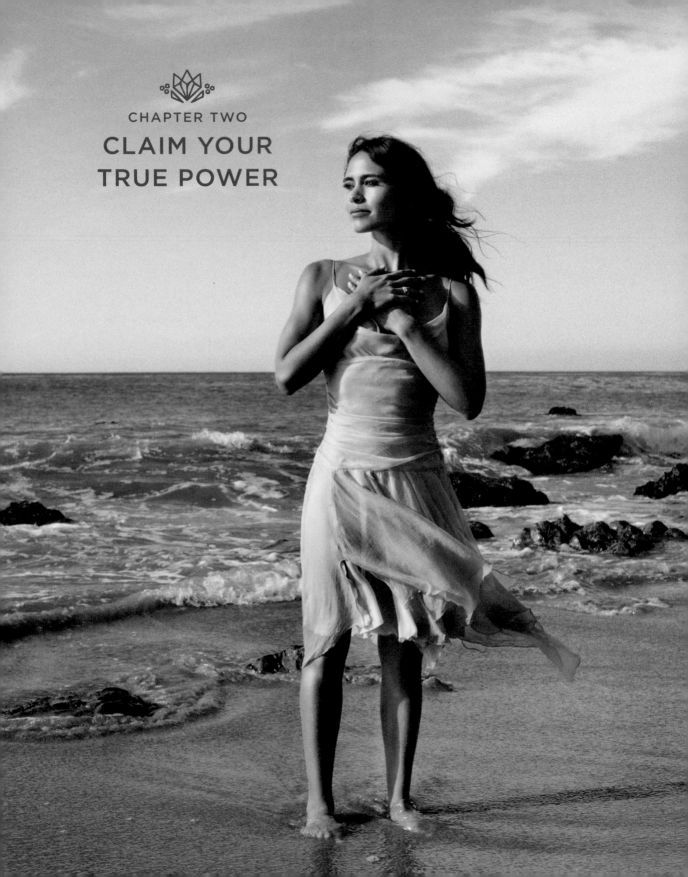

CHAPTER TWO

CLAIM YOUR TRUE POWER

Now that we've established that there are different aspects of your being, and that they are all interrelated and affect each other, you may be wondering, *What is the title of this book all about? What is "power" as it relates to weight loss and looking good and being happy—you know, Kimberly, the good stuff?*

True power originates in you. It is the result of unity within. Have you ever met someone who was so passionate about what they were doing—no matter what it was—that you could just feel the energy surging through what they were doing? They demonstrate a complete alignment of their will and the thoughts behind their actions, and consequently, there is almost an electric charge infused into anything they focus on. That is true power. True power is when there is alignment and consistency flowing through all aspects of you—your thoughts, core beliefs, words and actions. When you achieve this alignment, you become extraordinarily powerful, healthy and beautiful, and you can shape the body and life you want, surpassing perceived limitations.

On a recent trip back to Thailand, I met a jewelry maker on the streets of Bangkok. She was so absorbed in finishing threading the chain of a necklace that she didn't even notice all the people who were browsing through her finished pieces, which were draped over a small blanket at the edge of the sidewalk. When I asked her about the stones in one of her necklaces, she looked up and peered at me for a moment, as if she had been off in another world. Her face lit up as she explained the significance and properties of her jewelry and stones. Even though her English vocabulary was very limited, her vibrant energy told me a lot more than words ever could. And, of course, I would want to wear a necklace that she had made with so much care and passion, and I purchased one. She was completely aligned with what she was doing, and it was truly powerful.

You might be able to rattle off your weight goals in a flash. But you may also be dealing with a lifelong struggle to maintain your weight. There may be underlying beliefs you have been harboring and repeating to yourself, which keep you from achieving your goal weight, or even subconscious reasons you keep fat on your body as a form of "protection." I have designed each of the Power Alignment Shifts in this book to guide you on your journey to becoming conscious of the thoughts, beliefs and patterns that are creating blocks for you, and to removing them to allow your true power to shine forth.

True power and ego cannot coexist. Ego (which we'll talk about in much greater detail a bit later) involves focusing on achieving an outward goal that others can perceive, regardless of whether your means are aligned with your beliefs or whether they are nourishing for you on all levels. For instance, you might stay in a job you despise for the title and the salary, or you might stick to an overly restrictive diet focused solely on hitting a number rather than nourishing your body. Ego also creates habits and patterns that are rooted in fear. And fear takes away your true power.

Why Shortcuts Don't Work

In my work I see a lot of fear around eating any kind of carbs, which is perceived by many (due to information put out by mainstream diets) as a cause of weight gain, though unrefined carbohydrates are a macronutrient that make up many beautifying, natural foods. But fear and operating on the ego level can create a drive to just get to the weight "no matter what," and can result in extreme dietary imbalance by trying shortcuts. I define a *shortcut* as something you do in the belief that you are getting one up on the system. In this case, the "system" is your body, and the reality is that there is no fooling your body. Many people fall into the trap of *believing* that they've found the perfect way to eat as little as possible without being hungry or gaining weight, or *believing* that they've found a trick of eating processed foods that are designed to be low carb so they can prevent themselves from feeling deprived. They believe they can accomplish their weight-loss goals without having to do it the "real" way, which is by eating actual whole foods. But this dieting strategy is not aligned with the true needs of your body and thus will never provide lasting results.

When you choose a diet filled with artificial this and low-calorie that—meaning shortcuts rather than whole foods—your life will start to reflect that diminishing of consciousness, that disconnect between mind and body. Shortcuts do not work for long (if they work at all), and rarely if ever do they result in the magnetic, all-around beauty and health that come from living and nourishing yourself in an authentic way. When you embrace the practice of eating a whole-food, plant-based diet, there is no need for shortcuts. In Power

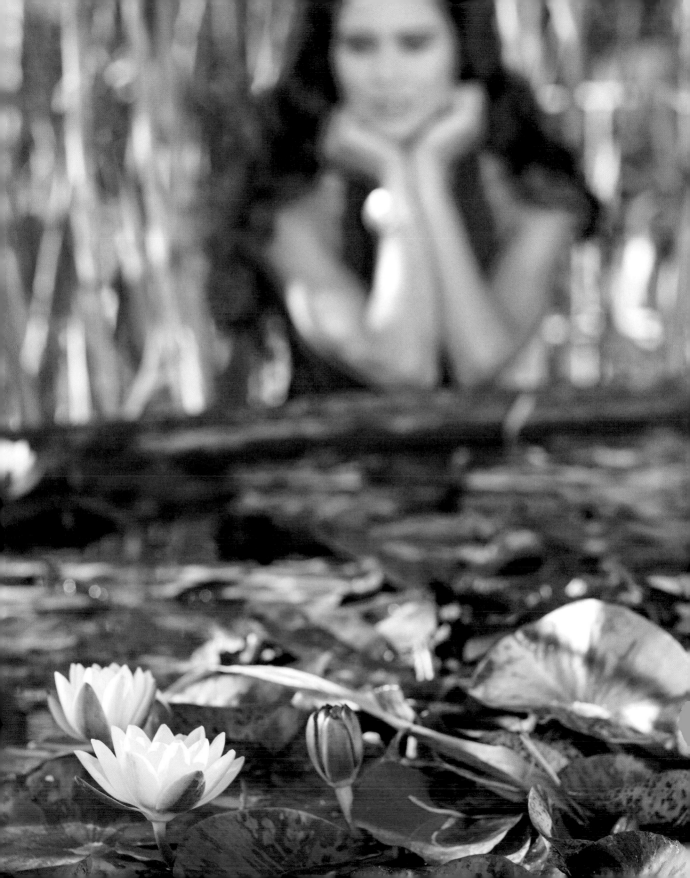

Alignment Shift 6, I provide over sixty delicious new Beauty Detox recipes to help get you on your way to living beautifully and authentically whole.

DITCH THE SHORTCUT	DISCOVER WHOLE FOODS
Processed protein bar	Almonds or chia seeds
Artificial energy drinks and shots	Glowing Green Smoothie (page 255)
Low-calorie microwave meal	Veggie soup and salad with avocado
Diet soda	Water with lemon, coconut water

Embrace Your Wholeness to Balance Your Weight

It is widely accepted that the mind and the body are connected, but the term *mind-body connection* is not quite right. The word *connection* implies that the two entities are separate and are joined at various locations. *Connection* is a form of dualism.[1] A mind-body *fusion*, on the other hand, implies that there are no areas of separation between one entity and the other, that one does not begin where the other ends. You can't isolate single waves from the sea; they are part of a unified entity. And there are similar fluid interactions between all aspects of the complex being that is you. Your mind and body are like two waves in the ocean: they flow from the same source and meet again at that source. They are not independent or disconnected in any way.

This pattern of wholeness is exemplified in every aspect of the universe. Australian physicist Paul Davies, PhD, illuminates this fundamental aspect of the universe in his book *Superforce*: "To the naive realist the universe is a collection of objects. To the quantum physicist it is an inseparable web of vibrating energy patterns in which no one component has reality independently of the entirety; and included in the entirety is the observer."[2] Similarly, David Bohm, a protégé of Albert Einstein's and one of the world's most respected quantum physicists, speaks of how everything in the universe is part of a continuum. In his 1991 book *The Holographic Universe*, in which he uses as one of his springboards Bohm's contributions to quantum physics and his model of the universe, Michael Talbot writes, "Despite the apparent separateness of things at the explicit level, everything is a seamless extension of everything else. . . . Things can be part of an undivided whole and still possess their own unique qualities."[3]

This aspect of "wholeness" includes you. You are an integrated system: all your parts are designed to function in a unified manner, not just on the physical plane, but also on the formless mental, emotional and spiritual planes. Most of your body, which seems solid, is actually space. In fact, every solid particle of matter is composed of more than 99.999 percent empty space.[4] What fills up this space? Energy. This energy is dynamic and fluid and can be shaped by you when you are in tune with your power.

Love is a formless energy, and the impact of love on the body has been well examined. In a study performed in 1987 at Yale University, men and women were surveyed before submitting to angiography tests. Using regression analyses, they found that those people who reported feeling loved and supported were far less likely to experience blockage in their arteries.[5] Dr. Dean Ornish, whose low-fat, plant-based diet is famous for reversing heart disease, conducted many studies on the power of love for his book *Love and Survival*. "The diet can play a significant role," Ornish concludes, "but nothing is more powerful than love and intimacy."[6]

There is clearly a physical response to emotional feelings. According to Jerry Kiffer, a heart-brain researcher at the Cleveland Clinic's Psychological Testing Center, when an individual experiences anger, there are more fat globules in the blood vessels and higher levels of glucose in the blood. In addition, the pumping of the heart increases and blood pressure surges.[7] An analysis of findings from forty-four studies published in the *Journal of the American College of Cardiology* supports the prevailing view that a link exists between negative emotions and heart disease.[8]

The wholeness of everything—including you—is rooted in an authentic Oneness that connects us all. Oneness and fusion are repeated all over the universe, as evidenced by the spiderweb that trembles when just one thread is jostled to the symbiotic ecosystems on planet Earth. The name of this Oneness doesn't really matter. Some refer to it as the Divine, God, the universe, cosmic energy, prana, Qi or chi. Tune into the collective, interconnected pulse of all the molecules and sub-molecules in the universe. It's beautiful and mysterious and amazing all at the same time. We don't have to understand how it all works to appreciate it and to benefit from acknowledging it.

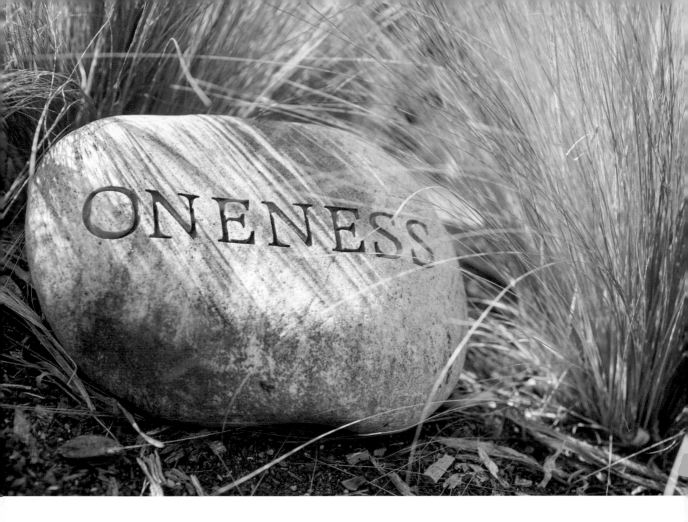

Unity Magnifies Your Creative Potential

The opposite of fusion is disembodiment, a practice that creates divisions in the oneness of your mind and body. Unfortunately, there is a pervasive undercurrent of disembodiment in modern society. At the gym, for instance, people read magazines or watch TV while using cardio machines to work out their body. They are actively trying to keep their mind from being fully present to their body's motions. This is not *wrong* per se, but it encourages the ever-widening split between body and mind.

Popular nutritional beliefs and weight-loss strategies generally place a strong emphasis on numbers: caloric counts, grams of carbs and grams of protein. Yet despite all the formulas out there that have come up with the perfect mathematical equation for weight loss, we still struggle. Why? Because our bodies are multidimensional. Strictly

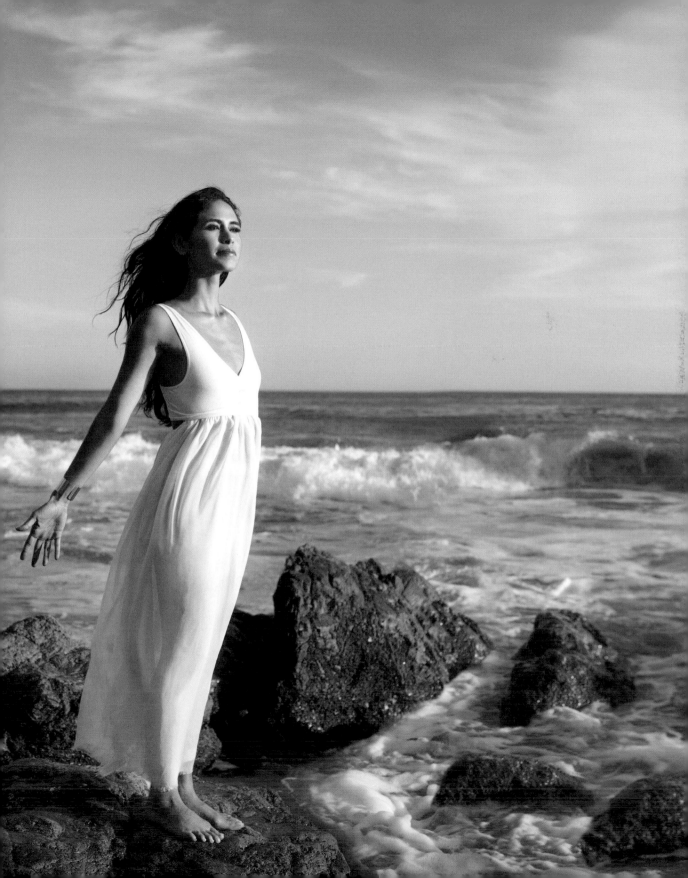

one-dimensional approaches are not in alignment with our bodies' optimal functioning, and trying to follow these approaches is a form of disembodiment, of misalignment.

The philosophy behind Western medicine is that medications cure disease by working purely on a physical, biochemical level. But there is research to show that our whole being participates in healing. One study found that when anesthetists verbally encouraged their patients to get over their postoperative pain, those patients needed fewer narcotics than those who did not receive the same encouragement.[9] In another remarkable experiment, a doctor held positive consultations with his patients, saying that he knew exactly what was wrong and then either telling them they needed no treatment or giving them medication. Then in his negative consultations, the doctor said he did not know exactly what was wrong. He either offered these patients no treatment or gave them a medication, stating, "I'm not sure that the treatment I am going to give you will have an effect." Two weeks later, there was a substantial difference in the health of the patients who had positive and negative consultations, but not in the patients who received treatment or did not. Their results seemed to depend largely on what they were *told* rather than on the treatment they received. Similar results have been achieved when treating depression.[10]

The mind and the body are not separate or merely connected. The mind and the body are *one*. But despite all the research supporting this accepted view, modern society encourages a disconnect between your body, your mind and even your spirit. Do you sometimes think of your body as a separate entity, as an object that you have to "deal with"? I hear my clients lament, "My belly is so fat." This declaration diminishes their feelings of self-worth. And by making such negative statements, even casually, you are identifying your body as your possession while equating what you own and who you are. When you reduce yourself to separate parts you lose your power to lose weight, find happiness and reach your full potential. Shift your focus to feeling your strength or your overall energy, which is much more empowering. Your power is in your wholeness.

Today, Western medicine is based on highly specialized physicians who focus on treating specific areas of the body. This approach has some positives, but also limitations, because some medical tactics and medications designed to support one bodily system can create an imbalance in, or even injure, another. That's why it is beneficial to treat your body as one integrated unit.

Vanessa's Story

When I first met Vanessa, she was recovering from bulimia and was ten pounds heavier than she wanted to be. Vanessa was very hard on herself, criticizing herself with extreme language such as "ridiculously bad," "the worst ever," "mind numbingly stupid," and "beyond horrible" if she thought she had performed less than great in her work as a hedge fund manager. She often told me she thought she was so ugly that she couldn't even bear to look in the mirror. Though she did tell me about the purging, she was embarrassed to do so, because she felt shame around it and that in turn made her feel worse about herself.

I did private yoga sessions and awareness work with Vanessa, including breathing exercises, nature hikes and guided meditations, which helped her to become really aware of her thoughts and words. She also worked with a psychologist who specializes in eating disorders. These approaches were far more important than just looking at her diet, which did need some balancing. We needed to address the emotional and mental roots of the binges, as these not only compounded her suffering, but were also the cause of the extra pounds.

It has been a long road, but one that is marked with vast improvement. Vanessa is more in touch with her self-worth, from doing no more than simply being the beautiful, whole being that she is. She's identified her emotional triggers for binging, namely, feeling overwhelmed and highly anxious, and she has tools to help her break the pattern, such as communicating her needs to delegate more of her work and take more breaks to step outside. When it comes to her diet, she chooses lots of filling whole foods. Nourishing, all-vegetable soups in particular have been enormously helpful in making her feel full and stabilized when she starts to feel really anxious. She has lost the ten pounds she wanted to shed, she has more energy, and she is a *lot* happier and less self-critical. She no longer has to hide or feel bad about some of her actions. She is now in touch with her true power.

Separation creates suffering. Separation also creates struggle. When you refrain from nourishing yourself on a whole level, this separatism cuts you off from your creative potential to manifest the body you want. Later we will discuss specific ways to embrace your unity. For now, focus on internalizing the idea that you are whole. You are truly complete. And you are perfect just as you are. It's exciting, and it may be hard to believe or take in (what are you saying to yourself right now?) but it is the truth. To realize this, you just have to tap into your power. Keep reading, Beauty, and you will learn to do just that.

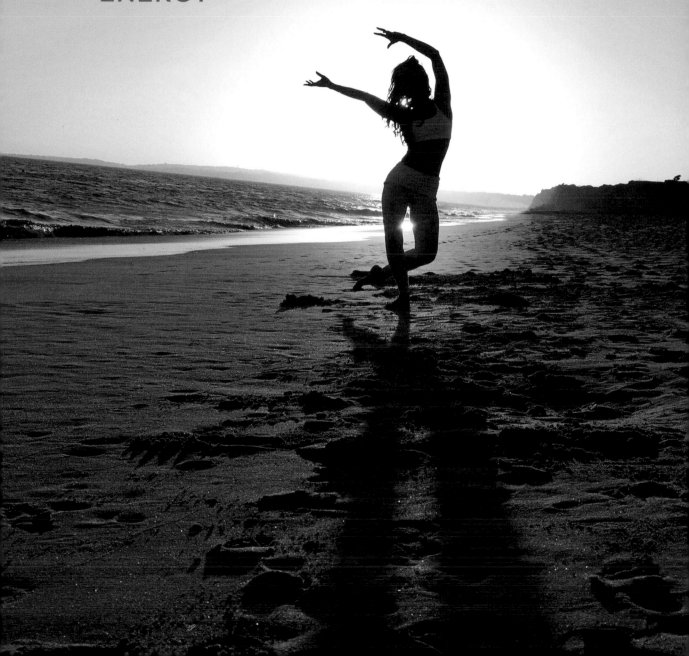

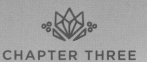

CHAPTER THREE

HARNESS YOUR BODY'S DYNAMIC ENERGY

Whenever I'm in the ocean, especially the ocean off western Puerto Rico, which is a heart-nourishing place I feel a strong connection to and where I have written the vast majority of the *Beauty Detox* books, I like to swim out a little ways and then just let myself float on my back. One time I floated for so long that I was a little startled by how far out I had drifted, but I just swam peacefully back to shore. The feeling of floating on your back in the ocean or in a lake is incredibly blissful. It allows you to be free of the weight of your physical body and just be.

You may experience this feeling during *shivasana,* the corpse pose at the end of a yoga practice, when you let yourself be still and integrate all the teachings of the practice. When this happens, you can feel your "aliveness," your energy beyond the weight of gravity and your physicality. When you allow yourself to be in such a space, it connects you back to the realization that you are so much more than your physical body.

Tune In to Your Body's Natural Flow

Your body is made up of a vibrating energy field of constant movement and is not a static physical structure. *Prana,* which is the Sanskrit term for "vital energy," pervades the universe at all levels and runs through you. No part of you is static. It's really a miracle, when you think about it. Within the seemingly solid, dense mass of flesh and bone is an ever-swirling plethora of billions of cells that are in constant fluid and dynamic movement.

Like water running through a river, atoms flow through you and constantly create new ones. Your skin is fresh every month. You have a new stomach lining every four days, and your surface cells that actually come in contact with digesting food are renewed every five minutes.[1] Fluids constantly circulate, carrying waste and toxins out of the body to

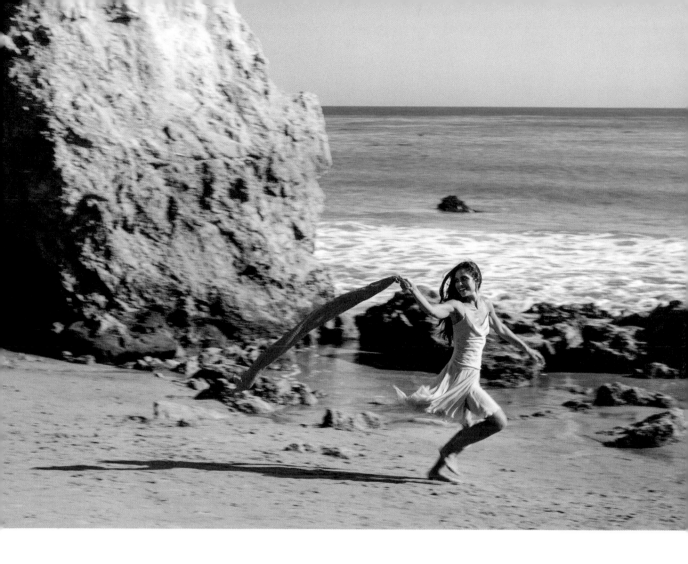

purify it and maintain a healthy internal environment. Some elements, such as fiber, help to support this movement.

Trying to stick to a static measurement when it comes to your body, such as your numerical weight, is completely out of tune with the body's natural flow. It's the opposite of dynamic movement; an outer, ego-based label that creates suffering and limitation if you obsess over it. It frustrates me that so many people feel the need to weigh themselves every day, or even multiple times a day. Your fluid levels are ever shifting, and minute discrepancies in weight are completely normal and natural! Attaching yourself to labels and static descriptions can create "holding patterns," and these are not in tune with our energetic flow. They can create chronic stress, sickness or dysfunction in the body, and they can cause the "storage" of excess energy, which can translate into excess weight.

Abandon Numbers for True Change

Here are some typical statements I hear from people when we start working together:

"I don't know if I can drink that Glowing Green Smoothie. I mean, how many calories are in it? Are there more than 150? I think fruit has too many calories. What about sugar? If there are 12 grams of sugar in it or more, I just don't think I can drink it. Sugar makes you gain weight, you know."

"Can't I just eat my protein bar in the morning? It has only around 230 calories. Oh, and 20 grams of protein! I know you said you don't like me eating them because of all the super-processed dairy and soy stuff they contain, and . . . oh yeah, vegetable oils, too . . . but I dunno . . . I just feel safer eating them."

"Since I'm almost 30—I can't believe I just turned 25!—my metabolism is starting to slow down. I can feel it already! I feel like I'm getting so many wrinkles! I wish I could be 21 again. It would be so much easier for me. I could stay skinny easier. Do my legs look big to you in these jeans?"

"I weighed myself again this afternoon, and I was up 2 pounds from last night! I know you say that water weight fluctuates, but don't you think I should weigh less in the afternoon than in the evening? I need to get below 120 pounds—by next week. I was 124 this afternoon, and I'm going to weigh myself again tonight. 120 is where I need to be! Okay, let me tell you how many calories I ate today. . . ."

I truly believe that one of the biggest issues with the Western world's approach to diet and nutrition is its obsession with numbers. Judging what you eat in terms of numbers is a form of strict reductionism, and that type of mentality cuts you off from the universal flow. It creates rigidity and stagnation.

If you fixate on the static number that shows up on a scale, you are reducing yourself to one label instead of feeling the full extent of your energy, strength and beauty. Stop weighing yourself every day or week and focus on how you feel. Your energy will open up and will flow freely, even down to the cellular level, as rigidities and stagnant energy diminish. When you don't obsess about your weight or beat yourself up about it, it becomes easier to lose weight and to create your ideal body in a healthy and sustainable way.

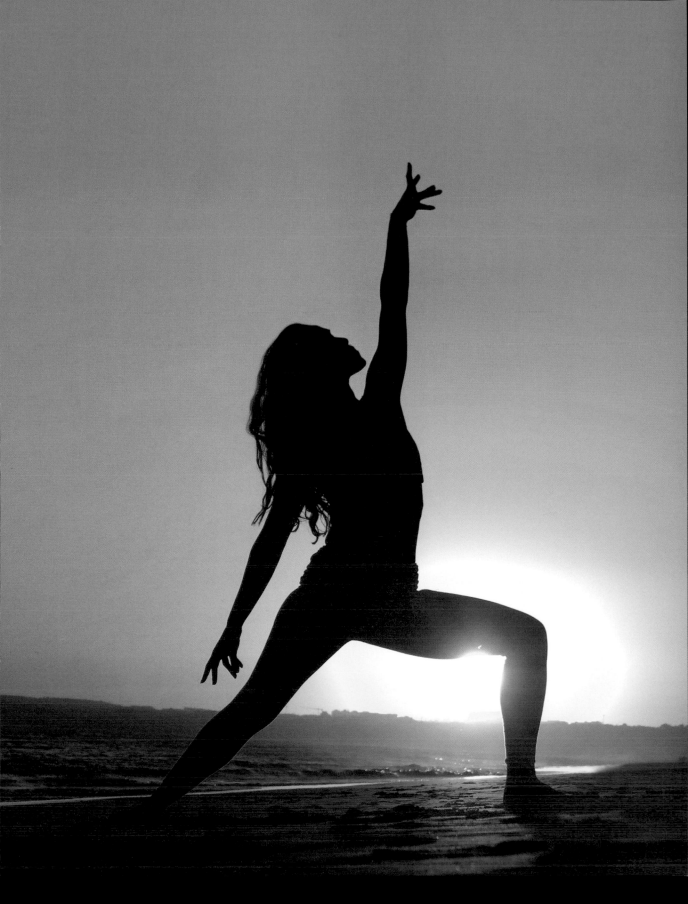

Asha's Story

Asha wanted to lose a few pounds and brighten her sallow skin tone, as she was looking tired and worn-out. She was a carb and calorie-counting addict and had been for years. She knew the numerical content of all the foods she ate, and she was very reluctant to eat foods if she didn't know their calorie count. When I asked her how she *felt,* all she could say was, "Pretty good," and I got the distinct impression that she really didn't pay attention to her feelings and energy levels. She just accepted what was, and she didn't entertain the notion that she could feel amazing every day, while at the same time slimming down and improving the appearance of her skin.

I asked Asha to pay attention to how she felt while and after eating certain foods, and what they did to her energy. While I was present, I had her eat a large kale salad with avocado and instructed her to chew really well. Then I asked her how she felt, and had her note and text me an hour later then later that afternoon. This lunch was a very different type of lunch than her usual tiny, measured-out piece of chicken with some limp broccoli. Little by little, she made the transition from a diet characterized by small portions of low-carb, nearly fiberless food, which left her starving, to one with an abundance of whole Beauty Foods. To make her feel safe while doing so, we did track her calories in general terms, but I kept weaning her off of obsessing about her calories and charting them and had her focus more and more on the nutritional aspects of her food. I reminded her over and over again that fiber is a natural form of calorie restriction, and that when you eat whole foods, you don't have to fixate on calorie counting or portion sizes.

Asha did slim down and lose the pounds she wanted, and she told me she was surprised that it was much easier than in the past. But it was her skin that dramatically changed, as it brightened and started looking more smooth, especially under her eyes, and her hair grew in thicker and fuller. Her overall vitality also increased. She went from fatigued-looking to energetic and radiant. Asha, reformed calorie counter, hasn't given it up completely, but is spending a lot more time shopping and sourcing in abundance in the produce section, where natural foods aren't labelled by numbers.

Food labels and mainstream diets place far too much emphasis on numbers. A fixation with numbers can increase stress and anxiety, which can lead to overeating. A study conducted at the University of Toronto concluded that threats to emotional tranquility can result in overeating.[2] The labels on packaged "diet" foods list isolated nutrients and their quantities. This makes you believe that the numbers on display are the most important ones to be aware of, but it is far more important to look at a food holistically.

Counting calories doesn't really work for the long-term. Not only are we complex systems, but counting calories also doesn't take the filling element of fiber into account. You can eat the same number of calories of fiber-free junk food as from a huge kale salad with drastically dissimilar results. Processed ingredients do not digest the same way whole foods do.

That number on the scale alone is not enough to encompass the vitality of your whole being. Likewise, if you live by the reductionist approach of constantly identifying with your age, you will forever be comparing yourself to the past or future and thinking that you are too old or too young to look this way or to do that. This is incredibly limiting and disempowering.

As the great yoga guru and spiritual master Paramahansa Yogananda advises, "Never tell people how old you are." It's not that your age should be a secret, but you don't have to volunteer it constantly and thus reinforce that ego-based concept at every turn. Many people say things to me like, "Well, I'm 38 now, so it's normal for my body to be breaking down and harder for me to maintain my weight," or "I'm so old. I'm 26 now" (you hear this a lot in Hollywood). So absurd!

Deepak Chopra suggests that we all have three ages: our chronological age (calculated according to the calendar date), our biological age (contingent on our cellular and organ processes and our health) and our psychological age (determined by how old we feel). Our biological age is influenced by our psychological age. In other words, the thoughts we feed ourselves directly influence how old we look!

Start looking at foods in terms of how nourishing they are to your body as a whole. Don't fixate over calories and grams of carbs and protein. Go back to trusting whole foods. The more naturally you eat, the more beautiful, slim and healthy you will become.

And stop obsessing over the number related to the year in which you were born, or in other words, your chronological age. Beautiful is beautiful. It is not dependent on looking "good" for a certain age. Being healthy, energetic and full of vitality is possible at any age.

Create the Body and Life You Want

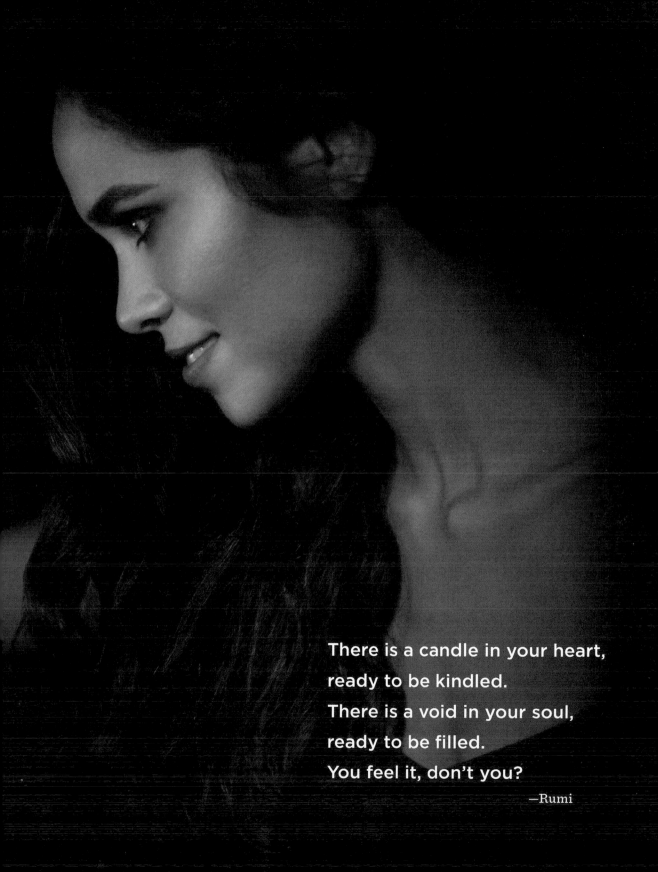

There is a candle in your heart,
ready to be kindled.
There is a void in your soul,
ready to be filled.
You feel it, don't you?

—Rumi

In the same way that Power Alignment Shift 1 acknowledged the connection between mind and body, opening you up to change, the information in this shift helps you to understand how excess weight can be a result of negative thoughts or protection against fear, or both. Many of us are not really aware of pervasive, repeated thoughts or underlying beliefs. But once you acknowledge negative thoughts, you can begin the process of reclaiming your power by replacing them with powerful affirmations and aligning your deepest thoughts and beliefs to support your goals. At the center of Power Alignment Shift 2 is the core concept of breaking free from the limitations of ego and reactive behavior, and focusing on living in the present.

Peace and power are already within you. You need not acquire either—you already have them. Just be present, and tune in to what you already have.

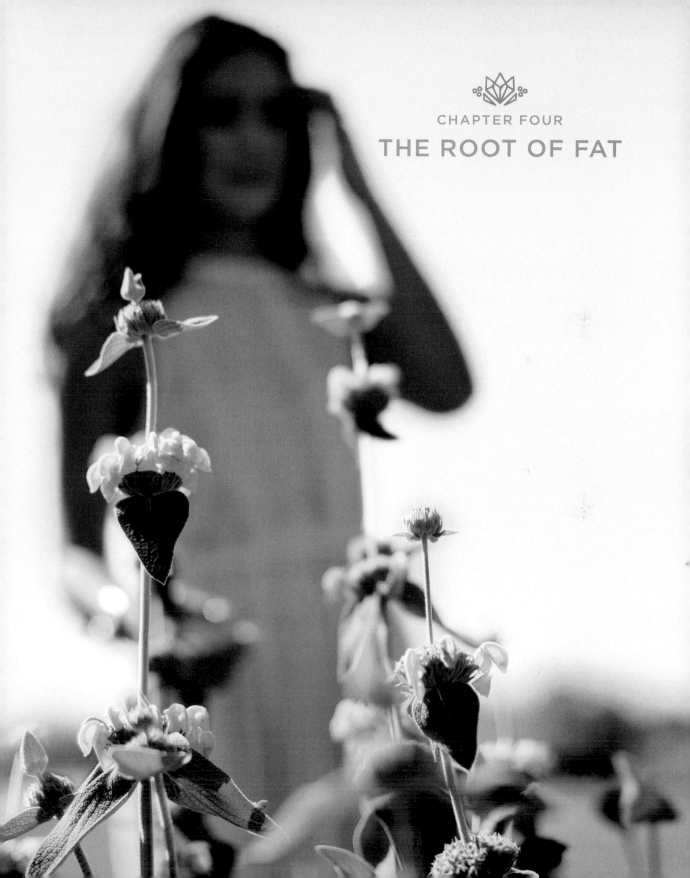

CHAPTER FOUR

THE ROOT OF FAT

Fat is a supercharged word for many people, especially us ladies. Sadly, one of the most common ways to belittle or criticize a woman is to throw the word *fat* in her direction. But it's just as easy and just as harmful to use this word on yourself. In a study of public perceptions of obesity-related public health messages conducted in 2011, researchers at Yale University found that the word *fat* creates shame, embarrassment and feelings of being stigmatized and blamed.[1] But now we're going to talk about fat from an objective, safe and loving place. It's okay. Don't be afraid of fat! As your understanding of fat grows, you will have more power over it and more power over your body.

The first thing you should know is that your fat is contained in your fat cells, which have the capacity to both expand and shrink. Fat cells themselves have some very interesting features. First of all, fat's natural quality is to insulate and protect. It helps to create warmth in your body and to cushion your nervous system from outside stresses. Every nerve in your body is coated in a layer of fat, called the myelin sheath, which insulates, protects and guides the electric impulses of your neurons. Your body also uses your fat cells as a place to store heavy metals and other toxins to keep them from circulating around the body via the bloodstream and damaging organs at the cellular level.

It is also in your fat cells' constitution to store energy. Of all the cellular components that make up our bodies, perhaps the most energy-holding element is fat. *Energy* is a very broad concept, and it certainly includes emotions and thoughts. As we've been discussing all along, the boundaries between mental and physical states are not that rigid, after all. Einstein famously showed that mass is a manifestation of energy. As part of his theory of relativity, he discovered what is called mass-energy equivalence. This principle explains the equal convertibility of a measured quantity of energy into a measured quantity of mass, and vice versa.[2] While mass-energy equivalence is certainly more complex than the notion of thoughts (energy) automatically being converted into fat (mass), Einstein's theory provides us with a scientific framework by which to understand the phenomenon of thoughts and emotions affecting the physical fat on your body.

Based on my reading of a Stanford paper entitled "The Equivalence of Mass and Energy"[3] and observing the behavior of people I have worked with and those around me, I hypothesize that if thoughts are tiny amounts of energy, and energy and mass are equally convertible, then repeated thoughts (or compounded energy) eventuate in greater mass, thus increasing the probability of physical manifestations. In other words, a "harmful" thought, such as "I'm fat," may start out with very little energy (which is equivalent to very little mass), but as this thought is repeated, it takes on more emotion, imagery and other connections, and so more energy (which is equivalent to more mass) gathers around this thought, almost like a snowball rolling downhill.

As the "harmful" thought is repeated, it is more likely to effect the visible physical reality and is harder to reverse. Fat can be one of the most visible physical expressions of energy patterns (or thoughts). Dr. Anita Goel, MD, who also holds a PhD in physics from Harvard University, states that "We're going to have to expand the language of physics to come to terms not only with matter and energy, but matter, energy, and maybe even consciousness."[4]

When you want to protect yourself from fear, insecurity, uncertainty, imbalance, hurt or abuse, or create more boundaries around you to feel protected or "insulated" from something, fat can appear as the physical manifestation of the protection you're seeking. If you cling to negative energies, including stress, anger, jealousy, resentment or hatred in your mind and do not process them or release them properly, they can become stuck matter. And stuck, stagnant energetic matter can manifest as excess weight. Repressed feelings are energy, too. If they are not dealt with, they can be pushed down and held in your fat cells. This is similar to the process by which your body attempts to push physical toxins away from your vital organs, into fat cells and deep into your digestive tract. If you are resistant to letting go, forgiving or moving on from something, stuck energy can manifest as matter, as fat. Toxicity blocks flow. It encourages entropy and weight gain by inhibiting movement. Toxins come in the form of food, but also in the form of toxic relationships, emotions and environments. Energy is healing, and when allowed to flow freely, it will balance out. The opposite is toxin-filled fat cells, which are encumbered, stuck.

At one time, I wasn't even aware of how often I complained that my thighs were "fat." Talking about my fat thighs became so annoying to my boyfriend (now my husband) that one day he said to me, "Do you hear how you are talking?" I paused and got clarity for the first time. I stopped complaining about my thighs and obsessing over them, took to jeans that had a bit of stretch, and just like that, my thighs stopped being a problem. That experience helped me become more aware of what my clients were saying to themselves. And, wow, was it eye-opening!

Negative self-talk is so prevalent and accepted that you may not even be aware of the negative messages you are feeding your mind and creating in physical form on your body. A study done at Brigham Young University showed that women with less than positive emotional health have a significantly increased risk of weight gain over time than women with positive emotional health.[5] When you have unhealthy emotions, it may not simply be that you consume more calories and gain weight. Your negative beliefs can manifest on your body in the form of unwanted weight gain.

Take a moment now to pause, especially if you are chronically heavier than you'd like to be or if your weight tends to fluctuate. Sit quietly and ask yourself what in your life you may be subconsciously trying to protect yourself from. Is there someone or something you are harboring anger or resentment toward? Or are you holding on to anger or regret about a past situation? Here are some charged words that might clue you in to the fact that you are harboring anger or resentment: *should, fair, unfair, blame.* Do you find yourself saying any of these words to yourself? Are you frightened of "messing up" at work or at home? Are you concerned that someone is going to discover that you aren't good enough in some way? Do you ever worry that you don't deserve what you have or the further good that is coming to you? Are you absorbing a great deal of negativity or stress at work?

Don't judge your feelings. Just take note of them so that you are aware of them and present. Try to be completely honest with yourself. I know it's not easy; otherwise that energy wouldn't be stuck there in the first place! Next, consider the following question:

What might I be trying to protect myself from?

Think about it and see what comes up. The answer might not present itself immediately, but if you focus on creating a safe space and staying open to it, it will come.

Honor the Intelligence of Your Body

Dr. Bernard Siegel, an acclaimed surgeon, a professor emeritus at the Yale School of Medicine at Yale University and an author, writes in *Love, Medicine and Miracles* that "Other doctors' scientific research and my own day-to-day clinical experience have convinced me that the state of the mind changes the state of the body by working through the central nervous system, the endocrine system, and the immune system."[6] The state of your body includes, by definition, your digestion, your organ functionality *and* your weight and appearance. Remember our concept of wholeness.

Stress is a great example of the fusion of the mind and the body because it leads to measurable physical outputs. During stressful times, blood is directed away from digestive organs, as digestion becomes a low priority when survival is at stake. This can contribute to issues like constipation, upset stomach and, eventually, weight gain. By analyzing dozens of published papers involving thousands of subjects, Laura Kubzansky, PhD, MPH, an associate professor at the Harvard School of Public Health, found that optimism cuts the risk of coronary heart disease by half, and that anger, high levels of anxiety and depression may contribute to the development of heart disease.[7] "They tend to co-occur," she says. "People who are angry a lot tend to have other chronic negative emotions as well."[8]

The stress response, which includes faster breathing, an accelerated heartbeat and the tensing of muscles, is only one manifestation of the body-mind exchange. Your body absorbs and reacts to *all* your internal thoughts, because there is a constant communication exchange between your inner self and your body. The body is highly intelligent, highly responsive, pliable and adaptable. Your thoughts become part of the sculpting process; they are materials that your body uses to create. Positive thoughts can be equally as powerful as the negative ones we just discussed.

Your thoughts not only affect your body but also *shape* your body. Now that you are becoming aware of the repeated thoughts and deep-seated beliefs that may be sabotaging your goals, you can begin feeding your body healthier thoughts. Take a moment to consider your own repeated thoughts. Thoughts like "It is so hard to maintain my weight" and "I am so fat" are not what you want to feed your body.

The best way to become aware of what you truly believe about your body is to go into a quiet room alone and turn off your phone and computer. Just be alone for a little while as you ask yourself this question:

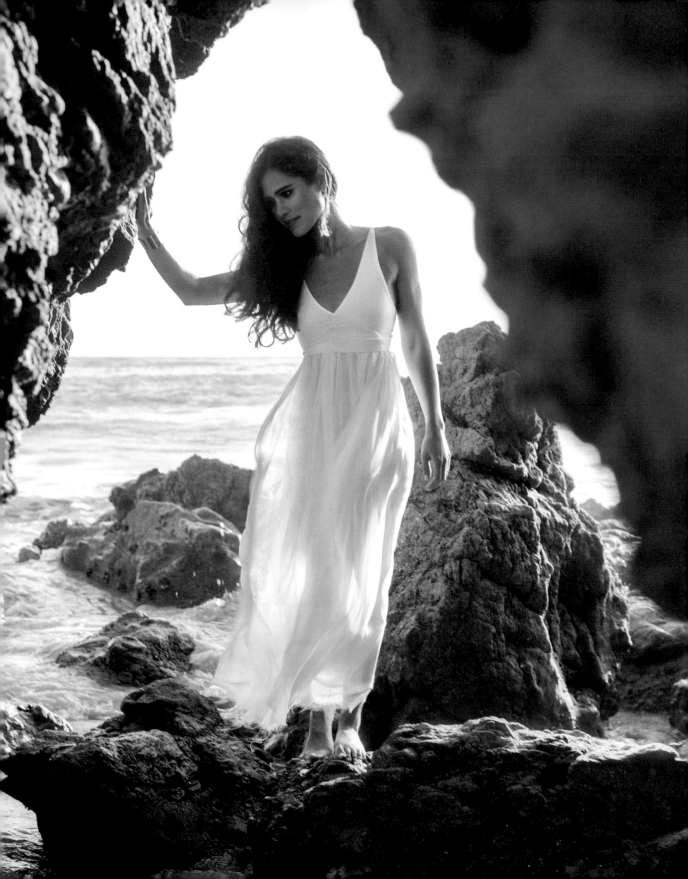

What do I think about my body and about the topic of weight?

See what comes up. Write it out—it's truly powerful to write things down by your own hand (don't type). Studies show that putting pen to paper helps you to process the information in a way that is advantageous to typing.[9] Come face-to-face with the thoughts that you are subconsciously thinking and reinforcing. They have become so ingrained in your being that you probably don't even realize that they are not the truth or reality.

Sometimes it can be hard to confront these thoughts for the first time and be honest with yourself. That's okay. This process can take days or even weeks, but just give yourself a safe space in which to think about your beliefs. For me, acknowledging the fact that I was constantly repeating "I am so fat," and even uttering this casually to my friends, helped me to realize that I actually believed it on some level. It was a revelation for me.

Once you identify any negative, deep-rooted beliefs, you can start to notice when they arise, maybe for the first time consciously, and change your thought pattern to something positive and simple. For instance, instead of thinking, *I am so fat,* you could choose to tell yourself, *I am strong and grateful for being healthy.*

Stop with the abusive self-talk right now and honor the powerful creative intelligence of your body. It is more powerful than anything you can get from the outside. Realize you have the power to be fit and happy.

Paul's Story

When I met Paul, a top accountant for a large firm, he was quite overweight, and I was told I was his *fifteenth* nutritionist. I wasn't sure if I could help him. After all, he'd never been able to sustain weight loss in the past. He was extremely hard on himself and constantly made negative comments about his shape ("I am such a slob") and lack of willpower, not to mention the fact that he felt "dumb at work" and "worthless." But now he was ready to try to lose weight again, not only to improve his health, but to be around longer for his wife and four young children, and so we began working together on an intense weight-loss plan. I created a nutritionally superior plant-based diet centered on lots of fiber, nutrients and chlorophyll.

Over the course of eight months Paul lost close to eighty pounds. During that time, not only was he following my diet plan, but we were also together regularly, as I helped cook some meals in his home and I also did private yoga sessions with him. And even when we were not together, we were constantly in communication through texts. In other words, I was able to provide constant emotional and energetic support and encouragement, and he was never left alone to fester in negative emotions or debilitating thoughts. Whenever he would say something negative, I would point it out, reflecting it back to him like a mirror, and then encourage him to say something positive right afterward. We worked on some positive affirmations, which he was especially open to after relaxing with a yoga session. With a lot of love and encouragement, I could see that he was moving toward self-love and better self-esteem.

When he had reached his goal and was ready to move forward without my constant guidance, I taught a chef and an assistant how to prepare foods for Paul so the program could be maintained after I left. Paul started off well, but then slowly started gaining back the weight. Although he was eating in accordance to the same overall dietary principles as when we were together, after I left, he stopped balancing his thoughts and emotions the way I had taught him. His self-love and self-esteem suffered, and he started wallowing in negative thoughts, which manifested in his continued weight gain. As he became increasingly negative, his weight gain increased. He also began to give in to some of his old eating habits. Within six months, he had gained back all the weight he had lost and then some.

Our bodies are a physical manifestation of all parts of our being, not just the food we eat. Despite this setback, I am still hopeful Paul will grow and learn from this experience and put the teachings and techniques we discussed and worked on together into practice for future success.

Why Attacking Fat Backfires

In our society there's a lot of fear surrounding body fat. We try to hide it with figure-squashing undergarments or under baggy clothes, or avoid situations where our body fat might be visible. People have told me that they avoid the beach and pool parties if they don't feel they are at the "right" weight.

Old stored energy receives less oxygen, less *prana* and less nourishment from both physical and psychic sources. Therefore, it becomes even more "stuck" and difficult to mobilize. It develops into a static form, rather than one that is fluid and dynamic. If you tell yourself and others around you that you are fat, whether it's in a casual conversation, silently to yourself in front of the mirror or in quiet mutterings, remember you are actively creating your outward form. Repeated thoughts become things. As the great yoga guru Paramahansa Yogananda states, "It is this creative force inherent in man's thoughts that makes them so formidable. The truth in the adage 'Thoughts are things' should be duly respected!"[10]

Some pretty incredible findings emerged from a study conducted at Harvard University. The study concluded that thoughts, influenced by information, can result in weight loss. In the study, eighty-four female room attendants working in seven different hotels were measured on various physiological health variables affected by exercise. Those in the informed group were told that the work they do (cleaning hotel rooms) is good exercise and satisfies the surgeon general's recommendations for an active lifestyle. They were provided with examples of what made their work exercise. Subjects in the control group were not given this information. Although the actual behavior of either group did not change, four weeks later the informed group perceived themselves to be getting significantly more exercise than before and showed an *actual*

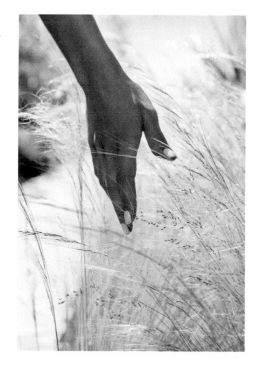

decrease in weight, blood pressure, body fat, waist-to-hip ratio and body mass index compared to the control group.[11] Their thoughts changed their bodies!

I have personally experienced the phenomenon of changing the shape of one's body by altering one's thoughts. When I moved to New York after my trip around the world, I joined a gym and worked out there for about six months (after that I just joined yoga studios). I had incorporated lots of dietary changes during my journey, and I was generally happy with my weight, but I was still frustrated by the lack of muscle tone in my arms, to the extent that I would often choose outfits based on which ones made my "flabby" arms look better. I loved yoga and practiced it, but I also tried other things, such as free weights, and I even asked a trainer to point me in the right direction with weight exercises.

It wasn't until years later that my arms became much more toned. In that time period, I did adopt other dietary changes, and these undoubtedly had an effect on my body. For instance, although my diet was already plant based, I decreased my oil intake, getting more of the beauty fat I needed from whole foods instead, and added some specific plant foods, such as dense green kale salads and chia seeds, as I discuss in *The Beauty Detox Foods*. In addition to these dietary changes, I also changed my mentality. I started to tell myself, first inaudibly and eventually aloud, "My arms are always thin and toned, no matter what." I didn't just blurt these words out. I needed to believe them, and so I said them out loud, with enthusiasm and authority, whenever I looked in the mirror. Over time, I noticed an improvement in the tone of my arm muscles, and to this day it is much easier for me to maintain my upper body muscle tone. I will share more about how to make affirmations work for you in the next chapter.

Negative emotional energy can show up physically—not just in the form of excess weight, but even as acne. Those who experience chronic acne flare-ups may find no relief after making dietary changes and investing in good skin-care products. If you engage routinely in self-criticism, you must confront the deep-seated negative feelings that you have internalized, or these thoughts may continue to show up in a physical form that others can see: as visible pimples and blemishes right on your face, which is front and center to the world. The body, including the skin, reflects your internal beliefs and thoughts.

By acknowledging the emotional energy that may be held in your fat cells or that gets dumped in them when emotional flare-ups occur, you can begin to bring movement back to that area and become unstuck. First, you must acknowledge this energy and work to discover its origins. This stuck energy is like the dormant life energy within seeds. Water is able to awaken seeds: when seeds are soaked with water, their energy starts to move. *Consciousness* is the water that can move the stuck energy within you.

Harness the Power of the Whole

Synergy is when the interaction of multiple elements in a system creates an effect that is greater than the sum of the elements' individual effects. In his book entitled *Whole: Rethinking the Science of Nutrition,* T. Colin Campbell cites a fascinating nutritional study on reductionism versus the power of the whole. The subject of the study is a whole apple versus one of its isolated components, vitamin C. Food scientist Dr. Rui Hai Liu found that 100 grams of fresh apple (about half a cup) contained the antioxidant activity equivalent to 1,500 milligrams of isolated vitamin C.[12] But when he analyzed the actual vitamin C content of the 100 grams of fresh apple, he found only 5.7 milligrams of vitamin C present, which is obviously *far less than* the 1,500 milligrams arrived at by measuring the apple's antioxidant activity.

In other words, the antioxidant activity of 100 grams of fresh apple was a whopping 263 times more potent than that of its isolated vitamin C.[13] The lesson in this is that you cannot derive the greatest nutritional benefits from a food by isolating its components; these nutritional benefits are conferred only through eating the whole food, in this case, the whole apple. In other words, the whole is greater than the sum of its parts.

When you connect to your synergistic wholeness, you can feel and even influence the constant exchange of communication between the physical, spiritual, mental and emotional parts of your being. Although you may have many descriptive terms for your body—too fat, not toned enough, flabby, too thin, ugly, good legs but soft belly, and so on—put them aside for a moment. Pause and try to feel the inside of your body, the energy inside you, your aliveness. This is the bridge to start connecting with who you really are, which is something beyond your physical form and more than any outward descriptor or limited qualification. You may be wondering, *Why should I care about this?* Because this is the beginning of being able to control your body and its shape.

When you take a pause, you start to shift your awareness away from your outer body. You grow aware of your consciousness and become anchored in the present moment. Let's practice tapping into your aliveness, your awareness of being, right in this moment. Eckhart Tolle offers a guide for doing this in his book entitled *A New Earth: Awakening to*

Your Life's Purpose.[14] He guides us first to become aware of our hands, to sense a "subtle feeling of aliveness inside them." You may sense this as a slight pulse or a tingling sensation or just a presence. Once you can feel your "inner hands," as he calls them, you can go on to your feet, then on to other parts of your body, and then, finally, you can move on to your whole inner body.

When you make contact with your energy of aliveness, you are beginning to tap into your tremendous, unlimited power. When you become connected to this power, you will be able to create the body (and the life) that you want. It's time to start living your journey to true power.

Starting in this chapter and going forward, I will provide you with what I call Power Tips, or recommended steps to take to move forward toward your goals. You can always turn to these Power Tips for guidance. They will be accompanied by a photograph of a rock stack so that they are easy for you to find. And this emblem will serve as a reminder that the Power Tips are grounding for you, in the same way that rocks are grounding elements in nature.

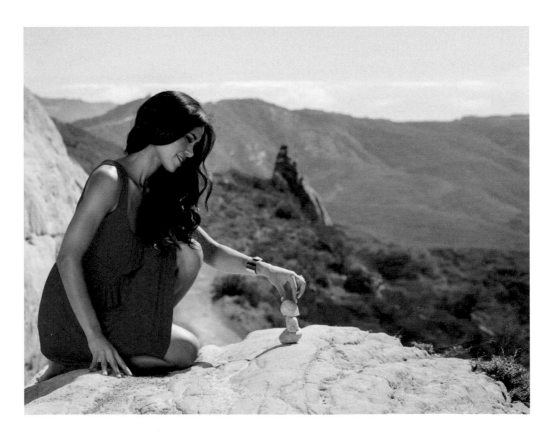

POWER TIPS

1. **Pay attention to what you say out loud and your inner thoughts about your body.** Start taking note of negative comments, and make a commitment to yourself to stop saying anything negative.

2. **Generate and reinforce thoughts of the body you want.** In your mind, focus on positive images of your body, as if you had your ideal body now. Concentrate on positive descriptions about how you feel, such as strong and capable.

3. **Visualize.** Your mind can't tell the difference between pictures and reality. Put pictures of a healthy and fit you inside your bathroom cabinet, where you can see them every day, to bring those images into the present.

4. **Begin to let go.** Create an awareness of anything you are feeling resentful about or are holding on to. These feelings don't serve you, and they don't make wrongs right. Awareness begins the process of letting go, which translates into relinquishing not only emotions but also weight.

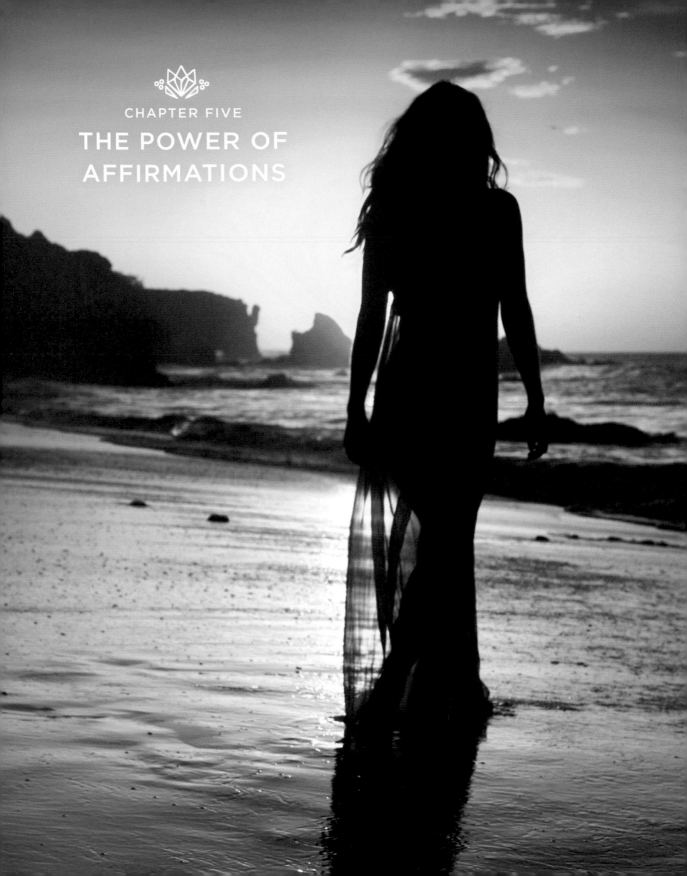

CHAPTER FIVE

THE POWER OF AFFIRMATIONS

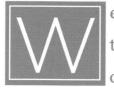We've already established how important your thoughts are to the process of healing, and we will continue to discuss this in the coming chapters. So what do you replace your negative thoughts with? Positive ones! Thoughts that support what you want to create. Affirmations are positive statements consciously stated and repeated.

I am a huge believer in affirmations. They can help to dislodge deeply rooted, subconscious negative beliefs and open up enormous potential positive energy to flow in. They are an important tool for creating unity in your actions, thoughts, beliefs and goals, the unity that is at the core of your true power. Affirmations influence the flow of information in your body, allowing new biological information to be produced by the mind-body fusion.

Stating affirmations doesn't mean babbling off statements written on a piece of paper with an underlying feeling of disbelief or "yeah right" in your head. You must be present for your new beliefs and generate enthusiasm and joy as you state them. To get the most benefit, affirmations need to be repeated regularly and with concentration. They should be declared and not stated as a question. Reading the affirmations that start in this chapter and appear throughout the book will enable you to begin the process of rooting out subconscious negativity, which is holding you back.

Deep down, many of us feel that we don't deserve to be beautiful or thin or happy. But this idea of "not deserving" needs to be reversed. Affirmations can help to create change in your body and appearance . . . not to mention in your overall joy.

We're so used to trying to isolate the *one* cause of what ails us and seeking the one remedy that we don't realize we are practicing disembodiment. We need to be aware of our fusion, and we must consider the multiple areas that may require change in order for us to heal ourselves. Affirmations help to align what you consciously want to create in the world with your subconscious beliefs, and they can cast a light on negativity, which you may not have even been aware of, based on what comes up. A practice related to affirmations (in terms of allowing you to create unity and access your power), and yet distinct, is authentic self-observation.

Gia's Story

When I met Gia, she had a healthy, trim and toned body. But her face was constantly breaking out. She tried to fight the acne with various creams and facial treatments, and she even made dietary changes in an effort to improve her skin. She omitted gluten, dairy, soy and other common allergens from her diet and took probiotics daily, but nothing seemed to help. Since she was also depressed, she saw a therapist from time to time.

What ultimately made a difference for Gia was looking at the problem as a whole. We worked on fostering her self-love, first by making her aware of her deep beliefs and then engaging in the power of affirmations. She faithfully recited such affirmations as "I truly accept myself just as I am." Since we began this work, her acne has gotten much, much better. It flares up, but not on a weekly basis, and now it appears in isolated patches rather than on most of her face. And whereas previously she would always look down due to her low self-esteem and her acne, she now holds her head up high and exudes confidence when talking to others. In general, she is a happier person, which also makes her more beautiful.

How Consciousness Leads to Change

Self-observation is truly powerful enough to create change on the physical level. Researchers at the Weizmann Institute of Science discovered a phenomenon called the "Observer Effect," which is the effect that an observer has on observed reality through the very act of watching.[1] The researchers demonstrated how a beam of electrons changes when it is being observed. Even more remarkable, they determined that the longer the observation period, the greater the change.[2]

In her book *The Brain Revolution: The Frontiers of Mind Research,* Marilyn Ferguson references research by scientists in the former Soviet Union on the effects of different stimuli (laser light, electrical stimulation and others) on electromagnetic radiation (called bioplasma) given off by the human body. These scientists found that when "a subject quietly directs his thoughts toward a specific part of the body, the bioplasma shows corresponding changes."[3] Think about it. Our thoughts are more powerful than lasers! The results of this study reinforce how important it is to become conscious of your thoughts, especially your repeated thoughts.

Such studies also offer insight into how meditation, which is rooted in self-awareness or "watching ourselves," can produce change in and of itself. By being present as we meditate and observing thoughts, emotions, sensations and other phenomena within us, we are actually able to shift and transform ourselves. The same is true when it comes to "observing" affirmations daily and repeating them.

Deepak Chopra states in *Ageless Body, Timeless Mind,* "Every thought you have activates a messenger molecule in your brain. This means that every mental impulse gets transformed automatically into biological information. By repeating these new statements of belief, affirming to yourself that your body is not defined by the old paradigm, you are allowing new biological information to be produced; and via the mind-body connection, your redefined sense of yourself is being received by your cells as new programming."[4]

Affirmations will help you to create your new reality. Research has shown that self-affirmation improves problem-solving performance in underperforming, chronically stressed individuals.[5] Self-affirmation leads to an awakening and creates the belief that you have something unique and meaningful to contribute, as we all do, because we are all part of the interconnected whole. Whatever you withhold, the universe withholds from you, as well. Deep down, perhaps you are withholding because in your heart of hearts you do not feel you are good enough or smart enough. But when you *do* believe you are good enough (and you are!), your body will respond with more vitality and focused energy to create the changes you want. Affirmations are an aid to get you there.

Mirror Work

It's helpful to say affirmations in the mirror anytime you pass one throughout the day. Mirror work, which is something I learned about from Louise Hay,[6] can be very helpful for increasing self-love. Whenever you pass a mirror, you come face-to-face with yourself. Whenever you pass or look in the mirror, get in the habit of gazing into it and saying to yourself aloud, "I love and accept you exactly as you are." Look yourself directly in the eye as you say these words. It may be difficult to gaze at yourself at first, as this sometimes elicits buried emotions, so be extra patient and gentle with yourself and observe all the feelings that surface.

It's great to say affirmations out loud. But my favorite method is to record them as a voice memo on my phone so that I can play them as I'm drifting off to sleep at night and as I'm getting ready for my day in the morning. I program my affirmations into my phone so I can listen to them after my home yoga practice and while I'm brushing my teeth. I play them on my speakerphone when I'm driving alone in my car and have some privacy.

What should you say? How should you word your affirmations? You should affirm the positive, as if it has already been achieved. Always use the present tense. Start with something along the lines of "I am fit and trim," or come up with whatever positive body description that you like. Then write down on a piece of paper all the areas in your life that you'd like to focus on, body related and otherwise, and create positive affirmations around them. Remember to affirm what you want as if you have it now, and make sure that your affirmations generate authentic enthusiasm. Concentrate on what you are saying as you speak, or record your affirmations and play them back.

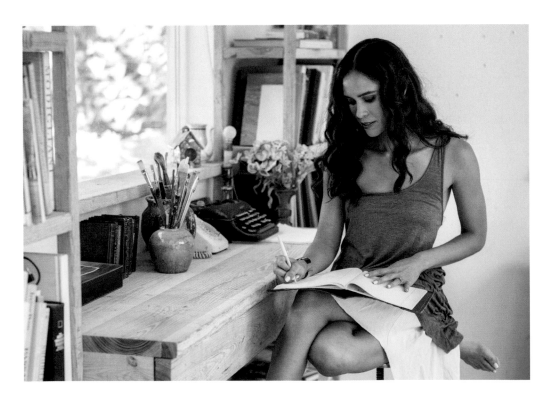

At first it may feel funny or unnatural to say these things out loud, but affirmations are the best way to begin creating energetic (and biological) change. Resistance is greatest when you are operating on the surface of your mind, which is bound up with ego. By declaring your affirmations, you can push past this surface level and delve into deeper levels, levels where change is possible. Affirmations are a way of saying yes to your true nature and essence. Remember, you are powerful, and your thoughts are powerful.

Here are some examples of affirmations:

It is easy for me to maintain the trim, fit body that I want.

I now make great whole-food choices to support my body and my health.

I now release any habits from the past. Now I am fully in the present.

I am powerful and beautiful.

I love myself and accept myself right now.

I am successful in all my endeavors.

My thoughts are powerful.

I now consciously use my thoughts to create what I want.

I deserve great [relationships, success, friendships, and so on], and I am open to receiving more of them.

Because affirmations are so powerful, we are going to use them throughout the rest of this book to foster positive change. Just by reading affirmations, we activate them, set them in motion as catalysts to create positive change. Keep an eye out for them as you explore the pages that follow.

My thoughts now support my goals,
and I am in touch with my true power.

I love and accept myself just as I am.

I have unlimited power to create
what I want and be joyful.

POWER TIPS

1. **Begin keeping a journal** in which you write down those aspects of your body and your life that you'd like to improve upon. Keeping a journal is a good exercise as it requires you to articulate your feelings and confront what you might be harboring or storing in your mind and body.

2. **Create positive affirmations** based on the themes in your journal. Record your affirmations on your phone or another recording device and listen to them in the morning and the evening, and whenever you have time during your day.

3. **Recite your affirmations regularly—** ideally daily. Saying them silently to yourself is still beneficial, and be sure to say some of them as you gaze into a mirror. Make them a part of your life in order to enact real change.

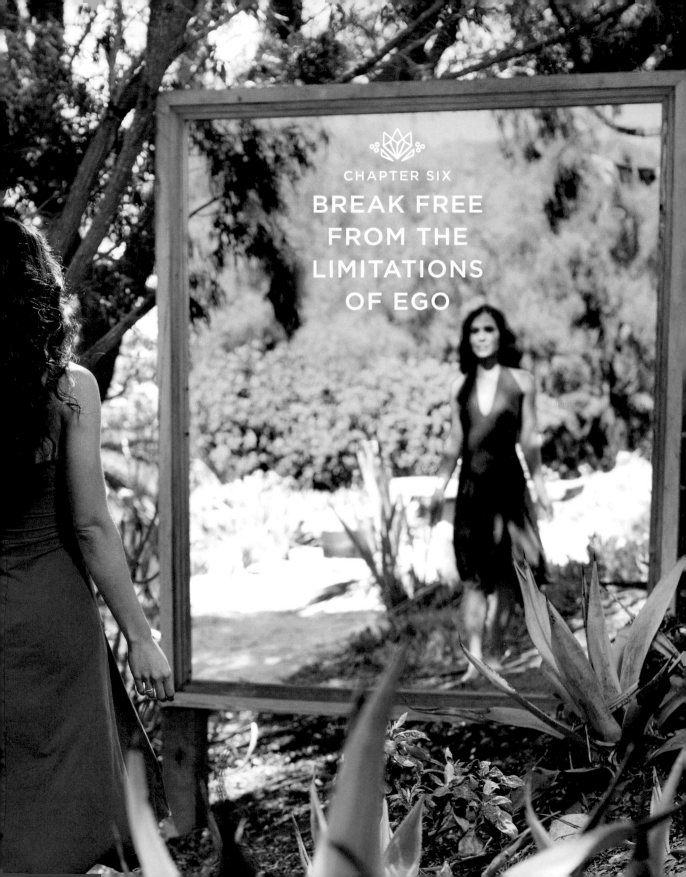

CHAPTER SIX

BREAK FREE FROM THE LIMITATIONS OF EGO

True power originates from within you, while ego involves clinging to outward labels (such as fat, skinny, pretty or old). True power and ego cannot coexist. If you live from your ego, which is the opposite of true power, you will be forever limited and it will make losing weight and feeling joyful a struggle. The ego creates habits and patterns that are rooted in fear. But as you take away those limitations and abandon ego, the struggles dissolve and your true power comes forth.

I grew up in an almost exclusively white town in the northeastern United States, and since my ethnic background is mixed (my lineage has been traced back to Asia and Western Europe), I was labeled "ethnic." As a small child and an adolescent, the last thing I wanted was to stand out. I longed to fit in with the crowd, but the one question people always asked me, much to my annoyance and embarrassment, was, "What are you?"

I have a vivid memory from when I was six years old. It was early fall, and I'd gotten quite tan over the summer thanks to my olive skin tone. One of my blond-haired, porcelain-skinned teammates told me during a soccer game, "You're dark like the devil!" I ran to my mother's car and sobbed to her and my aunt. I equated who I was with how I looked, and I was ashamed to be me.

Throughout my childhood, I loathed the attention I got from looking different, even if that attention was positive. All I wanted was to look like the other girls. The first time I got my hair and makeup done at a local salon was for a homecoming dance during my freshman year of high school. I remember feeling a sense of great optimism when I asked the makeup artist to make my eyes look more "round." I was hoping she could help me fit in and look more like everyone around me. When the redheaded makeup artist responded, "Impossible. That's not what your eyes are like," I was crushed.

Because the world around me put so much emphasis on how I looked on the outside, I came to identify who and what I was in terms of my appearance. I was a very insecure teenager, and in high school my hyperawareness of my differences turned into an obsession with my weight and body shape. I worked every day to control my weight through running and counting the calories I ate. If I couldn't control my skin tone or the shape of my eyes, I was determined to control my weight and my body shape.

Over the course of my life, I've probably been asked hundreds (if not thousands) of times, "What are you?" I realize that the persons who have asked me this question were simply attempting to classify me so that they would have some categories to cling to, something most of us do. At first when I was asked this question, I usually said something along the lines of, "I think you're asking where I come from, not what I am. I come from the East Coast." (Or, if I was abroad at the time, I'd say, "the States.") Finding this answer unsatisfying, most people replied, "No, I mean where are you *from* from? You know, what *are* you?" It became tiring to watch these people try so hard to attach a label to me. Eventually, "I'm a human being," became my standard answer.

Though you may or may not be able to relate to this type of racial ambiguity, I'm sure you can relate to the idea of how you identify yourself. While constantly fielding the race/ethnicity question was exasperating, it's also what provoked me to start thinking about the idea of identification. I didn't believe that a list of countries from where my ancestors came was an appropriate response to the question "What are you?" I didn't define who or what I *was* in terms of those places. But it was easier for those in the outside world to conveniently tack labels on me so that they could compartmentalize me in their mind. Most people want to identify everything in their world. Assigning labels to people and situations is a form of ego, and many people cling to this form for the sense of safety it imparts. In other words, they feel better when they organize things in their mind and try to make sense of a confusing and at times chaotic world.

But while these types of identifications may be comforting, they are inherently limiting. The realization that I didn't have to identify myself with any outer qualifications gave me a tremendous sense of freedom. I felt freer and freer mentally as I adventured to the farthest corners of the earth, to dozens of different countries and all the continents (except Antarctica) with a true joy, adapting easily to all the different cultures and feeling alive and joyful in each present moment of my daily existence.

I didn't know it yet, but it was my decision to give up outer identifications that allowed my power to grow. As I continued on my journey, I refrained from rattling off all label identifications that pertained to me—where I had been working, my age, details about my education, and where I came from—as I now considered them irrelevant. I was able to relate to the people I met on a much deeper level by setting these outer or ego identifications aside. Of course, none of this information was "secret," but I no longer identified with those labels, which seemed exceedingly limiting. I finally realized they had nothing to do with what I *was*.

Around this time I also completely stopped weighing myself and counting calories. I began to enjoy learning about local foods, and I became aware for the first time, in an authentic sense, of how eating foods actually made me feel. I thrived. I'd come a long way from my former food addictions and behaviors, which I'll discuss more in Power Alignment Shift 3.

How Ego Diminishes Your Power

When most people hear the word *ego,* they associate it with arrogance. But ego also encompasses any label or description that you identify with or identify others by. These include age, physicalities (pretty/ugly, thin/fat, etc.), possessions, fame, occupation and education. For instance, when you identify with what you own, with your possessions, and you use the word *my,* you are operating on an ego level. Try to become aware of yourself claiming your possessions. Take note of how often you use the word *my:* my car, my hair, my purse, my legs, my house, my this, my that.

Many people identify who they are by what they do for a living. They often introduce themselves by stating what they do professionally, and then they immediately ask you what you do. But what you *do* is not who you *are*. Others identify themselves more strictly based on numerical facts about themselves. These numbers are often presented as a qualifier, such as in the statements, "Now that I'm 30, it's harder for me to lose weight" or "I'm 43, so you know, now I'm getting to the age where your body starts to break down." Often, clients, friends or just random people I meet tell me repeatedly in the course of a conversation how old they are and sometimes how much they weigh, even though I never asked them. It's easier for many of us to cling to numbers than delve into how we're really feeling or what's going on with us as whole beings.

When you identify with ego-based labels, you limit your own power. You constantly try to improve or defend those labels, which may seem safe but in reality are completely limiting. Adherence to labels is a form of disembodiment, which creates weakness, because it separates you from the whole. Labels and labeling disempower you, prevent you from creating the body and the life that you desire.

When your actions support an ego-based identification, you end up playing a "role." For instance, I hear so many women remark (lament helplessly, really) that they feel less vibrant or have more flab around their belly, "Because I'm 40 years old!" By fixating on a number, you make all the associations attached to that number a reality. In fact, many of your habits and thoughts may be a function of your attempts to maintain those associations.

If you identify closely with the numerical amount that you weigh, the slightest deviation (which could simply be due to water weight) can throw you into a panic. In this case, you waste energy trying to adhere to a limitation, a number. Ironically, the more you become fixated on a number, a label, the more you create toxic energy around it. In other words, it will be more difficult for you to attain the weight and the beauty you are seeking if you identify yourself based on ego constructs, which is all that labels, numbers, are. When you do this, you aren't aligned in your whole being anymore and your connection to your true power is severed.

A study conducted at the University of Minnesota found that 64 percent of the twenty-eight hundred adolescents surveyed employed unhealthy weight-loss tactics when their mothers specifically discussed their weight with them.[1] Perhaps these adolescents would have turned to healthy ways to reach their ideal weight if their overall health and well-being had been discussed rather than just their actual weight.

Another problem with identifying who you are in terms of labels, or ego constructs, is that no matter what position or condition you are in, you will always feel inferior to some people and superior to others. Let's say you are at the associate level of a company. If you consider your job title an integral part of who you are, you will feel superior to those who are assistants, but you may lack confidence when meeting people who are in higher management positions or who are vice presidents. Instead, if you can separate your job title from who you *are*, you will feel comfortable just being yourself and contributing in your unique way. You don't have to feel inferior or superior to anyone.

If you think your body is your identity, deep down, you may very well feel superior to those who are heavier than you. But if you go to a party where the other girls are in better shape than you . . . Whoa, is that a blow to the ego! Your body is not what you authentically and completely are, but it does reflect your deepest thoughts and beliefs. It is when

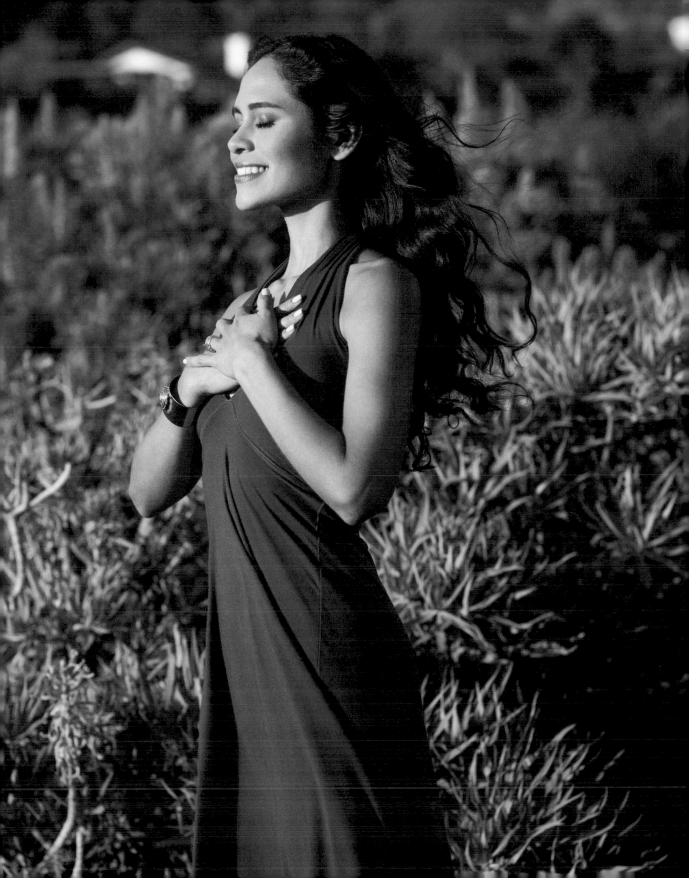

you put your ego aside and tap into your true power that you'll be able to shape your body as you desire.

It's perfectly fine and wonderful to enjoy your possessions as long as you aren't attached to them or feel that your self-worth is tied to them. You can have a Birkin bag or a Mercedes and enjoy them, but if owning them makes you feel even a slight sense of superiority to others, that's your ego peeking out. The ego likes to equate having things with who you are. If you *have* a "perfect" body, will that make you finally accept yourself? Do you feel a sense of superiority when you are thinner than your coworkers? Do you feel you are not good enough because you can't lose those last ten pounds? Just as what you do is not who you are, how you look or what you own is not who you are. If you believe that the opposite is true—that you are how you look or what you own—you will always suffer and struggle. The truth is you are so much more powerful than that.

What You Truly Are

If you are not a label, such as your race or ethnicity, your age, your weight or your personality traits, then *what are you?* Finally, I get to answer the very question that plagued me for so many years in my childhood! What is left if you discard the ego-based labels according to which you have identified yourself and others your whole life?

You are pure, unrestricted, formless energy. You are not your body, your emotions or your mind. If you were your mind, how would you become aware of your thoughts, which are generated in your mind? Your mind, your personality and your body are parts of your experience here on earth, but they are not what you *are*.

If you subscribe to any of the labels that have been affixed to you, to your mind or your body, such as your personality, your numerical weight or your age, you are placing a limitation on your power. And if you keep limiting yourself, you will never be able to express your full potential, which includes the ability to create and maintain a beautiful body, the energy you want, and happiness and joy in your life.

Ego-based labels will never be able to describe you adequately, and the limitations they impose will create a constant struggle and unhappiness in your life. As Paramahansa Yogananda states, "Unless a wave dissolves itself and becomes one with the ocean, it remains inordinately limited."[2] While watching a vivid sunset one day by myself in Puerto Rico, the full meaning of these profound words finally set in for me and shifted my outlook.

Yogananda goes on to state, "When the soul is identified with Spirit, it feels itself as one with the joy of limitless space.... The soul, identified with the body, loses its consciousness of omnipresence and becomes identified with the trials and misfortunes of a small ego."[3]

Most everyone I meet suffers from self-hatred and guilt to varying degrees. They believe that they are not good enough or that they are too small to matter. These are all thoughts that you have to become aware of so that you can separate from them. You don't have to believe any limitations as truth. When you start to realize and accept that you are pure awareness and consciousness, the intensity with which you measure your looks and your bodily struggle begins to diminish. You realize that as a divine spark, how you look, how you age or how your weight fluctuates in no way affects what you *are*. You are already perfect, because you are pure consciousness and you lack nothing.

You may be rolling your eyes right now and scoffing to yourself, *Perfect? Not me!* If that's what you are thinking, it's because you are doing just that: thinking. To realize these truths, you must allow yourself to feel and experience them rather than trying to think them through. It's not unlike the inexplicable joy or sustained energy you feel when you start drinking the Glowing Green Smoothie (page 255) regularly. In both cases, you experience something that you may not be able to explain fully to others, as no specific thoughts have formed in your mind. But you can feel on a deeper level that what you're consuming, or thinking, is giving you the best nourishment. You have to experience this for yourself. Reading this book will help you to foster more consciousness and introspection. The affirmations in these pages can help you to better receive this experience, while the Power Tips will guide you to actions you can take now.

The more you integrate the truth that you are pure consciousness, a whole being that is more powerful than any ego-based labels, the easier it's going to be for you to lose weight, look younger and find joy. Why? Because lessening your identification with ego frees up extreme amounts of energy. Old, stuck energies will become unattached and will dissolve. This includes energies held in your body, such as in your fat cells. This includes the psychic energies that contribute to cravings and emotional eating. This includes rigidities of the mind that manifest as poor long-term eating habits, which until now have seemed nearly impossible to overcome.

The more conscious you are, the easier it is for you to tune in to the true needs of your body and avoid confusing them with mind-induced cravings or habitual thought patterns. The need for counting calories or any other numbers as it applies to food becomes obsolete

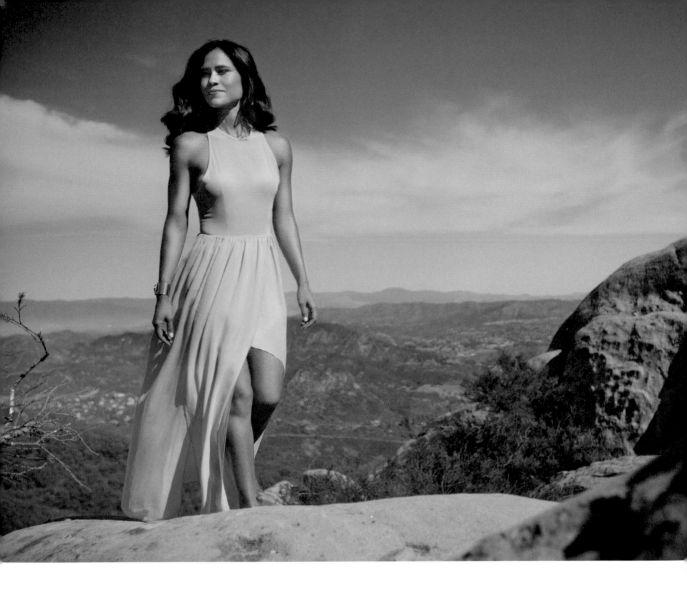

and unnecessary because you are so in tune with your body that you know what to eat and how much.

As you feel your power more and more, you will become increasingly attracted to pure, unprocessed and natural foods. Such foods are in attunement with consciousness. You won't feel like you're "missing out" when you avoid your old vices, because you won't want them as much. You'll experience freedom from habits that are linked to negative emotions and thoughts. You simply won't want to regularly put crap or processed food in your body. And you will become more youthful and energetic, and you'll possess more vitality and vigor.

The reason most people have an ongoing struggle with their weight is that they are out of alignment. Their ego has taken over, and they overidentify with their body. Since they aren't in tune, they become unsure about what to eat and, as a result, overanalyze their diet. They are not aware of their body's needs, because they are confusing labels or thoughts with true needs. But you don't have to struggle or be confused anymore.

As you improve your lifestyle, you will have to put forth an effort and perhaps spend more time than you have been sourcing, stocking and preparing more nourishing foods. And there may be a transitional period when you may feel some intensity with the dietary changes. But over time the changes you are making now will become second nature to you. Be patient, Beauty, because your power will continue to grow in a huge way.

Shift into Awareness

Pause for a moment and see how you identify with your ego. For instance, do you spend a lot of time thinking about what you're going to eat next, feeling guilty if you ate too much at a previous meal or adding up calories? How much of your self-worth do you identify with these factors? Do you feel bad about yourself if you don't lose as much weight as you wanted, if you overeat or if your body doesn't look the way you want it to? If you endlessly obsess over your body or think your life will be perfect when you weigh a certain amount, look thinner and more toned, have better hair or skin, or even make more money, the message you are sending yourself is that you are not good enough.

Eating is one of the most basic processes of living. Treating food as the enemy, being chronically frustrated with food and thinking hostile thoughts about your diet mean that you are fighting life itself. The good news is that you can start to alter that erroneous thinking right now. Remember that you are already perfect. You have unlimited power. You are pure consciousness, and pure consciousness needs nothing external to "complete" or "better" it. As you realize more and more that you are pure spirit and that nothing can diminish that, you will start to feel a tremendous sense of relief and freedom. And as you become comfortable with accepting your wholeness, you will have an easier time in all your relationships, including your relationship with food.

Hal's and Deborah's Stories

When I started working with Deborah, I could sense right away that she was a sweet but very insecure woman. She made condescending remarks about herself and her appearance in passing, but they really struck me, even more since she didn't know she was making them. I went to meet with her in her home, as I do with certain clients, to really see what's going on. Her kitchen shelves and her pantry were packed with diet products with labels shouting out their numerical values. "Zero-calorie powdered drink mixes!" "Low-carb bread!" "Sugar-free protein bars!"

While the rest of Deborah's home was relatively neat, her bathroom was also jammed full with products, as if she was preparing for a devastating natural disaster that would wipe out all beauty stores. The counter and every drawer held an untold number of tubes, bottles and jars containing antiaging, anticellulite, antiwrinkle and anti-frizz products. With all of those "anti-" products, it was no wonder that there wasn't a lot of "pro," or positivity, and that she had low self-esteem.

Can you see the parallels? Deborah was trying desperately to acquire a "perfect" body, not only by buying diet food products but also by stockpiling an overwhelming number of beauty products, in an endless quest to find a miracle in a bottle. She didn't trust that her body had the intelligence to create a beautiful self and healthy skin out of "real" foods. Buying more and more stuff was Deborah's way of dealing with the fact that she didn't accept herself.

Another client of mine, Hal, also couldn't shake the feeling that he needed more stuff to make himself feel whole. Hal was a successful, wealthy businessman in the shipping business. In his family home, expensive decorations (clutter, really!) were piled on every table and surface area, every closet was jammed to the brim with knickknacks, coats, old magazines and old toys, and there were more than a few "junk rooms" in the house, all of them completely filled with boxes of more stuff. To combat his fear that he might need something one day, rather than give old things away, he rented out two storage units, and these were just as packed with things as his house. Meanwhile, more stuff was delivered in the mail daily, as Hal and his wife continued to buy, buy, buy.

Not surprisingly, Hal had a major weight problem. His attempt to fill his life with stuff, whether material objects or food, was clearly not working. No matter how much matter he packed in, he couldn't make the void he experienced go away. It was clear to me that the unhappiness Hal felt was the result of identifying with his ego, and a lack of self-love.

With Hal, I felt that easing him into the program was not the right approach. I had to do something more extreme. I wanted him to experience as soon as possible feeling amazing in his body, a sensation that no amount of acquisition of goods could ever give him. I put him on a strict twelve-day detox. He stuck it out, and by the end of the twelve days he had lost ten pounds. But more importantly, he had incredibly high energy and felt less pain in his ankles and lower back, and he was inspired to continue with better eating habits. Feeling so much better was something that stuck with

him. Since completing that detox, he has made some important long-term changes, such as trading in diet sodas for water, greatly reducing his meat intake, and forgoing binging on cheese. He still binges, but at least it is now on gluten-free crackers and not dairy products. Unfortunately, I can't say that his storage units and his closets have all been cleared out, but at least the toxins in his body have!

As for Deborah, it took some effort to pry her away from counting every calorie and carb she ate. I started her on a regime that involved eating lots of baked veggies and big salads—foods that I knew she would feel comfortable eating and that would not make her gain weight, while she started to shift her perspective. I also asked her to ditch all artificial sweeteners. Before long she was thrilled to see an improvement in her skin, which had started to glow. I'm sure she still uses lots of those beauty products— don't we all love at least a bunch of products?—but now she realizes that she also has powerful beauty products in her kitchen, ones that come right from nature.

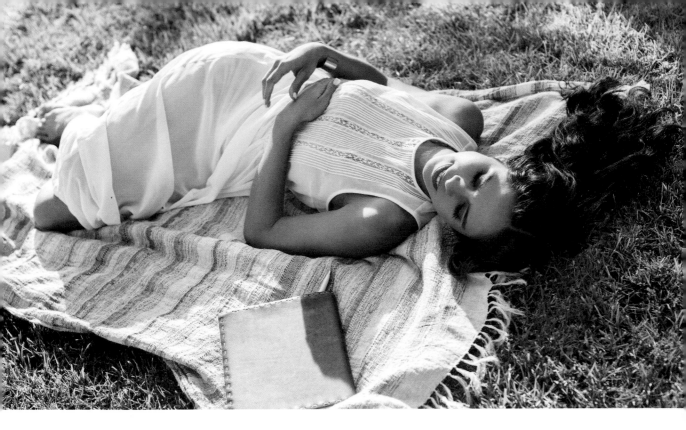

Emotional Eating and Reactivity

Years ago, I used to get a lot more riled up when people would argue with me about my philosophy or beliefs. But now I realize that not reacting is the most powerful thing you can do. Not reacting takes the emotional charge out of the situation. I focus on supporting those who are inspired to evolve and live their best life, not on people who are not in alignment. It's important to be aware of how and when you react. Your emotional reactions may take the form of anger or an urgency to prove yourself, which go back to reinforcing ego. You don't have to have the same emotional reactions that you've had in the past. You have so much more to offer.

You may be wondering, *What do my reactions have to do with my weight?* Well, your reactions matter in *all* situations. Remember that all parts of your life are related. The more reactive you are in any area of your life, the more you are pulled out of the present and away from your goal of realizing yourself and your power. Emotional reactiveness is petty and limiting. When we experience emotions like anger or fear, we tend to eat in a more reactive way, and we eat more in general.[4] In a more direct sense, emotional eating is one way of reacting to situations, and it is a way that clearly leads to weight gain.

Taking a Deliberate Pause

When you feel you are being reactive and, as a result, are about to engage in emotional eating or some other activity that doesn't serve you, take a deliberate pause. Take at least six deep breaths, holding each breath for a moment and then breathing out through your mouth. As you do this, try to focus your mind on the breath alone and imagining stress and tension leaving your body with each exhalation. Taking a pause weakens the link between whatever is causing you to react and the reaction itself. Consciously deciding not to react and then practicing calmness is a surefire way to combat reactiveness.

One time when I was in Cambodia, I had to cross a flooded road in a bus. The bus was packed with locals, some caged chickens and a few travelers like me. The roof was weighed down with countless plastic bundles fastened with string and backpacks, and halfway across the water the bus got stuck. Everyone had to evacuate the bus and wade through the muddy water and then wait nearly five hours for help to come.

The locals were all completely calm as they waited. The adults sat in the shade of some nearby trees, while the children played in the newly formed muddy river, their sweet, high-pitched and almost birdlike laughter punctuating the atmosphere during those hot hours. In contrast, the other tourists on the bus became increasingly agitated as the hours ticked by. Some rolled their eyes and threw their hands in the air, complaining about how this delay would upset their travel schedules. I sat a bit to the side and witnessed these two extremely different reactions to the same situation. It was such a contrast that it was quite amusing to me, and when I look at photos from that day, I still chuckle. When you choose peace over agitation, you realize that a joyful inner state is worth more than gold.

Your ego wants you to react immediately and take some kind of automatic action. But being calm is like a placid lake. The lake is a pure, unblemished canvas upon which you can create what you'd like. Reacting creates ripples, leading images to become distorted, and there is no space to let the light shine through. It's not that you are expected to be perfectly calm all the time, starting right now. Think of calmness as a state of being that you strive toward. It's certainly an area that I am personally working on, as I am a pretty passionate person and sometimes I have to corral that passion. But the calmer you are, the more powerful you are. True power is within you.

The awareness and acceptance of the fact that you are not your thoughts, your emotions or your body bring forth the power to shape your thoughts, emotions and, yes . . . your body.

POWER TIPS

1. **Observe those around you** while actively refraining from trying to label everything.

2. **Reduce your use of ego-based labels,** such as your age, your weight and so on, in conversations. Resist the urge to identify yourself with labels, and focus on how you feel.

3. **Shift your focus from external forms to internal bliss through breathing.** The reason so many people feel so wonderful after a yoga class is that they are brought into the present and out of the ego by breath awareness. Breathing exercises, a simplified term for the branch of yoga known as *pranayama,* are a tool to dive deeper into consciousness, as your breath is the connection to that consciousness beyond your physical body and the greater whole. But don't wait for a yoga class to experience some of the benefits of breathing exercises. Start by becoming aware of your breathing throughout the day, no matter what you happen to be doing (washing the dishes, answering emails, playing with your kid, shopping and so on). Each time, deliberately slow down your breaths, breathing in and out more deeply.

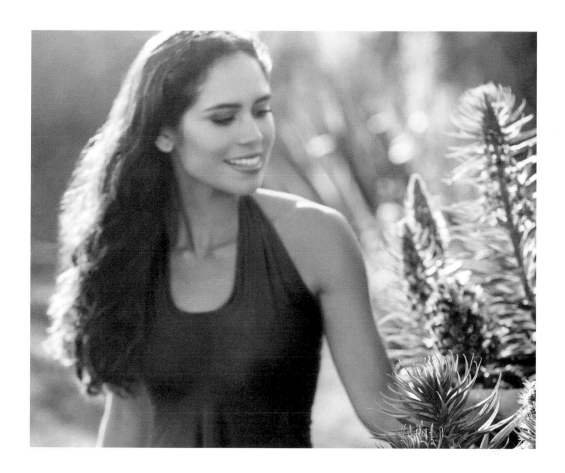

I pause regularly to just be.

I am more and more aware of my true needs.

*I choose to slow down and enjoy
each moment of life.*

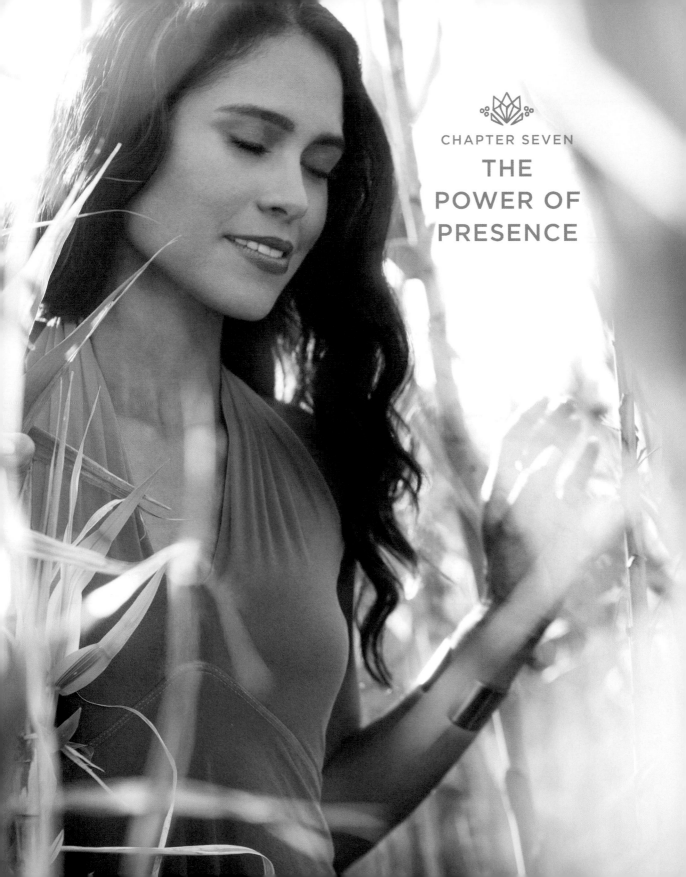

CHAPTER SEVEN

THE
POWER OF
PRESENCE

In high school I was an astute calorie counter. The calculator that I brought with me everywhere was for my calculus class, but I also used it to keep constant tallies of the calories in the pretzels, apples and other foods I allowed myself to eat. This information was jotted down in the back of my notebooks so that I could keep track of how many calories I had "left" for the day. I was always starving, even after I'd "used up" the number of calories I deemed okay for me to eat in a day, and I was endlessly frustrated. Sometimes I was so hungry by mid-afternoon that after track practice I would come home and raid the fridge. But if I ate "too much," not only would I make myself skip dinner, but I might also skip breakfast the next morning, in an effort to get the total number of calories within a twenty-four-hour period to add up.

Unfortunately, teenage Kimberly isn't the only one who has ever exhibited this type of behavior. With the excessive number of calorie-counting apps available nowadays, it has become common practice to think of what we eat as part of a large mathematical equation, something that is to be charted, studied and critiqued. I see this type of behavior in women all the time. Instead of thinking about what they need to nourish themselves in the present, they might tell me, "I ate *way* too much last night. So today I'm just going to have the Glowing Green Smoothie and juice all day." Or someone might say to me, "I was really bad and ate too much fruit (or some other food that's actually healthy and nourishing), so today I'm just not going to eat for a while." In other words, this individual might skip dinner or eat nothing after 3:00 p.m. Periodic, properly administered cleanses can be helpful, as they accelerate the release of toxins for better general health and energy and they can help reinforce long-term habits. But what we're discussing here is clearly a self-imposed starvation day because of guilt, which is vastly different from a cleanse.

If I could go back and tell teenage Kimberly anything, it would be to throw away that calculator (or keep it for math class only!) and learn to eat in the present moment. I would explain that regretting what you ate in the past and using this regret to justify not eating in the future is a sure way to keep your diet (and your entire life) out of balance. Mentally staying in the now can help you better achieve your goals. In 2011, Harvard Medical School published an article entitled "Mindful Eating May Help with Weight Loss" in its newsletter. The article comments on the growing body of research that suggests that mindful eating, which is based on "being fully aware of what is happening within and around you at the moment," can help with weight loss.[1]

Staying present beats calorie counting hands down in every possible weight-, health- and beauty-related way. Researchers at Indiana State University and Duke University conducted a study whose participants included 150 binge eaters. They found that the group that received mindfulness-based therapy, including meditation at mealtimes and throughout the day, seemed to enjoy their food more and to struggle less when it came to controlling their eating.[2] If you stay present, you'll be able to get in touch with what your body actually needs at any given moment, you'll make more authentic and nourishing choices, ones that feature whole, fiber-filled foods. Not only will this help you lose weight and keep it off, but it also will allow you to nourish your body and enhance your beauty in a deeper, more fulfilling way.

Pause to Move Forward

There is a subtle pause between each inhale and exhale. There is a universal pause in nature right before sunrise and right after sunset, when the earth transitions into a different phase of the daily cycle. The moon pauses as a new moon between the waning and waxing phases. These pauses, which are intrinsic to nature, are also essential for you to take regularly so you can tap into your body's true needs, which are beyond anything ego-based. Thoughts produce feelings, and feelings create emotions, which can lead to mindless eating. Pauses help to sort out the thoughts and emotions so you won't be tempted to soothe your mind by stuffing yourself with food.

When you pause, you create an opportunity to become aware of your thoughts, which may be influenced by your ego. You can then choose to identify with them or see them for what they are—perhaps a remnant from the past, a habit passed on to you from someone else, or the remainder of an old childhood wound. By choosing not to identify with these thoughts, you can break the pattern of turning thoughts into emotions and then into eating habits. But if you don't even take the opportunity to pause, the pattern, including eating habits, will just repeat itself again and again. The world is getting faster. You can play games on your phone anytime you have a free moment, or you can race through different websites while surfing the internet. Pauses seem simple, but taking them requires your conscious effort.

Staying present with your body will be the most effective part of your weight-loss strategy, far more impactful than the countless fad diets or the mental mathematics you may have expended incalculable amounts of energy on over the years. Pauses create space, and space directs your awareness inward, which is where your real power lies.

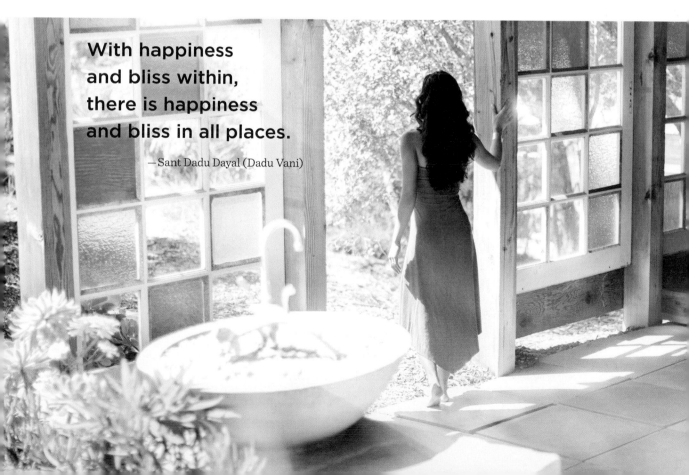

With happiness
and bliss within,
there is happiness
and bliss in all places.

—Sant Dadu Dayal (Dadu Vani)

Make the Best Choice You Can in the Now

Remember that power is always available to you in the *present* moment. The best way to become present is to begin eating with attention and care. When I visit a client at his or her office, I am always shocked to see people eating at their desks, in front of their computers or while talking on the phone *and* answering emails! This is a clear example of disembodiment. Trying to save time by completing as many tasks as possible while eating means there's no presence to the act of eating, no respecting or helping the intricate process of digestion so it can be performed most efficiently. Sometimes, more time is allotted to watching a favorite television show than to focusing on mindfully eating a meal.

When I traveled back to India and stayed at ashrams outside Calcutta and throughout the country, I took part in certain dining rituals. Before entering the dining hall, you take off your shoes and add them to the neat rows outside the front door. The women and the men sit on opposite sides of the dining hall. And absolute silence is maintained during meal times. At first, I thought that sitting in silence would take away from the joy of meal times and that I would miss out on an opportunity to interact with some of the Indian devotees. But soon I realized that I was present while eating, and that was quite remarkable. I could be with my food, pay attention and truly appreciate it. Not only did it start to taste better, but I also started needing less of it, as the silence allowed me to tune in to what my body truly needed at that moment. I also realized that gratitude is one of the strongest energies. Having gratitude for daily gifts, such as having access to nourishing foods, infuses your life with energy and brings more joy to you.

If you take the time to focus while you're eating, by refraining from performing other tasks, you will have so much more power over what and how much you eat. On the other hand, bartering with time never works when creating a balanced body *or* a balanced mind. If the past and the future are in the foreground of your thoughts more than the present moment, you are creating hidden agendas, whether you are aware of this or not. This focus on the past or the future, which are not in existence, creates a dysfunctional relationship with your diet.

Many of us do this unknowingly. One clear sign that we are not present while eating is our use of the word *should*. So often I hear women fret, "I should have eaten a salad last night at dinner, instead of another sandwich" or "I should already have lost five pounds by now." The word *should* implies regret about the past, and living in the past pulls you away

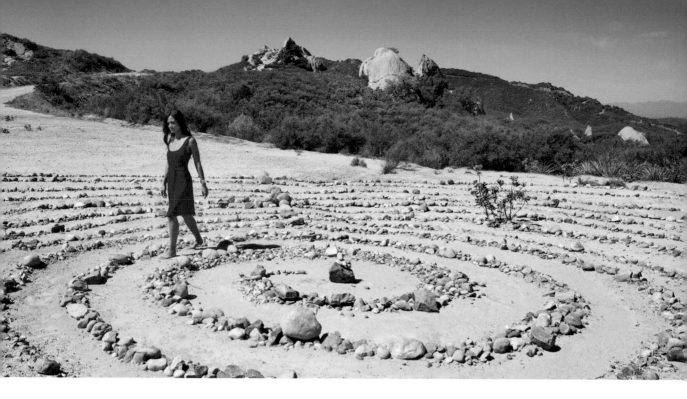

from the present and is disempowering. If you had an "off" day or went out with some friends and overindulged, so what? You want to make better choices overall, but you don't have to worry that you have to eat 100% ideal foods all of the time. Let it go. Some less than ideal choices here and there aren't going to make a big impact.

On a recent trip to Amsterdam I was in a pub, watching the World Cup, and I was starving from walking all day. I really needed to eat something, and I didn't want to miss the match and go trolling around, looking for the perfect snacks, so I ended up eating a whole bunch of chips. Not a tiny little bag, but a big ole serving. And you know what? I didn't stress about it. I don't eat chips regularly, I didn't worry and I didn't gain weight.

Stay present and make the best choice you can in the now. Start asking yourself, "What will serve me best right at this moment?" This is not the same as saying, "I want that candy bar right now," or not planning ahead and coming home, starving, to an empty fridge and succumbing to fast food as a result on a consistent basis. These choices are made on the surface level of ego, and they are reactive.

I want you to take a pause before you choose what to eat so you can feel what your body authentically needs at the moment. Not what taste you are craving, not what the fastest option is, but what will provide true nourishment. When I take the time to do this, I can feel if I'd rather have hot soup, a hearty salad or another smoothie at that time, and I feel more deeply satisfied, because I'm making a choice based on what my body is really telling me it needs. I can also tell when I need something more substantial than just a raw salad to carry me through, like, say, Comfort Chili (page 239).

To be prepared, you have to take the right steps: grocery shopping, thinking through your day, making large batches of certain dishes that keep well for a few days, keeping your freezer stocked for emergency meals and being strategic when eating in restaurants. Some simple tips you can apply anywhere are always order a big salad to start your meal no matter what else follows, choose veggies over fried or heavy sides or sides containing dairy, and go into the meal hydrated so you minimize your consumption of liquids, which can slow digestion by diluting digestive enzymes.

Tracey's Story

Tracey was a human resource manager who felt like she had to have every meal planned out days in advance. She would create a schedule for the week, and everything she ate had to be precisely measured for its calorie, fat and carb content. During one of our conversations I learned that her father was in the military and her mother was a strict schoolteacher. She grew up in a household where discipline was favored. As a child, she was taught to try always to be "perfect." Growing up, Tracey was super hard on herself. She strived to get good grades and to be "the best" at everything she did, whether it was playing field hockey, playing the clarinet or engaging in any other activity.

Together we realized that this need to be perfect had manifested in Tracey's relationship with food as a rigid eating schedule. She felt the need to control everything she ate. If she went out to dinner and ate what she deemed was too much, she wouldn't eat much of anything the next day. Or if she was hungry and ate a bigger lunch, she'd make herself skip dinner (even if she went to the gym and was hungry), chugging copious amounts of water to try to quell her rumbling stomach. When she came to me, her body was very thin, but she wasn't satisfied that she was skinny enough.

I began to prepare food for her, packing it in the portion sizes I deemed ideal for her for lunch *and* dinner. At first, she balked not only at not knowing the exact caloric count of what I made for her, but also that the amounts seemed like "way too much" to eat in one day. I explained to her that the large salads I prepared, topped with avocado or hemp seeds, and the whole vegetables I baked, such as yams and winter squash, were going to fill her up but not make her heavy, and that she had to get present and eat well now, not try to plan with the future or the past in mind.

It took months for her to trust me and to start eating most of what I gave her. We had constant text and phone exchanges, as she needed encouragement all hours of the day. I don't think she ever ate it all, but I saw a huge improvement. Slowly but surely, she was able to let go of micromanaging her meals, doing away with the eating schedules and the measurements. She now rarely skips meals, and focuses on choosing whole foods in the now.

By shifting your thoughts away from shoulds and regrets, you'll be able to stop the cycle of extremes and move toward balance. Avoid binging at dinner and then starving yourself the next day, eating a huge brunch with a friend and then eating only a packaged protein bar the rest of the day "to make up for it," or having only coffee or juice all day so that you can eat a big dinner. Once you stop dipping between the extremes of regretting the past and planning for the future, you will live in the present moment, you will start to relate to your body on a much deeper level, and you will get the results you are looking for without the struggle. In fact, your whole life will change.

POWER TIPS

1. **Plan your day with balance in mind.** Ensure you get in your Glowing Green Smoothie (page 255). Stock up on good staples to have at home, such as

greens, lemons, avocados, apples, pears, bananas, sweet potatoes and winter squash (you can just throw the sweet potatoes and the squash in the oven when you get home from work), quinoa, lentils and your favorite spices, as well as ingredients for dishes you can make in bulk and have for lunch, such as The Twiga Salad (page 321), the Shakti Power Salad (page 243) or the Cauliflower Gnocchi with Walnut Pesto (page 279). When you are prepared, you protect yourself against binge and starvation cycles.

2. **Eat for nourishment at every meal.** Listen to your body and honor it by giving it the best possible choices. Avoid "diet" foods, and seek out fresh, wholesome, fiber-filled meals, which provide nourishment and won't leave you hungry. It's a great idea to construct your lunch every day around a large salad with add-ons, like avocado, sweet potato and other veggies, a large vegetable-based soup or a veggie wrap. Try to avoid consuming too much oil, which can make you feel sluggish.

3. **Be present.** When you eat, do not regret the past or think of the future or future meals. If you ate less than ideally at your last meal or are in a slump, don't worry or obsess. Let it go! Focus on the act of eating with gratitude, right in the present moment. Be grateful for your food, and it will be digested better and will be more nourishing.

4. **Ask your body what it really needs.** Before you make a meal choice, pose the question and see what comes up. If you find it hard to do this at first, start by taking stock of how you feel after eating certain foods at certain times. You may become aware of eating something because it was what others ordered; or eating something out of habit, even though it wasn't what you really wanted or needed at that time; or feeling overly full or lethargic after a meal. The more you tune in to your body, the easier it will be to be more in tune with what your body needs.

I claim my power in the now.

*I listen to my body and nourish it
with what it truly needs.*

I am loving and forgiving of myself.

*My diet is now beautifully balanced,
because I am present.*

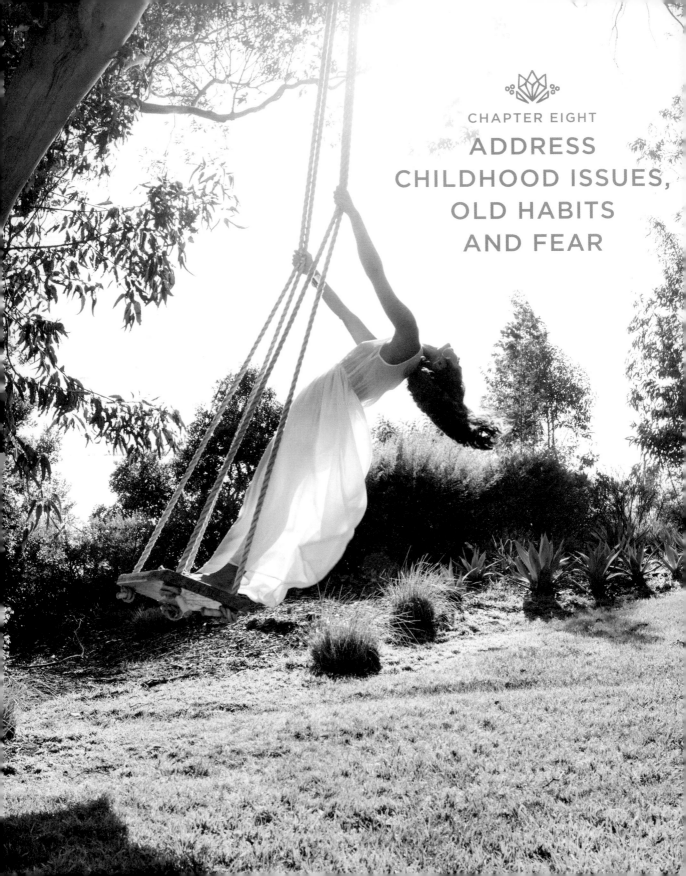

CHAPTER EIGHT

ADDRESS CHILDHOOD ISSUES, OLD HABITS AND FEAR

Research shows that eight out of ten women are unhappy with what they see in the mirror. While this may not come as a huge surprise, I do find it shocking how young many girls are when they start to diet. Surveys have found that at least 50 percent of girls are unhappy with their body by age 13. After 18, that number increases to 80 percent. One American survey showed that 81 percent of ten-year-old girls had already dieted at least once, and a recent Swedish study found that 25 percent of seven-year-old girls had dieted in an effort to lose weight. Similar studies in Japan concluded that 41 percent of elementary school girls (some as young as age six) think they are too fat. Even normal-weight and underweight girls who were surveyed said that they want to lose weight.[1]

These young girls are already suffering from body-image distortion, meaning they estimate that they are larger than they really are. Distorted eating habits and a distorted body image can show up early, as the statistics above indicate, or they can be revealed later in life. Our early life and family structure might have revolved around family meals and homemade food—or a lack of them. As a result, many of us have childhood issues with eating and with food that need to be healed.

Beyond our experiences with food itself, there are so many emotions and so much pain that can get pushed down into our bodies if they are not dealt with properly in childhood. These can then manifest later as dysfunctional eating habits, cravings and deeply rooted self-esteem issues, which may keep you reaching for more food when certain feelings come up, or trying obsessively to control what you eat when you can't control other parts of your life.

I have a distinct childhood memory from when I was eight years old. There was a pop quiz in class based on a reading assignment. Most of my classmates hadn't read the assignment and failed the quiz. Being a voracious reader, I had read it all and scored a 98 on the quiz. My teacher had written the 98, which is emblazoned in my memory, triumphantly at the top of the page, had circled it with a red marker and had drawn a small smiley face off to the right.

I waited all afternoon and into the evening for my mother to come home from work, and when she did, I burst into the kitchen to show her the quiz. "Mom, I got a ninety-eight and scored the highest! Almost everyone else failed, because it was a surprise!" My mother, who was probably exhausted and still in her work suit, glanced at the page briefly and asked, "Why didn't you get a hundred?" When we talked about it later, I learned that she thought it was obvious that she was being facetious. But I was a tiny and fragile child, and what I heard was, "Nothing you do is good enough." A big shift happened within me at that moment.

Feeling completely deflated, I shrank from the kitchen to my room. I made a silent vow to myself that I would never show my mother anything having to do with my grades again. Throughout middle school, high school and college I earned a near perfect GPA, getting A's and A⁺s nearly the entire time. I think I got a few B⁺s in all those years, much to my dismay. My striving to be "perfect" and to get perfect grades was nearly relentless. But I never showed my report card to my mother in person. I would just leave it on the counter for her to review on her own and sign.

Before long, this need to be "perfect" and to prove I was "good enough" was evident in the way I approached food and diet. As I mentioned earlier, I was also coping with the question "What are you?" which others constantly asked me. What a combination! It was then that I started carefully counting the calories in everything I ate and running obsessively. Being on the track team was a good excuse for all my running, but no matter what else was going on or even if I was on vacation, I felt that I *had* to run a certain amount every day.

Take Stock of Your Food Habits

The way you think about your body may have been influenced by your childhood and the way your family members and friends talked about their bodies. If you grew up in a negative, guilt-filled or anxiety-filled environment, you may have picked up a lot of negative

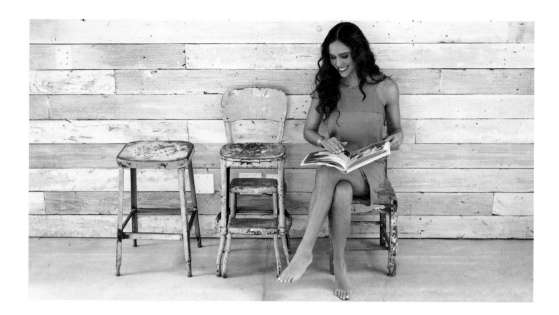

thoughts about yourself and your body. The Adverse Childhood Experiences (ACE) Study, which began in 1995 and is still ongoing (having surveyed more than seventeen thousand adults at present), found that child abuse, including emotional abuse or other traumatic experiences, is linked to obesity and a myriad of diseases in adulthood.[2]

Many people come to me with body issues and emotional issues, and when we start digging around, it's clear that the food and dietary dysfunction stems from something in their childhoods. As adults, they are trying to get comfort from food or to control food because they never dealt adequately with a lack of attention or love from a parent or some other negative experience from their childhood.

All our dietary and body beliefs are influenced on some level by our childhood. These beliefs may have come from our environment, our parents, or an influential teacher, sibling or other family member. Food is a form of tangible energy, and one that we have to engage with every day. Habits and deeply held beliefs are established during our formative childhood and adolescent years. For some of us, a healthy relationship with food and good dietary habits were fostered during that time, while many of us developed bad habits, which hold us back in our adult lives.

A dysfunctional relationship with food doesn't always stem from a specific moment. If you grew up hearing idioms like, "You have to finish everything on your plate," or, "If you are good you'll get a treat," you may have learned to equate being "good" with feeling the need to reward yourself with a goodie. But food should not be seen as a method of reward or punishment. It is not a mechanism for control. Food is simply a source of nourishment.

It can be hard to see it that way if you grew up spending time with a mother, sister or other family member who dieted regularly, struggled with her or his weight, and frequently proclaimed, "It's hard to lose weight." Accepting this belief can set you up for a lifetime of seeing food as the enemy, which leads only to struggling with weight and body image.

But the awesome, liberating truth is that you can let go of all the old beliefs about food that don't serve you. You are free to go forward and create the life you want. I did not have a truly healthy relationship with food until after college, when I relinquished the need to be perfect and took back my power. In order to let go of negative thoughts and emotions surrounding food, you first have to become aware of ingrained beliefs that might be affecting you today and put space around them so you can start the process of letting them go.

Food for Thought

Take a moment to write down in your journal any beliefs you have about food.

Here are a few examples:

If I'm good, I can have a treat.

Food is so frustrating. I always feel guilty for eating too much or I'm starving.

It's hard to lose weight.

Food is the enemy.

I'm just going to gain the weight back eventually, no matter what I do.

As you do this exercise, take the time to uncover your own true beliefs about food, no matter how deeply hidden they may be. Don't try to come up with something that sounds good, and don't worry about how well you do. No one is going to be grading this! Once you've written down your beliefs, think about how they manifest in your current relationship with food.

By simply identifying these beliefs and remaining conscious of them, you can create your own reality. Allow yourself to acknowledge which beliefs you may have picked up from others around you and which may have formed in your head as a coping mechanism. None of these beliefs have to hold true in your present life. They do not have any power over you.

Forgiving yourself, and anyone else who may have contributed to these beliefs, and releasing the past is so incredibly important in your quest for optimal health, and yes, for your ideal weight. When you have weight issues that won't go away no matter how many diets you try, you have to work on loving yourself. Dissolving resentment and anger can help you dissolve the excess weight, which may be a physical form that your body created to deal with the pent-up energy of resentment within. Letting go of negative emotions, and thus releasing energy, can also help you release energy on the physical level, in the form of dropping weight.

Old, stuck emotions and pain you suffered in the past can keep you reacting in the present to certain triggers. Perhaps you always feel that you have to be right, or perhaps you feel unhappy at certain times without really realizing why. These old upsets can also manifest as chronic emotional eating and an inability to move past other harmful eating patterns.

Replace Childhood Beliefs with New, Healthy Beliefs

An awareness of what happened in your childhood will give you the power to create different beliefs and nourishing, healthy eating patterns. Here is a list of some of the most common negative perceptions of childhood, the unhealthy eating habits that may arise from them, new beliefs you can create now, in the present, and affirmations to reinforce those new beliefs.

Whatever happened in your childhood simply happened. It may hurt even now, but you can heal and move forward in a healthier way. It will do you absolutely no good to blame your parents for the past. This will only keep the problem in the present, as it will feed new energy into old issues. Stay where your power is—in the present—and forgive the past. Take the radically compassionate and liberating viewpoint that your parents did the best they could at the time with the knowledge and the skills they had. In fact, they were most likely repeating the same beliefs that their parents passed on to them. If you can, try to find out more about their childhoods. This might foster further healing for all of you.

CHILDHOOD INCIDENT/BELIEF:
Not receiving enough love as a child. What's important is the child's perception, not the adults' intention, so if you feel that you didn't receive enough love as a child, then you didn't. It's as simple as that. This is not to say that it's right to blame the adults, as they probably did the best they could at the time. But it is what it is. This can translate into a lack of self-love or feeling "unlovable" as an adult.

EATING HABIT:
Binge eating or starving yourself. You are trying to control your body in order to be "perfect" and therefore lovable. Unrelated to food, not receiving enough love in childhood can also manifest as always having to be "right" in conversations.

NEW BELIEF:
Realize that you are whole and wholly deserving of love and nourishment in all areas of your life. Make a concerted effort to consciously accept yourself now. It seems radical, but letting go of anything that happened in the past is what is required to move forward.

AFFIRMATIONS:
I love myself.
I am perfect as I am.
I deserve proper nourishment.

CHILDHOOD INCIDENT/BELIEF:
Being abandoned, ignored or overlooked. This can create a sense of inferiority, of not being "good enough."

EATING HABIT:
Food cravings, failing to make nourishing or healthy choices. These habits stem from trying to replace the lack of love you felt with food. Making healthy food choices is also difficult for those who believe they aren't worthy of being taken care of or nourished.

NEW BELIEF:
Realize that you can lovingly nourish and take care of yourself, starting right now. Your past experiences can be valuable in building strength. Try to see them in a positive way. Learn and let go.

AFFIRMATIONS:

I love and accept myself fully as I am.

I choose to take care of myself, because I honor myself.

CHILDHOOD INCIDENT/BELIEF:

Being put down. Being told that "you'll never amount to anything" or that "you're stupid" can lead to low self-esteem.

EATING HABIT:

Lack of confidence when making food choices, susceptibility to diet fads and easy weight gain. If you have low self-esteem, your confidence is shaken at your core, to the extent that you may not even feel confident about what to eat. For the reasons described in Chapter 4, those exposed to debasing messages in childhood can be easily swayed by the latest "lose weight quick" plan or product.

NEW BELIEF:

Realize that the negative comments about you do not define you and are certainly not the truth. Go forward now and take care of yourself by making some foundational dietary swaps, such as eating more whole fruit instead of candy and drinking water rather than soda. Also, begin the Beauty Detox long-term dietary program outlined in *The Beauty Detox Solution*.

AFFIRMATIONS:

I deserve all the good in life.

I have all the power to create the life I want.

Ernesta's Story

Ernesta, a mom, had no problem preparing food for her husband and her son. It wasn't her favorite thing in the world, but she did it. However, when it came to herself, she was at a loss as to how to prepare anything remotely healthy. Instead, she would wait until she was starving, and then she would just buy something fast and easy (and cheap) out on the road. These poor choices were contributing to her weight gain and her lack of energy.

I learned that Ernesta's father abandoned her and her mother when she was very young. Her mother was not very affectionate or loving toward her, and this affected her confidence and many other areas of her life as an adult, including her ability to make healthy food choices for herself.

When Ernesta came to me for help, I realized that the key to her healing was smoothies. Smoothies such as The Cedric Smoothie (page 262), the Glowing Green Smoothie (page 255) and the Zanzibar Shake (page 247) were fast and easy to make, and therefore she could mentally accept preparing them for herself. The smoothies helped her have more energy and start to lose weight. As she experienced her own strength, she felt more empowered. Since then she has moved on to eating more salads and preparing simple plant-based dinners, and the weight continues to pour off. She has also started a job search, which is something that she had wanted to do but until now didn't have the confidence to pursue. While her mother has not become any more affectionate, Ernesta is able to visit her without feeling angry or resentful by affirming that even without her mother's explicit approval, she is wonderful.

My mother didn't exactly have a cushy childhood. She was the oldest of six children (after an older sibling died in infancy), and the whole family was crowded into a small house. My grandparents, a carpenter and a schoolteacher, were very honest, hardworking people. They were determined to feed all those hungry mouths and provide the best education possible, and they were probably more pragmatic than overtly affectionate. Learning about my mother's childhood has helped me to understand her and forgive past childhood issues around communication.

The incident when I got a 98 on the pop quiz had always bothered me, and it was just a few years ago that I brought it up to my mother. She laughed and recalled that her response was a joke, a compliment, really, that she'd meant that the teacher was being too nitpicky and should have given me a 100. I explained to her how much her response had bothered me, and I told her that I wanted to create a new memory. I asked her if we could role-play the situation and change the outcome. So I pretended to be eight years old again as I ran

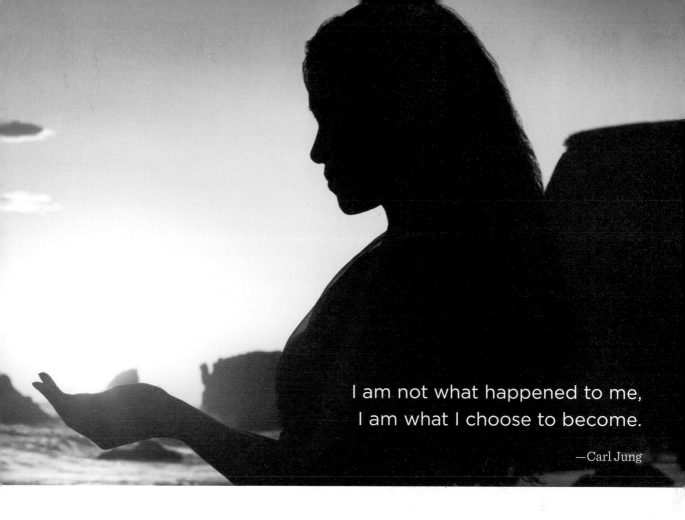

I am not what happened to me,
I am what I choose to become.

—Carl Jung

to her and showed her the 98, and this time she hugged me and told me how proud she was of me. This helped me get over the incident completely.

You, too, can create peace around situations from your childhood that have directly or indirectly led to eating issues. If a family member isn't able or willing to help you create new memories, you can visualize the moment in your mind, with an outcome that brings love and forgiveness. I know past hurts can be very deep, and this might not be the easiest thing, but be loving with yourself and remember you are powerful enough to choose to live your best life *now*.

The only way to get past emotional baggage is to become aware of it, allow yourself to be with it and then consciously release it. If you feel it would be helpful to get formal counseling, explore that option. Do whatever you need to come to terms with old hurts so that you are willing to let them go. They don't have to be a part of your life anymore. How do you release them? Try saying (out loud or inaudibly) to your parents or anyone else who has hurt you, "I forgive you for not acting toward me the way I wish you would have, and I am now free from any emotional attachments or pain."

Once you have released old wounds, if triggers come up or old patterns start to rear their heads, you can exercise your point of power in the present and choose not to react. You can see the past hurt and feel it, but you don't have to identify with it.

The past holds no power over you. Your true power is in the present. You can now release the past and live each moment with power, creating the life and the body you desire.

POWER TIPS

1. **Create a space of awareness about what happened in the past.** The space does not deny that any events took place but rather affords you the freedom not to react with the same emotions that you have in the past.

2. **Write down all the food-based beliefs you may have picked up from others.** Sit in a quiet private space and be really honest with yourself during this exercise. By acknowledging these beliefs, you will be able to be free from reacting to them with the same patterns.

3. **Learn about your parents' childhoods.** Understanding the place they were coming from when they were raising you can help you to gain perspective.

4. **Use the space and knowledge that you have to forgive fully.** This is the most powerful thing you can do to move forward. Forgiveness doesn't mean the past didn't happen, but it stops you from being imprisoned by it. It is a form of love, and the more love you have in your life, the more your power will come forth.

I choose to release the past, and
I choose to create in the present.

I release all past limiting ideas and beliefs. I choose love.

I forgive everyone and everything in
the past, because I am moving forward.

I am whole, complete and perfect just as I am.

Transform Your Cravings

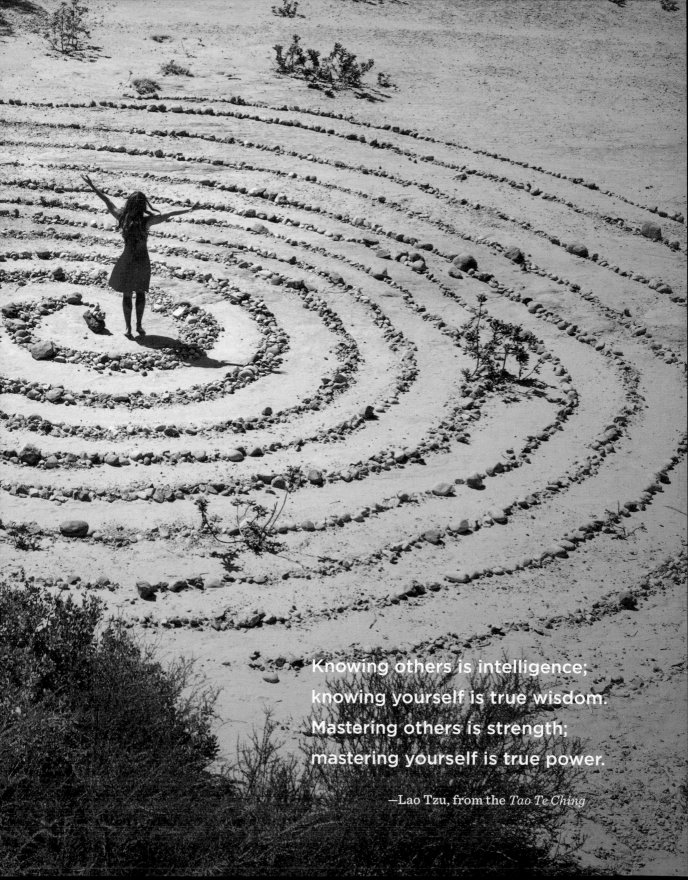

Knowing others is intelligence;
knowing yourself is true wisdom.
Mastering others is strength;
mastering yourself is true power.

—Lao Tzu, from the *Tao Te Ching*

Diets never work for the long term, because they do nothing to get to the root of what caused the mental, emotional or dietary imbalance in the first place. If you find yourself either giving in to cravings or constantly using every ounce of your willpower to avoid eating what you are craving, you are just suppressing your appetite . . . and your feelings.

But this can change. You deserve to feel empowered in every moment. To reclaim your power, we need to get to the root of what is creating your emotional hunger or craving, which has nothing to do with your true physical appetite. It is only then that you can begin to shift your energy, be in tune with the incredible power within you, and choose what will be truly nourishing for you in the present.

CHAPTER NINE

REALIZE THE UNDERLYING CAUSE OF FOOD CRAVINGS

There is more to a food craving than a simple preference for a certain taste or food. There are commonly used food additives known to keep you coming back again and again for more, but as we covered earlier, there is also a tremendous amount of emotions woven into the context of our dietary choices. So when you reach for that bag of chips, that chocolate bar, or whatever you crave, know that it may not be "just because you feel like it." There is likely a deeper reason for your craving.

Taking a pause before eating is key to determining what is really causing a craving. Try writing at least half a page in your journal about how you are feeling before eating, especially before dinner, when you may be decompressing from the stress of the day, and food can seem like an easy outlet. If you are just starting to get into the flow of writing or don't have a lot of time, even jotting down a few adjectives to describe how you feel (sad, annoyed, anxious, worried) can be very insightful for you and can foster a growing awareness of your emotions and how they impact the food choices you make. Find a friend you can text with, and support each other by taking the time to check in before eating. It is in these pauses that real awareness begins.

Taking pauses, which we've already touched on, is an important practice for breaking the pattern of food cravings, where you may feel X and automatically start craving Y. They help prevent mindless mental chatter and thought chains, a phenomenon that is referred to as the "monkey mind" in Zen Buddhist writings, as well as in Taoism and Neo-Confucianism.[1] One thought leads to another thought, which reminds you of something in the past or future, and suddenly you're craving the same old food.

But the pause interrupts the habitual pattern and can give rise to genuine knowing, not from a fleeting sensory perspective, but from a more authentic place: "Ah, the Glowing Green Smoothie will provide me with nutrition and make me feel good all morning." This is not to say that you'll eat perfectly every single time or that adapting this simple but powerful method will automatically negate all the less than ideal foods and snacks that may be in your life right now, but if you are more present with your needs and what you choose to nourish your body with, your ability to make better choices will grow stronger.

Cravings and Nutrition

A long-standing theory that's been passed around is that cravings are both your body's signal that you have a nutritional deficiency and your body's way of telling you what you need. According to this theory, if you crave a burger or a steak, you need iron or protein. If you crave chocolate, it's because you are low in the mineral magnesium. But is this really the deal with food cravings?

Recent research has destabilized the premise that food cravings are nutritional red alerts from your body. In an article entitled "How to Fend Off a Food Craving," which appeared in the *Wall Street Journal* in 2012, the author states, "But a growing body of research casts doubt on the nutritional-deficiency notion.... Instead, studies show that food cravings involve a complex mix of social, cultural and psychological factors, heavily influenced by environmental cues."[2]

I tend to agree with this. Some research connects nutritional deficiencies with cravings. But if nutritional gaps were at the root of most food cravings, wouldn't we be craving nutritional superstars, like vitamin- and mineral-rich kale and broccoli, instead of pizza and cheeseburgers? A study published in 2000 in the journal *Psychology & Behavior* found that a monotonous diet, rather than nutritional deficiencies, was more to blame for food cravings.[3] This is another great reason to incorporate a wide variety of veggies and other foods into your diet, as recommended in the Beauty Detox lifestyle.

Some researchers have speculated that chocolate consumption may be driven by a magnesium deficiency[4] and that low magnesium levels may contribute to PMS symptoms.[5] But if this nutritional issue were the central reason for chocolate cravings, then nuts, which contain comparable amounts of this nutrient, would be craved in a similar way.[6] And this is obviously not the case, as chocolate lovers everywhere can personally attest to.

Furthermore, researchers have found that while Western women often report that their chocolate cravings are highest around their monthly period, women from other cultures do not report similar cravings,[7] which suggests that culture influences cravings.

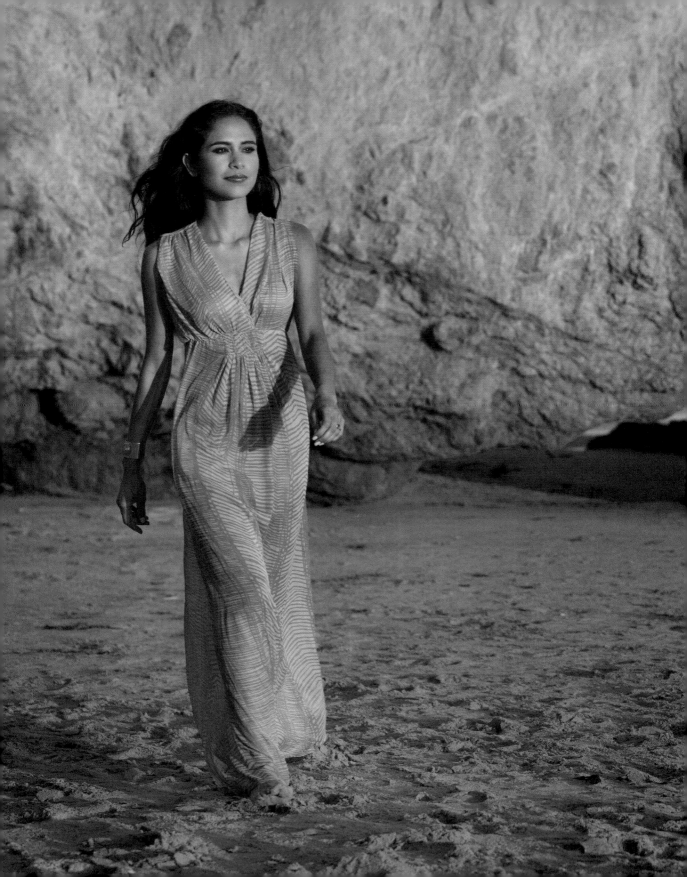

A 2009 study of pre- and postmenopausal American women conducted at the University of Pennsylvania found that self-reported chocolate cravings did not appear to decline after menopause to the degree that would be expected if the cravings were hormonally driven.[8] In alignment with what we're going to discuss in the specific cravings sections, some psychologists suspect that women may consume sweet treats and refined carbohydrates as a form of "self-medicating," as such foods prompt the release of serotonin and other feel-good brain chemicals.[9]

So the bottom line is that if you're eating the well-balanced Beauty Detox way, your cravings mostly likely stem more from emotional and mental needs.

My Story

I can still remember the crispy, velvety taste of the Rold Gold pretzels I used to binge on as a teenager. Oh no, I wouldn't settle for just any old pretzel! My favorites were the large, thin ones in the classic twisted pretzel shape, not the brittle ones that were as thick as a carrot or the long stick varieties. I used to fill a soup bowl with them and chomp on them while I was at my desk or on my bed. An insatiable desire for the pretzels would compel me to drift back into the kitchen when no one was around to replenish the bowl again and again. The predictable crunchy, salty texture acted as a best friend, and sometimes it was the only friend I had to soothe me when I was feeling particularly lonely or isolated. The pretzels also fit the bill because they were fat free and relatively low in calories, and back then I was not only a strict calorie counter, but also an extreme fat-phobe. With the extreme amount of gluten I ingested on a daily basis, it's no wonder I became bloated and constipated and my skin broke out. And that sure didn't help my loneliness!

For me, age 13 was a time of anguish. I look back and say a prayer of gratitude that I don't have to relive it. My Auntie, who had lived with my family since I was born and who was someone that I looked up to and confided in, left our house and moved to New York City to pursue some of her own personal interests, since, at 13, I was no longer a child who needed constant watching over. While I also lived with and loved both my parents,

Auntie was the one who had been home with me the most. Her departure happened during the precarious juncture between middle school and high school, that ultra-confusing time between girlhood and womanhood. I felt like I was left dangling in emotional isolation. It was around this time that the pretzel gorging sprung up, and it continued for nearly a decade. I consumed my beloved pretzels ritualistically, in my bedroom with the door closed, sitting cross-legged and hunched over the bowl. Safe in my room, I could crunch my feelings away in solitude without judgment from anyone else.

It wasn't until years later, when I made the space to become aware of the pervasive underlying feelings and beliefs I had had at the time—the constant anxiety that I didn't fit in and that I wasn't good enough—that I started to heal the bingeing. I went through a period of self-exploration, especially during my around-the-world trip, where I filled journals with writing, spent hundreds of hours on trains and buses, gazing out the window in silence, studied with teachers in formal and informal contexts, and started to really look within. As my body moved around physically to the farthest corners of the earth, my mind actually became more and more introspective and centered. I experienced extraordinary internal growth, particularly in the countries of Thailand, Laos, Nepal, Zimbabwe and India, and these countries will always have a very special place in my heart for this reason.

I remember a long journey down the mountains from Kashmir, India, that I spent in the very back corner of a super-crowded minivan, wedged between a small window that was jammed shut and a woman holding a sniffling child on her lap. I spent the entire ride quietly alert but relaxed, listening to some music. When I stepped out of the minivan, I had the incredible feeling that I had emerged from a profound experience. I can describe it as a reassuring, deep feeling of "knowing" that I was connected with everything around me. I hadn't really *done* anything except let myself be still. Yet I felt like I had really worked through something inside, on a deeper level of consciousness.

But if we backtrack to the beginning of my world journey, I still remember the extreme levels of anxiety and fear that were present right as I embarked. I had just quit my job and broken up with my boyfriend at the time. I was far away from my family. *How will it be, being alone so much?* I wondered as I got my tickets and got ready to leave. *What am I going to do in the future?* Much of my fear at the beginning of the journey was not about the journey itself, but about getting a future job and what I would do with myself down the road. Some might think the traveling alone aspect of my journey would be the scary part, but that part didn't really worry me. The future did!

My journey started in Thailand. I flew into Bangkok, but it was too frantic for my restless state of mind at that time. I continued all the way north on trains and then buses, past Chiang Mai and a smaller city, called Pai, to a small village. Exhaustion had already begun to weaken my anxiety, and when a wrinkled, happy-faced tuk-tuk driver pulled up to me in the bus station and asked if I needed somewhere to sleep, I happily conceded and hauled my backpack onto the floor of his tiny one-seat motorized machine and climbed over it, resting my legs on top of the backpack because there was no space to put them anywhere else.

He took me to a small, family-run guesthouse. I was the only guest staying there. The owners' son took one look at me and said in broken English something along the lines of, "There is something wrong with your eyes. You need to learn how to meditate." From that greeting, I guessed he sure could sense my extreme anxiety. He was my first teacher on the road. That afternoon he took me on a hike to a local Buddhist temple, which I found mysterious and intriguing. And the next morning I packed a small bag and got on the back of his motorcycle. We drove to some kind of forest monastery he knew about, where monks sat in caves and walked along paths in the forest, meditating. It was the first time I was forced to confront my thoughts and anxiety, because there were no distractions and it was so astonishingly quiet. My journey, both outer and inner, had begun.

About a month after that experience, I stayed on a small Thai island called Ko Pha Ngan for a few weeks. At that time, parts of the island were still unpaved. Now it's shockingly much more built up (from one year to the next there's radical development in Thailand) and filled with tourists, but I got to see it when it was still a wild place off the beaten path, a place filled with fire poi–slinging locals, full moon parties in the jungle and plenty of eccentric backpackers from all over the world.

This was the first time I was in an environment where no one cared about my past or my future. No one asked where I'd gone to school or what I was going to do in the future for work. One warm, star-filled night, I experienced an epiphany that changed my life. I was coming back from hanging out on the beach, listening to some music. My bungalow was close to the ocean's edge, and I could hear the waves gently slapping against the shoreline, as if making another form of music. As I stepped onto the first concrete step leading up to my bamboo bungalow, I suddenly felt as though heavy boulders were being lifted from my shoulders and mind. It was a sensation charged with energy, but it also felt physical. The weight had been there for so long that I didn't know what it was like to be without it.

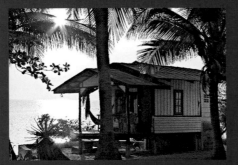

The actual Thai bungalow where my epiphany took place.

In that moment I recognized that this pressure, which I thought was being exerted on me from the outside, was in reality self-imposed, and I had the power to be rid of it. On that night, years' worth of worrying about what I was going to do next, where I was going to work and what people were going to think of me all dissolved in one clean instance. By the time I reached the top of those bungalow stairs, I felt rebirthed into a new state of freedom, even though absolutely nothing on the outside had changed.

I started living in the moment and not worrying about the future. I was free. My travels wove me through years of adventures as I traveled across Asia, Australia, Africa, Eastern and Western Europe, and South America. I met mind-changing teachers all along the way, and they all helped shape my perspectives and beliefs. I kept going deeper and deeper, even in everyday experiences, such as during that Kashmir bus journey.

There was certainly no direct or preplanned path. But I can see now that everything that has led up to this present moment was perfect, was an essential part of the journey, and contributed to my purpose, which is to create and share a health and wellness lifestyle that I love, and to inspire others to live their best life through this lifestyle. The epiphany I had that night on Ko Pha Ngan and my ensuing experiences showed me what being present really meant and helped me to understand the importance of becoming aligned, centered and authentic.

You do not have to experience a dramatic epiphany, and you certainly don't have to travel or seek out mountain

> excursions in crowded minivans like I did to tap into your own power. My experiences have helped me discover the techniques and tips that I share in this book, which we can all benefit from.
>
> I believe that I was meant to experience these journeys because I was meant to share what I learned from them with you. Because we are all one, we are *all* meant to share and learn from one another.

We are all born with a driving desire to access a deeper bliss and joy. The amazing truth is that right now you have access to the deep joy you are looking for, because it's within you. Though there may be some internal work to do in order to tap into feeling your wholeness and power, it's comforting to know that you already have everything you need to experience the joy you've wanted so badly, and you don't need to acquire anything else. This new understanding, and the increased mental and emotional balance it creates, will give rise to a balanced weight, a balanced body and an increased level of inner peace.

Uncover Food-Craving Triggers

You, too, are probably intimately familiar with food cravings, especially if you are a fellow woman. In one study, researchers compared food cravings in women and men and concluded that more than twice as many women than men experienced food cravings. They also discovered that the women felt negative emotions when they indulged.[10] This isn't exactly shocking, right? When you're flying high and feeling awesome, you probably aren't going to drown your sorrows in a bottomless bag of chocolate chip cookies or a mountain of potato chips. A study conducted in northern Finland that examined stress-driven food cravings found that a lack of emotional support was a significant trigger for women who overate.[11]

Research suggests that cravings are linked to cognitive, conditioned and emotional processes, rather than to masked nutritional needs.[12] Consistent cravings overwhelmingly represent imbalanced emotions, an unmet emotional need crying out for attention. A person with cravings is similar to a woman who always dates the wrong guy. Until she gets to the root of why she chooses men who don't treat her well, her underlying attraction to these men will remain. And until you get to the root of why you crave foods that don't nourish your body, the cravings, too, will remain.

When a food craving hits, nourishment is the last thing on your mind. The food you are craving pops into your mind, and your mouth begins watering in anticipation. You feel an urgent need to consume the food . . . now! Food cravings can be triggered by specific events, underlying feelings of loneliness or anger, or a series of small annoyances or occurrences that cause a buildup of frustration and anxiety. A study published in 1999 in the *International Journal of Eating Disorders* measured the amount of ice cream female college students consumed as stressful situations were introduced.[13] The researchers determined that the food was indeed used to "mask" or "distract" as the students' distress and feelings of helplessness increased.[14] So if you have tried to eat away your stresses with ice cream in the past, you can be assured that you have company! In fact, you have so much company that ice cream bingeing has been deemed worthy of a scientifically conducted study.

A 2003 study from the *Proceedings of the National Academy of Sciences* that attempted to discover why individuals crave comfort foods found that the subjects consumed high-energy foods twenty-four hours after their stress response systems were activated.[15] While the impact of incredibly stressful events, such as a divorce, is easy to measure, the effects of chronic stress—about work, finances, relationships, even one's physical appearance and weight—add up over time in a sneaky way and thus may be harder to detect. Losing weight is especially difficult when chronic stress is the cause of the weight gain in the first place, because most people find trying to lose weight stressful. The anxiety triggered by the thoughts around the process of losing weight starts the cycle of stress all over again, and so the cravings keep coming back.[16]

When I was in Tanzania recently, I learned that each banana tree flowers and bears fruit only once. But each tree automatically nourishes a new tree stalk, which grows from the creeping underground stem. If you don't unearth and target the roots, the banana trees will continue to regenerate and spread. Think of your persistent and enduring food cravings in the same way. You need to dig deeper to the root emotional cause of the craving to create and sustain powerful change. By following the advice and the Power Tips in this book, you will discover the root cause of your cravings so that you can overcome them once and for all. (Once in a great while, I still let myself have some pretzels when I really feel like eating some, but I don't feel the need to binge on them anymore.)

How to Target Your Cravings

The journey to end emotional eating once and for all isn't necessarily easy. But recognizing the issues that are causing the eating will allow you to create space and increase your awareness, and over time this will weaken the cravings. Food cravings entail using particular foods to feel better emotionally or to shift your energy level when you feel restless, ill at ease or imbalanced in some way. So the more peace you have in your life, the more peace you will have with your food cravings.

Keeping a Food and Emotions Journal

I find writing in longhand therapeutic, and I encourage you to explore it as part of your regular *sadhana,* or practice, in personal growth. I like to use completely unlined notebooks, as these enable me to express my feelings without limitation. Sometimes I write out words in large block letters, and other times I make sketches or draw stick figures next to my thoughts, since I'm a visual person.

An excellent exercise is to jot down everything that you eat. Simply writing down what you eat can help you with your weight control over the long term. According to Jack Hollis, PhD, the author of a study on the concept of keeping track of foods, which appeared in 2008 in the *American Journal of Preventive Medicine,* "The more food records people kept, the more weight they lost."[17]

Along with noting what you eat, write down what you are feeling when you experience food cravings and when you eat specific foods. This can force a confrontation between you and your emotions, which is key to your ultimate freedom from cravings. You may start to notice that you experience a general sense of unease or simply feel "off" when you find yourself eating lots of chocolate or sweet treats. And if you are honest with yourself, you may realize that the craving was triggered, for example, by dwelling on Suzy from the office, who looks super thin in those skinny jeans and has a perfect boyfriend. It turns out it isn't *really* about the cupcakes in the pantry. The cravings have everything to do with the frustration you feel about being single. And if you boil it down *even* further, the true emotional root of these cravings is feelings of loneliness and unmet love.

Such pauses and moments of reflection allow your emotions to come forth for resolution. When you are not ready to admit these feelings to others and thus make yourself emotionally vulnerable, your notebook can be your sanctuary to be authentic to yourself.

Do not fear that your cravings will be impossible to overcome or that they are hard-wired in your brain. The Power Tips in this chapter and your daily affirmations can and will help! Herbert Benson, MD, a professor of medicine at Harvard Medical School and the coauthor of over two hundred scientific publications, writes in *Your Maximum Mind*: "If you focus or concentrate on some sort of written passage which represents the direction in which you wish your life to be heading, this more directed thought process will help you to rewire the circuits in your brain in more positive directions…and before long, the pathways or wirings that kept the phobia or other habit alive are replaced or altered…Changed actions and a changed life will follow."[18]

You are incredibly powerful, and you *can* change your actions. You *can* change your life!

POWER TIPS

1. **When you feel a craving arise, engage in a twenty-minute cooling-off period.** Go for a quick walk, run a quick errand or throw yourself into a cathartic bathroom-cleaning session, and stay out of the kitchen, the break room, or wherever the snacks or other food may be lurking. You are strong enough to do this, so be strict with yourself here. A great practical way to implement this is to use the timer on your phone or watch, and create the space and integrity within yourself to not forgo this period of pause. Tune in to what you really need, and allow the cravings to pass.

2. **Use mental imagery as a diversion.** Studies have linked cravings to specific mental imagery. The more vivid the image of a certain food in your head, the stronger your cravings for that particular food may be.[19] Cravings take up cognitive space and make it difficult to concentrate on anything else. When cravings show up, think of your favorite scene in nature—a field of wildflowers, a tropical beach, whatever. By creating a vivid mental image of something else, you can distract yourself from the cravings long enough for them to dissipate.[20]

3. **Purify your mouth.** So many emotional food cravings begin with intense feelings in your mind and then are transmitted to your mouth. By having a mint or some herbal tea or by brushing your teeth, you can purify that part of your body and bypass the craving.

4. **Love yourself.** It may sound or feel silly at first, but perform for yourself a simple act of self-love. It could be smiling at yourself in the mirror, treating yourself to a hot shower or a quick hand rub with your favorite cream, or taking a moment to sit and breathe. I personally love physical demonstrations of love, like literally wrapping your arms around yourself to give yourself a comforting hug. Don't

worry. If you need to, you can do this while hiding out in a bathroom stall, where no one can see you. Self-love and internal peace are powerful "medicines" for eliminating emotional eating. Anything you do to foster self-love and acceptance is healing.

I create balance in all aspects of life.

*I love and accept myself because
I know I am already complete.*

Joy and peace come from within me.

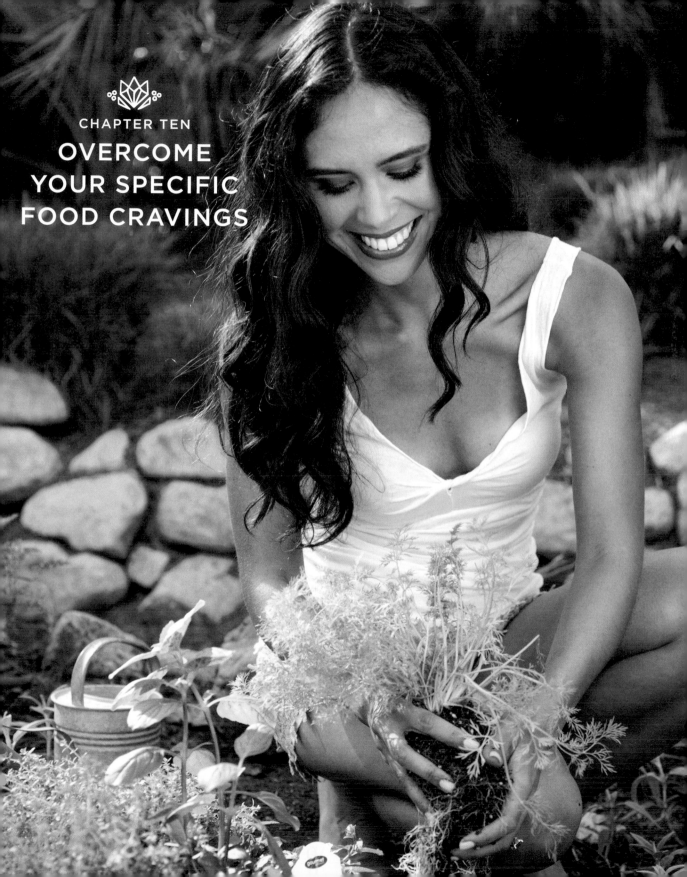

CHAPTER TEN

OVERCOME YOUR SPECIFIC FOOD CRAVINGS

When your emotions and thoughts are not dealt with adequately, whether that means simply confronting the past or seeking counseling for more serious issues, your body will use its infinite intelligence to self-medicate, to take advantage of the mood-altering properties of certain foods. Every food you crave corresponds to a specific emotion or issue calling for your attention.

There are biological and psychological reasons you crave certain foods at particular times. When you feel depressed or low in energy, you will crave foods that brighten your mood. When you feel tense or irritable, you will crave foods that are calming and soothing. Boredom will produce cravings for foods that provide pleasure and are synonymous with excitement in your mind. Each food is a unique conglomeration of smells, textures, amino acids and other mood- and energy-influencing properties. Similar to drugs, foods have different qualities that can act as stimulants or depressants. These mood-altering food properties were recognized in ancient Chinese medicine and food therapy, which is believed to date back as early as 2000 BC (though documented evidence goes only as far back as about 500 BC).

Bernard Lyman, PhD, a university professor from British Columbia, conducted a survey in which he asked subjects to imagine themselves experiencing various emotions, such as anger, boredom, depression, loneliness and joy. While the subjects imagined each emotion, Dr. Lyman asked them which foods they liked to eat. When merely *thinking* about feeling anxious, the subjects overwhelmingly picked junk snacks as their food of choice. This survey clearly illustrates how specific food choices correspond to specific emotions.[1]

While there, of course, may be some individual preferences, people are remarkably similar when it comes to moods and correlating food cravings. Based on my personal experiences and observations of clients and people all around me, as well as on the work of other researchers and experts, such as counseling psychologist Doreen Virtue and Bernard Lyman, PhD, I have rounded up the eight most common food cravings, examined them and designed specific power tools for each of them to empower you to better understand food cravings on your way to overcoming them!

The 8 Most Common Food Cravings

SWEETS

....

The most natural food for humans to consume, and the one that is most readily available in the wild, is fruit. We instinctively choose ripe fruit, which is not only the sweetest but also contains the most vitamins and nutrition. Sadly, today most commercial, nonorganic fruit isn't really sweet or tasty enough to satisfy our sweet cravings, plus the onslaught of refined sugars in processed foods makes us crave an artificially high amount of sugar and a supersweet taste. Many of us simply forgo natural fruit and choose to eat refined, processed sugars instead. It's also amusing to me that some people avoid fruit because they believe it has "too much sugar," but then they eat large amounts of chocolate, candy or baked treats! (If you're interested in learning even more about this topic, see the discussion of fruit, fat and ongoing cleansing in *The Beauty Detox Foods*.)

Since many of us have come to view food, especially sweets, as a reward, for many of us sugary treats are like a hug—soothing, comforting and reassuring. The sugar gives us a temporary boost in energy and has the capacity to make us feel happy or comforted, especially if those feelings are lacking or if we are experiencing stress in some form.

The very anticipation of a reward triggers the neurotransmitter dopamine in our brains. For example, during the dry season, thirsty elephants can walk for miles in search of a water hole. When elephants spot fresh water in the distance, dopamine surges in their brains as energy is released to propel their journey to the water. Dopamine makes you alert, enables you to focus your attention on the task or object that meets your needs, and motivates you to pursue whatever it is that meets your needs.[2] Dopamine has been linked to food addictions (especially an addiction to sweet foods), and a correlation has been shown between low levels of dopamine and overeating in women,[3] possibly because food serves as an immediate, readily available reward and eating is easier than dealing with true needs.

But you have the power to define and address your needs. Your habit may be to seek out sweet treats to stimulate the good feelings that dopamine brings, but you can create new pathways. Establish a new goal in your life, such as learning a new skill, pursuing a hobby, branching out within your profession or exploring anything that you feel passionate about. As you take steps toward your goal, your brain will reward you with dopamine along the way, just as elephants feel the effects of dopamine as they near the water hole and then right before they take that first thirst-quenching sip. The step you take could be small, like starting to do some research or reading a book on a given subject. Any step is wonderful! As you follow through with this step and move forward toward your goal, you will feel a diminished need to reward yourself by eating sweets. The added benefit is more passion in your life.

Lilly's Story

Lilly had a major sweet tooth. She came to me looking to lose weight, but the high-protein diet she used to follow had convinced her that all foods containing sugar—even natural fruit—needed to be avoided to achieve weight loss. During the day she wanted to consume only green juice, and she often skipped meals if she was on the go. She avoided the Glowing Green Smoothie because there was some fruit in it, and she would make the Power Protein Smoothie (in *The Beauty Detox Foods*) without banana for the same reason.

Despite her aversion to sugar, she would frequently consume large amounts of dark chocolate and vegan desserts, such as cashew ice cream, in the evening! What's ironic is that she ended up consuming *way* more sugar by eating those desserts than she would have if she had just eaten some of the fruit that she worked so hard to avoid. Fruits are among the most beautifying foods of all, packed with vitamins, antioxidants and powerful cleansing properties. Lilly's unbalanced dietary pattern—being overly disciplined all day and binging on sugar in the evening—was creating real problems. She had a candida imbalance and suffered from mood swings. Her poor diet showed on the outside, too—her skin looked dull and unhealthy and she experienced regular acne flare-ups.

Lilly dealt with high levels of stress on a daily basis. She worked in the highly competitive sales field, where she very often faced rejection. Sweets became a reward to help her deal with the pitfalls of her daily life. I urged Lilly to focus on developing her own personal regimen to combat the sugar binges. She wanted to know what I ate, even though I urged her to focus on what her body was telling her she needed. But she was really interested in my diet, and when I told her how much fruit I ate regularly, her eyes grew as big as saucers.

"But what about the sugar?" she asked me. Isn't it funny when someone has such tunnel vision that she or he can't really see the whole picture?

"What about *your* sugar?" I asked her. I went on to explain that as her digestion improved and her diet became balanced, she, too, would handle and digest fruit efficiently.

We started slowly, because of the candida, introducing some low-sugar fruits back into her diet, such as blueberries and green apples. I encouraged her to consume whole foods and added the Glowing Green Smoothie to her diet. These became the foundation for her new regimen. I strongly urged her not to skip meals during the day and always to eat lunch and dinner. She was disciplined at first, but after a few days she went back to skipping meals and partaking in her sweet indulgences.

When she realized that she didn't feel good, she returned to the regimen that we had established. It was a process.

I encouraged Lilly to explore a passion she had outside of her job, since she didn't feel she expressed her creativity at work. Jewelry-making was something that she could pour her passion into, and she realized that she could create each piece for its own sake. Sourcing her stones and materials and designing unique pieces were part of her healing process, part of her creating new pathways for rewards and new patterns of feeling good. She started out making necklaces and earrings for her friends, but then acquaintances and contacts saw her work and started seeking out her pieces. She has enjoyed so much success that she is even thinking of turning her jewelry-making into an online business.

Nowadays Lilly still consumes sweets most days, if not every day, but it's usually just a little square of dark chocolate, versus half a chocolate bar or a whole chocolate bar or a huge bowl of cashew ice cream, which is what she used to consume in a single sitting. She enjoys the fruit in her Glowing Green Smoothie without fear. Her digestion is operating much better, and her skin is beautiful and smooth, (mostly) acne-free, and glowing.

POWER TOOLS FOR CRAVING SWEETS

▸ Become aware of incidents in your childhood when you were rewarded with sweets. It can be helpful to recognize the sweet/reward connection and to pinpoint where and how your sweet craving originated. Do you still associate the smell of baked goods with comfort and feelings of love? Through awareness of the association, you can help create space around it and weaken it.

▸ Try rewarding yourself with scents instead of tastes. Scents are very powerful and can help shift your moods. Essential oil-based aromatherapy candles, diffusers, soaps and massage oils can be incorporated into your daily life. Try the satisfying and soothing scents of lavender, clary sage and neroli oil.

▸ Eat more whole, ripe fruit, which satisfies our natural desire for sweets in the most nourishing way. Choose organic whenever you can, and if you are just beginning to reintroduce fruit into your diet, choose fruits that are lower in sugar, such as grapefruit, raspberries, green apples, blueberries and blackberries. As your diet becomes more balanced, fruit will play an even more important part, and you will be able to metabolize and process the fruit sugar better.

▸ Consume the right kind of probiotics, which help balance yeasts that feed off sugar and help create balance in your system overall. I offer a very effective form of probiotics based on soil-based organisms (like the kind our ancestors used to consume from veggies fresh from the garden, coated with a little bit of soil) which you can check out on my website if you're interested, at www.kimberlysnyder.com.

Nothing can enhance me or
diminish me, for I am already whole.

There is sweet joy all around me.

I discover and pursue my true passions.

CHOCOLATE

Okay, chocolate is a sweet, too, but as an admitted chocolate lover myself, I feel it deserves its own category. Research has found that chocolate is the number one food that people, and especially women, crave.[4] And it's no wonder why! Chocolate has a well-known reputation for promoting feelings of love, intimacy and romance. It can even act as a temporary antidepressant when one is feeling sad. There are scientific reasons why chocolate makes us feel so good. It contains phenylethylamine (PEA), a chemical in the brain that improves mood and even mimics the feeling of being in romantic love. The stimulatory properties of chocolate are due not only to PEA, but also to theobromine, a bitter alkaloid that is similar to caffeine. Pyrazine, a chemical in the odor of chocolate, can trigger the pleasure center of your brain.[5] During their menstrual periods, women may crave chocolate in an effort to balance their moods, since chocolate consumption stimulates the production of neurotransmitters, such as serotonin.[6]

Intense and consistent cravings for chocolate may indicate you have unmet needs for love, whether you are single or in a relationship. Before I met my husband, one of my former long-term relationships had some upsides, but overall, the relationship left me feeling lonely and empty much of the time. He was a great guy. But we didn't communicate in a way that made me feel emotionally supported. I felt like I couldn't really talk about things that were important to me, and this left me feeling suppressed and unsatisfied. I realized that I felt happier in the company of friends or even acquaintances from yoga class, which was a big warning sign.

Right before we broke up, I became aware of how much chocolate I was actually going through. And, oh, boy, it was a lot. We used to keep one dark chocolate bar in the house, which we'd get at the market about once a week. But in between trips to the market, I started picking up chocolate at the deli all too conveniently located across the street. Then I started noticing how quickly one large chocolate bar would be gone. Like in twenty-four hours.

"Babe, did you eat a bunch of this chocolate?" I would ask him.

"No, I haven't even touched it," he would shout back from the shower or the other room.

Then it sunk in: *I* was eating all the chocolate. I hadn't even realized how much I was eating. He always went to bed a few hours before me, since he had to be up early for work, and that was when I would keep going back into the fridge and breaking off more and more pieces of chocolate. I didn't even notice it anymore, I was just stuffing myself to feel better, to feel the love I wasn't getting in the way I needed from my relationship.

There was an even lonelier period once the relationship ended. This loneliness is part of what makes breakups so hard. During that time, I indulged in even more chocolate (as well as lots of vegan pad thai and gluten-free pretzels). But soon enough, the healing from the breakup was complete, and I got back into the world and poured myself into my passions of learning and sharing with renewed vigor.

It is always better to be single than to be with the wrong person, because then you have the space to grow. So I allowed myself to enjoy the rebalancing time of singleness, but then I got into a relationship with my husband, John, and we communicate deeply about our feelings and thoughts. We enjoy chocolate together, but I don't feel a need to gorge on enormous amounts anymore.

POWER TOOLS FOR CRAVING CHOCOLATE

▸ As an immediate tool to subdue a chocolate craving, take a quick sniff (not a drink!) of some fresh coffee beans. The pyrazine contained in the coffee's odor will affect your brain's pleasure center[7] much like the odor of chocolate does.

▸ Exercise is a great way to boost serotonin levels and improve mood in general. Go for a hike or a quick stroll in nature, at a local park, or even just around a patch of grass next to your home or office.

▸ You may notice that you crave chocolate less when you feel love, which, unlike chocolate, is genuine nourishment. The good news is that you don't need another person to experience love. Be in love with life and with yourself. Using all the tools we've introduced up to this point will help you feel more connected to your true power and will enable you to experience unlimited love, found in embracing your unity to the whole. If you are in a relationship, being clear on what you will and won't accept from your partner is a way to garner self-love.

··

I always have access to unlimited love.

*I attract and keep only loving
people and relationships in my life.*

I am so grateful to be me.

CHEESE & OTHER DAIRY

In *The Beauty Detox Solution* and *The Beauty Detox Foods,* I go into great detail regarding the health and beauty benefits of giving up dairy. So while we're not going to go deep into that information here, I can't help but touch on it just a little bit. A study that appeared in the *American Journal of Clinical Nutrition* in 2000 showed that dairy has no real benefit for bones,[8] contrary to popular belief. And for the men reading this, and for the women with beloved men in their lives, please note that research chronicled in the *Asia Pacific Journal of Clinical Nutrition* in 2007 "suggest[s] that the consumption of milk and other dairy products increase the risk of prostate cancer."[9] These two studies are just the tip of the iceberg.

Dairy is not produced in nature to be consumed by humans, and cheese does not even exist in nature. Yet it is one of the hardest things for many of us to give up. That most definitely includes me. When I started eating a plant-based diet, it took me over two years to give up cheese. I loved eating it on my salads, cutting it into little wedges, and wrapping it in lettuce leaves while sitting on the floor of my New York City kitchenette. I can still remember the last time I bought cheese. It was a ball of fresh mozzarella, and I purchased it from a local shop in New York's Little Italy that made it by hand. Staring at the ball of mozzarella on my kitchen counter, I had the sudden realization deep inside me that cheese didn't serve me anymore. I threw that mozzarella in the garbage and never ate cheese again. *Sayonara, Mr. Cheese!*

If you have not arrived at a similarly definitive end to your cheese eating, don't worry. It may come in a more gradual fashion, or different form altogether for you. Keep going, and remember it took me two years to transition fully away from dairy. It was also difficult for my husband, John, to give up dairy. He is Italian and loved (and I mean *loved*) pizza his whole life. When I gave up dairy, I didn't push him to do the same, because I believed the inspiration had to come from within him. But over time he, too, felt the urge to give up dairy, and now he recognizes that he feels so much better without it. During our recent trip to Rome, he didn't even have the urge to eat cheese, though he did indulge in some fresh bread and pasta as a treat (as did I).

Yes, I know all too well how good cheese tastes, but there are other factors that make it so darn addicting. Cheese contains a great deal of tyramine, which is a stimulant. Milk contains L-tryptophan, which triggers the production of the brain chemical serotonin and thus makes you feel good. The choline in the milk has soothing properties, and the lactose can feel energizing.[10] Furthermore, cheese comes in a variety of textures: soft and creamy, which may feel comforting, and harder blocks, which give you something to bite down on when you're feeling angry or tense. With all these mood-altering properties, it's no wonder so many of us have a hard time giving up dairy! But if you work on balancing your diet and your mood, eventually you will no longer need a boost from Brie or cheddar.

POWER TOOLS FOR CRAVING CHEESE & OTHER DAIRY

▶ When you eat cheese and other dairy, commit to taking stock of how you feel afterward. Note in your journal how you feel after an hour, a few hours, and then the following day. Note any changes in energy, any sluggishness, any acne, and any bloating or other digestive issues that may arise. As you work to cut down on dairy or to cut it out of your diet altogether, note any improvements you begin to witness in your skin and energy. Having more energy and clearer skin can serve as great motivation to keep transitioning to going dairy-free.

▶ Nourish yourself with fresh foods, such as bananas and avocados, which are naturally energizing and can help boost your mood. Bananas are rich in vitamin B6, minerals such as magnesium, and the essential amino acid tryptophan, which helps to keep you in a good mood. Avocados are also a source of tryptophan, as well as beneficial beauty fat. Eat lots of greens, which contain folate and thousands of other nutritious compounds.

▶ Engage in activities that make you feel good. Yoga and hiking are two of my personal favorites. Explore the ones you love!

▶ Transition off dairy with delicious dairy alternatives, such as almond and coconut milk and yogurt. And you're in for a real treat with the new, delicious recipes you'll find at the end of the book, including Vegan Beauty Ranch Dressing (page 289), Italian Walnut Parmesan Cheese (page 292) and Beauty Food–paired Vegan and Gluten-free Mac 'n' Cheese (page 275). They will make you forget about even missing dairy.

....

*I stay authentic and trust
the path will keep unfolding.*

Everything now is as it should be.

I feel powerful and choose nourishing foods.

FAT

Stuffing yourself full of fat can be a way to prevent feeling empty. Often there is fear involved or an avoidance of making changes. Insecurities can be subdued with a consistently plugged stomach. A study published in *Health Psychology* in 2003 showed that adolescents engaged in a higher consumption of fatty foods and more snacking during stressful times regardless of gender, socioeconomic status, weight and ethnicity.[11]

If you are stressed, you may find comfort in eating fat. Research has found that "both chronic and acute stressors induc[e] the consumption of candy, peanuts, chocolate, and ice cream by obese subjects."[12] As you can see from the foods listed here, a lot of the high-fat foods that people turn to when they are under stress are also sweet. But it is their fat component that can make you feel heavier and grounded. Fat imparts a sense of stability when you're dealing with a whirlwind of activities, responsibilities and pressures.

I often find that fat cravings occur in people who feel empty and lonely, even if they are in relationships, as those relationships may not be fulfilling. Fat, as we discussed in Chapter 4, has energetically "protective" qualities. Fat is more than twice as calorie-dense as protein and carbohydrates, with fat containing nine calories per gram and protein and carbohydrates four calories per gram. Fat remains in the stomach longer and can even "plug" the bottom of your stomach, providing satiation.

No matter where you are or what's going on in your life, you can always rely on this truth for comfort: you are connected to the whole. Because of that, you are never truly alone, and you need to do nothing to be "enough," because you are complete just as you are.

Carolina's Story

Carolina always binged on a very specific thing: toast with loads of butter melted on top. The fact that she switched to gluten-free bread was the very first step in solving her issue. Why did she feel this extreme need to consume so much dense fat in one sitting? She didn't long for sweets or anything else. Only butter.

When she came to me, she had not been in a significant relationship in over four years, so the unfulfilling relationship dominating her life and her perceptions was the one with herself. She didn't really want to talk about her upbringing or her past, but I could sense that there was a lot bottled up in there. Her eyes darted around a lot when we talked, revealing a restless nervous system. And she apologized profusely for things that were not her fault, such as a deliveryman accidently knocking her purse off the back of her chair as we sat talking at Glow Bio in Los Angeles, where I love to meet people when possible.

She usually indulged in her toast and butter load late in the evening. She lived alone, and she told me she would never dream of letting anyone see what she ate. I had her begin a simple three-minute meditation practice in the mornings, and I told her to take a deliberate pause, to separate herself from her work, and to start tuning in as soon as she got home from work in the evening. I also encouraged her to foster more social connections by joining a local chapter of a cultural organization that was affiliated with the country she was from, as this was of interest to her. There she was able to speak her native language, to which she felt a strong bond.

Carolina enjoyed going to the gym, and I encouraged her to try some group fitness classes. This way she could spend her evenings engaging in various types of dance cardio while also connecting with the energy of others and working on rebuilding her confidence and self-love, which were at the root of the issue.

Carolina started drinking a lot of the Glowing Green Smoothie, which made her feel "whole" and full from all the fiber. She made a big batch at home every other day and drank a full twenty ounces each morning. I also had her pack some GGS for work and drink another 16-ounce serving in the late afternoon or early evening, before she came home, to help quell some of the physically empty feelings. Over time, she found that the combination of drinking the second serving of GGS and then going straight to the gym, rather than home, helped her break her pattern of butter binging.

Since we started working together, Carolina has lost about nine pounds, which puts her right where she needs to be. Her goal was to "lose a little weight," but mostly to become more balanced. And now she is.

POWER TOOLS FOR CRAVING FAT

▶ Create a meditation or other spirituality practice into your routine, as this is the most powerful way to overcome feelings of loneliness and isolation. Meditation or another spiritual practice will enable you to start tapping into and feeling your expanded connection to everything around you. See some beginner's meditation tips in Power Alignment Shift 5.

▶ Connect with like-minded beings in a healthy environment on a regular basis. Volunteer at the local botanical garden, at a museum or at a yoga studio (perhaps do some front-desk duty), or join a book, cultural or historical society (may sound nerdy, but it's not. I actually love these groups, and joined one while in London!), a moms' support group, or any group or organization that calls out to you (and that perhaps you previously pushed to the side).

▶ Focus on preparing healthy meals and eating more slowly so that you feel gratitude and appreciation for what you are eating. Such practices promote the feeling of being more connected to your food as a source of nourishment and lessen the need to binge on foods high in fat. Pause to give thanks for having access to fresh and nourishing foods. We are so blessed. You can also pause to offer some silent gratitude to the elements of nature (the soil, the rain, the sun) that nourish plants and to all the beings (the hardworking farmers, the bees, the worms) that cultivated the soil and offered their energy up in order for that fresh food to be present in front of you.

▶ If you're feeling like you really need something grounding, try consuming some avocado, which is a whole-food beauty fat that nonetheless contains water and digests well. Check out the BLT Stack with Avocado-Miso Spread (page 303).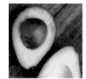

I am grounded with limitless love and peace.

I am full with the joy of life.

I now let go of all that doesn't serve me anymore.

SALTY, CRUNCHY FOODS

Sometimes people tell me they crave salt. But if I were to put a plate of salt in front of them, I highly doubt that they (or anyone else) would just start lapping up piles of salt. Of course, we need sodium to maintain our blood pressure and proper muscle and nerve function, as well as to maintain balanced electrolyte levels in our bodies, but it's very rare to have too little sodium in our modern diet. In fact, the vast majority of us consume more salt than we really need. We've *all* felt the bloating that accompanies eating out too much in restaurants or while on vacation, and this is at least partly attributable to excess salt.

The truth is that for most of us, a craving for salt is a craving for crunchy snack foods. When you think you are craving salt, you are probably really craving the crunchy foods themselves. We often crave foods with specific textures—crunchy, soft, creamy or smooth—and these textures correspond to particular emotions. When you crave crunchy foods, it may indicate that you are coping with frustration, anger, stress or resentment. Crunching down with your jaws is cathartic, almost like punching a wall. Remember yours truly, the reformed pretzel gorger? When I binged on pretzels, I was completely stressed out. On the other hand, soft, creamy or smooth foods can provide comfort or reassurance, and you often crave them when you are feeling fear or are ashamed of something.

When you are stressed, one of the easiest and most available outlets is food. After all, it is a physical entity that you can control and reach out for in a stressful moment. In one study, subjects were given a very difficult task to perform. They were also given unlimited access to free snacks. As the subjects' stress levels increased, so did the amount of snack foods they consumed.[13] And a great number of snack foods are crispy and crunchy!

Cravings for crunchy foods can also signal anger. If there's a situation in your life that is creating anger you aren't completely facing, chomping down on crunchy foods can be a way to temporarily appease those feelings. You may not express anger at the situation in the moment, but, girl, can you chomp down on that corn chip! Repressing anger or frustration is a sure sign that you need to shift your lifestyle. Something in your life is causing discomfort. If it is something you have the power to change, face it. If it is something you cannot change, the dignity of acceptance and surrender can also help to resolve those feelings.

After my Auntie left, I often felt that I had no one to really talk to when I got home from school, and this led to frustration mixed with anger and lots of crunchy pretzel eating. If I could go back and teach myself something then, it would be to let go of my attachment to ego-filled validation from the outside world, to do my very best and to be okay with any result that followed. Today I don't have those same attachments to validation, and I don't feel that pressure to please everyone, which I used to find so stressful. But if I do sense those old feelings rising up, I have a great support system in my husband and close friends and therefore the opportunity to talk it out and keep my perspective. And I'm delighted to say that I'm not a pretzel binger anymore.

You, too, have the power to choose to be present and to come from love, not ego. You are more powerful than your mind could ever comprehend. Relax. Take a deep breath. Release all tension stemming from expectations you created yourself, and from trying to control and plan everything. Stay calm, analyze what needs to be done in any situation and then do it. It can be *that* simple. There's nothing at all to fear.

POWER TOOLS FOR CRAVING SALTY, CRUNCHY FOODS

▶ Keep apples or crunchy veggie sticks around for a healthy way to chomp out frustrations. You can even enjoy the veggie sticks with salsa or Zucchini Beauty Sauce (page 300) if you feel the need to emulate your previous chip-and-dip habit! If you really feel the need to chomp out frustrations, at least you can do it with healthy, beautifying veggies.

▶ Exercise to deflate stress, anger and frustration. If you practice yoga, do a series of 12 or more sun salutations (even up to 108, if you have some stuff to really work out), and focus on your breath until you feel the frustration ebb.

▶ Become conscious of who or what in your life is causing you stress or anger. Create some space to think about how to deal with these issues without relying on food. Commit to taking one simple action to eradicate that stress, whether it's having a phone conversation or writing a constructive email.

Depending on the situation, you might need simply to summon grace and acceptance, one aspect at a time.

I remain calm and peaceful.

I have all the power I need to deal effectively with anything that arises.

I communicate and express myself authentically.

BEVERAGES

While there are so many different beverages that may trigger cravings, the three I have found to be the most prevalent are soda (including diet soda), coffee and alcohol.

SODA:

One of the most disturbing trends I've noticed when traveling internationally is the universal consumption of soda. I've seen farmers and children popping the tops off Coke cans in remote villages in Rwanda, Mongolia, the Philippines and Morocco. I'm often tempted to swipe the soda out of their hands and replace it with plain tea or fresh coconuts, which are commonly available in such places. It seems this obsession with sugar- and caffeine-filled drinks is ubiquitous.

Diet soda is a very popular stimulant and is often consumed in large amounts by people who are trying to lose weight. Others who have some form of imbalance in their lives often crave diet sodas, too. They get an "up" from both the caffeine and the sweetness provided by refined or artificial sweeteners. As I discuss in *The Beauty Detox Solution,* artificial sweeteners, such as aspartame, can trigger cravings, while the carbonation in sodas can feel "exciting," mood-altering and, therefore, addictive.

Furthermore, there are components in sodas (namely, aspartic acid and the isolated amino acid phenylalanine) that have a stimulating effect by triggering excitatory neurotransmitters.

COFFEE:

Coffee is widely known as the world's most common drug, but there are psychological as well as physical reasons for coffee cravings. If you dread going to work each morning, your morning coffee can become a little perk or something to look forward to. Coffee can also be a welcome break from your desk, as going to fetch some java is a workplace custom your boss won't question.

Excessive coffee drinking is something I often see in my clients who work in a job that they don't absolutely love. Guzzling coffee, with its large amounts of caffeine, becomes their way of gearing up, of summoning artificial energy or enthusiasm so that they can tackle daily responsibilities they don't really feel passionate about.

ALCOHOL:

Alcohol in small amounts can be a stimulant, and many people use regular, moderate amounts of alcohol to help manage stress. Alcohol contains a great deal of tyramine, which raises blood pressure and stimulates the production of the brain chemical noradrenaline. This can boost serotonin levels in the brain, though this effect is rather temporary. Beyond one or two drinks, though, alcohol acts as a depressant. Over time, alcohol depletes serotonin production, and a greater amount of alcohol becomes a depressant. For some people, wine enhances feelings of love or affection or prolongs the mood.[14] But the resulting wine hangovers aren't quite so mood-enhancing!

Sure, you may just really like your one cup of coffee each day, or you may sometimes enjoy a nice glass of wine at your favorite restaurant, but if you experience a persistent need to consume these drinks, there may be imbalances in your life that need to be addressed.

Stay true to your feelings and make a move to meet your genuine needs, instead of soothing them temporarily with beverages. Determine what you would like to create, then, like an archer, take aim and go for it. Authenticity, passion and focus infused into whatever you do is the key to your limitless success and joy.

POWER TOOLS FOR CRAVING BEVERAGES

▸ Drink the Glowing Green Smoothie (page 255) to stay hydrated and energized. A source of natural energy, the GGS will reduce your desire to feel stimulated by caffeine.

▸ Check out the recipes for awesome soda and coffee alternatives in the Beverages section (pages 331–335), to help you ease off your prior go-to drink fixes.

▸ Try to keep a regular bedtime hour. Cut out extraneous activities in the evening that prolong bedtime, such as watching TV programs you don't really care about or following a chain of links on the internet. Get thy beauty rest!

▸ If your casual alcohol indulgence has turned into an addiction, it's important to get professional support to get back on track. Check out counseling options and your local AA chapter. There is support and help available, so please take advantage of it.

▸ Tune in to what really inspires and motivates you. Whether it's making a major lifestyle shift or carving out more authentic space in your current situation, you can create ease and contentment through pursuing your true passions. Don't overthink or let fear get in the way. Start making moves toward living your dream.

I live with passion and joy.

I now create a path that is in tune with my dreams.

I have access to infinite energy from within.

CARBS

Sliced bread, crackers, fresh rolls, pasta . . . As you read this list of foods, did you start dreaming of the bakery on the corner or the market where you can't help but notice the stacks of sliced bread, like the kind you used to eat in sandwiches in school? Or are you thinking of your favorite Italian restaurant, the one that serves the best linguine? The joke in my family is that my father's middle name is Roland, which was also my grandfather's name, and as a huge carb lover, he never met a roll he didn't like.

Carbohydrates have a particular smell, texture and taste. Their mood-altering properties can make you feel euphoric, so we often crave carbs when we're feeling down and in need of a pick-me-up. Of course, whole, unrefined and gluten-free carbohydrates, such as sweet potatoes and quinoa, are important for optimal brain functioning and overall energy. Carbs are a macronutrient, after all. But cravings for refined, junky carbs are another thing altogether. Sorry, but you can't play the macronutrient card with those!

Carbohydrate cravings are especially common when you are overly stressed. As your tension levels increase, your body assumes you are in danger and secretes cortisol, a stress-induced chemical produced by your adrenal glands. Too much of it can leave you feeling even more anxious and frazzled. So when you are sad or emotionally hurt, you may turn to carbs literally to anesthetize yourself and numb the pain. Refined carbs break down very quickly into sugar, which can give you a short-lived energy high.

There are also psychological associations at play when it comes to carbs. Baked goods may remind you of your childhood, back when Mom comforted you with cookies or Grandma made you fresh bread. When life starts to feel complicated and you get agitated, you may go back to indulging in these carbs for instant feelings of comfort and ease.

Though binging on carbs may have felt comforting and soothing in the past, as you go within and identify events or conditions that trigger either stress or a desire to feel reassured, you'll find more sustainable ways to achieve emotional balance. A balanced life results in a balanced diet.

POWER TOOLS FOR CRAVING CARBS

▸ Work to *prevent* the overdrive mode as much as possible. Notice how when you get stressed, your breaths get shorter and choppier, and then your whole system goes into overdrive, which leaves you feeling like you need to be soothed afterward. On page 210 I offer some beginner's meditation tips, which include a basic *pranayama* breath technique.

▸ Focus on the positive in any situation, and offer up genuine compliments and recognition of others' gifts. Notice how others start responding to you in more positive ways, too. These are simple daily reminders that you are not isolated, but are connected to all others.

▸ Remove unnecessary stress from your life. Leave for work twenty minutes earlier so that fluctuations in traffic won't make you tense about the possibility of being late. Schedule fewer activities after work and on the weekend so you don't have to rush around as much. Avoid going often to stressful, crowded venues, such as loud, overly packed restaurants and bars. I'm not trying to sound like Grandma Kimberly, and I know that crowded social events at such places are unavoidable sometimes, but if you choose more relaxing spots more often than not, your nervous system will thank you!

▸ Carbohydrates are a macronutrient that your body needs, so do not deprive yourself completely from carbs, which can create more imbalance. Rather, focus on incorporating whole, unrefined carbs like winter squash, sweet potatoes, quinoa, millet and buckwheat into your diet. Check out my tip about probiotics in the Sweets section, which can help balance your system against refined carbs, which quickly break down to sugar.

· ·

I am calm and relaxed, and I trust the universe.

I know there is infinite love around and within me.

I have all the time and all the resources I need.

SPICY FOODS

Over the years, I've noticed certain clients use an excessive amount of hot sauce. They want their food to be as spicy as possible! One of my clients had a whole collection of hot sauces to choose from based on his exact mood at any given moment. (While he touted their flavor variations, they all seemed sort of the same to me.) Indeed, intensely flavored foods can feel novel and exciting, as if you are experiencing something exotic right at home. But if you are constantly craving spicy foods, it may be a sign that your life has become mundane or too routine, or that you feel you are not authentically expressing yourself in some aspect of your life.

Perhaps you feel your life is all work and not enough fun or play, and you need some outside stimulation. Spicy food, such as chili peppers and hot sauce, raises your body temperature and causes a burst of adrenaline,[15] which provides that stimulation. For some people, excessively spicy foods act as an anesthetic. They alleviate their emotional pain by purposely creating physical pain in their mouth and stomach. I worked with someone who had recently lost a loved one and had a lot of unresolved childhood issues she had not dealt with. In restaurants she would constantly ask that her food be as spicy as possible, and then, when it arrived, she would add more spice on top of the spice. I believe that the physical pain caused by the spice distracted her from the emotional and mental pain she was feeling. It took a lot of working through and filling her diet with satisfying foods to which you simply can't add hot sauce (such as the Chocolate and Sprout Love Shake, page 323) for her to begin to disengage from that spice habit.

If you are not used to acknowledging your feelings openly, it can take some effort to do so. But working toward sincere expression will afford you a great deal of relief and immense satisfaction—without the use of external stimulants. You have the power to live a life filled with freedom and fun, one in which you don't have to be anything other than yourself.

POWER TOOLS FOR CRAVING SPICY FOODS

▸ Express yourself honestly in all areas of your life. For instance, if you feel that you are taking on more than your fair share at work and you're not even able to take an adequate lunch break, you might approach your supervisor and arrange a meeting to discuss revising your schedule so that there is more balance or allocating more work to colleagues. If you have a friend who, in your opinion, talks only about herself and never listens to you, have an honest conversation with her about the communication you need in a friendship.

▸ Find ways to move your body in a free and spontaneous way, as the energy of your free body movement can help free up emotional and mental energy. It works! My favorite ways are allowing myself to move spontaneously on my mat during my home yoga practice, and dancing. If you're shy about dancing in public, just dance to a favorite song at home when you're getting ready in the morning, as I do. Let your spine and your hips move around, and don't try to move in a specific way.

▸ If you are really *not* into dancing, at least rotate your spine in wide circles in both directions daily, while standing or sitting in a chair, to help create more circular, rather than linear, movement and energy in your life. You can also try the Spine-Opening Yoga Sequence (see my YouTube video on this), or find time to play more games, such as Ping-Pong, pool or softball.

▸   Take the time to write down your life dreams in your journal. Under each dream, write down small but tangible steps you can take to achieve it. Go for it! Start today.

....

I find fun and freedom in every day.

I know I am safe to express myself genuinely.

I am free to just be me.

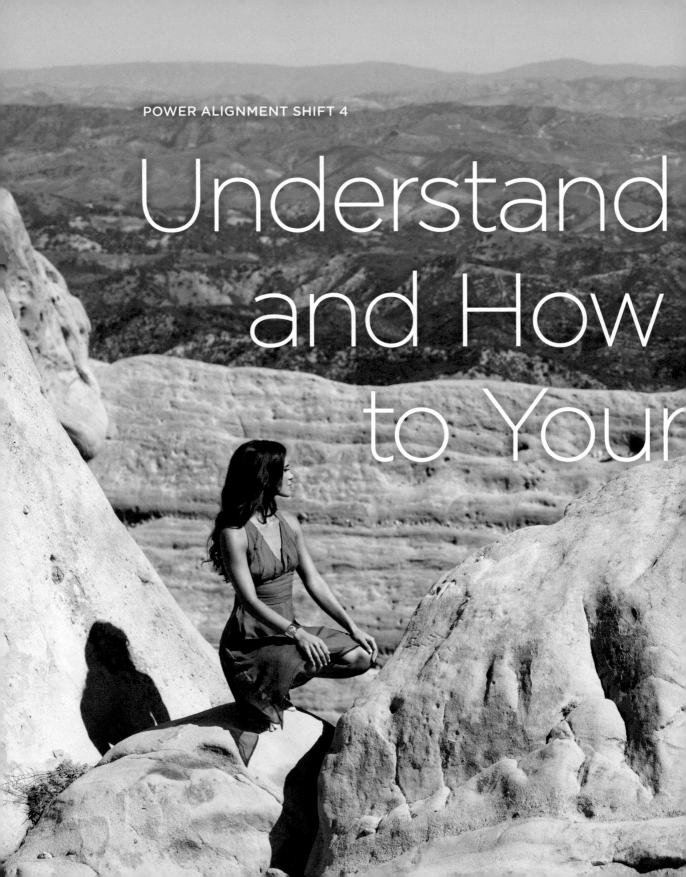

Understand and How to Your

the Chakras

They Relate

Body

We shall not cease from exploration,
And the end of all our exploring
Will be to arrive where we started
And know the place for the first time.

—T. S. Eliot

Sometimes we think we know all there is to know about something, and when we learn to see it in a completely new way, it can be shocking. New is awesome. It's like traveling to another country, where you see people eating with their hands, shouting at each other as part of a normal conversation or living happily in stilted bamboo huts in the jungle. Experiencing new cultures and concepts can drive you to learn more about yourself.

Perhaps you are familiar with many aspects of your being but have never heard of chakras. You don't have to journey to India to learn about chakras and reap the benefits of this knowledge. Integrating this knowledge simply requires you to remain open in your mind and heart. Though you may have never heard of them, the information in these chapters can have tremendous benefits for your health, your appearance, your energy and even your weight.

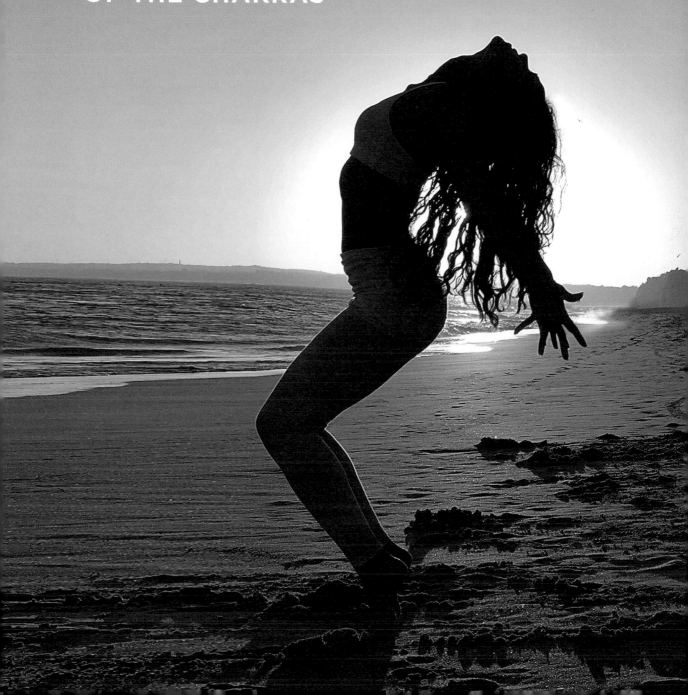

CHAPTER ELEVEN

THE IMPORTANCE OF THE CHAKRAS

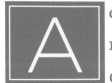ccording to the Western approach, the body is made up of physical entities that can be touched, dissected and/or seen on an X-ray: bones, cartilage, the cardiovascular system, the digestive tract, and so on and so forth. But that doesn't mean that this is all there is to the body. Beneath these physical aspects is the chakra system, which was discovered in Asia at least twenty-five hundred years ago.[1]

Chakra is the Sanskrit word for "wheel." The chakras are spinning energy "wheels." According to the most widely accepted chakra system, there are seven energy junctures along the spine (including the crown, which is technically more expansive, but which we will refer to as a chakra). These serve as connection points between the physical body and consciousness. You can't see them or touch them. Think of them as areas of concentrated energy. These energy centers receive, process and express your vital life energy.

Your chakras are analogous to motors. If you have a blender with a weak motor, you can't adequately break down the vegetables to make a Glowing Green Smoothie. And if you keep your blender on high all the time, you can burn out its motor. In the same way, if there is a deficiency or an excess of energy in your body, it can create a dissonance or a blockage of energy flow in one or any of the chakras, and physical, emotional, spiritual (consciousness) or mental imbalances can occur. The different aspects of your energy are interwoven and affect each other. Emotional or mental imbalances can create physical imbalances and so on.

From the Western perspective, an upset stomach means an upset stomach. But according to the chakra-based approach, an upset stomach could stem from too much mind-created anxiety, which creates an imbalance of energy in the third chakra, also known as the solar plexus chakra, which is associated with your fire element. This chakra is positioned right above your navel, and when imbalanced, it can contribute physically to chaos in your stomach. Constant nervous anxiety in the stomach can eventually manifest as ulcers and other forms of digestive distress. And hindered or inefficient digestion can cause one to hold on to wastes and matter in general, making it harder to lose weight.

Read on carefully, because balancing your chakra energies is crucial to reaching and maintaining your ideal weight.

Discover Your Energy Centers

If you're still trying to grasp what chakras are, instead of trying to think intellectually about them, I want you to *feel* what they are. Put your hand on your heart for a minute. Feel the physicality of your heart beating. Now close your eyes and remember when you physically felt a pang of love for your first crush, your current love, your mother or your favorite teacher right in that same area of your chest. When you feel extreme gratitude or the heartwarming grace of a child, you might instinctually touch your heart with one or both hands.

In Western science there may not be an explanation for feeling the emotion of love in your heart, but in the chakra system it is because your heart is the site of the *Anahata* chakra and is the place in your body where the emotional energies of love are centered. All our emotions and feelings are concentrated in different energy centers, which are located along the spine, and these are the chakras.

I definitely know something about chakra imbalance—in particular an imbalance of the third chakra, or the solar plexus chakra, which rests over the digestive organs. Oh yes! Or I should say, "Oh no!" because I experienced years of being constipated. That was a huge downer in every way, as it contributed to lots of health and beauty issues, like low energy, weight gain and acne. When I made major dietary changes, such as increasing my fiber intake and cutting out clogging foods, such as dairy and gluten, it helped tremendously, but even then I continued to be somewhat backed up. I felt like there was a lot more "in there." When I learned about chakra work, I realized I had major blockages in my *Manipura* chakra (third chakra), located right in my gut. I held anxiety there from the past, as well as insecurities about my future. This translated into "holding" in all parts of my life, which eventuated in constipation.

It wasn't until I went to India during my world journey that I really learned about the chakras. This new knowledge helped me to realize that I worried constantly, overanalyzed situations, and ran through what-ifs over and over again in my head, which blocked my energy and kept me from flowing with the present moment. Having physical issues in my gut that corresponded with my third chakra motivated me to investigate the underlying

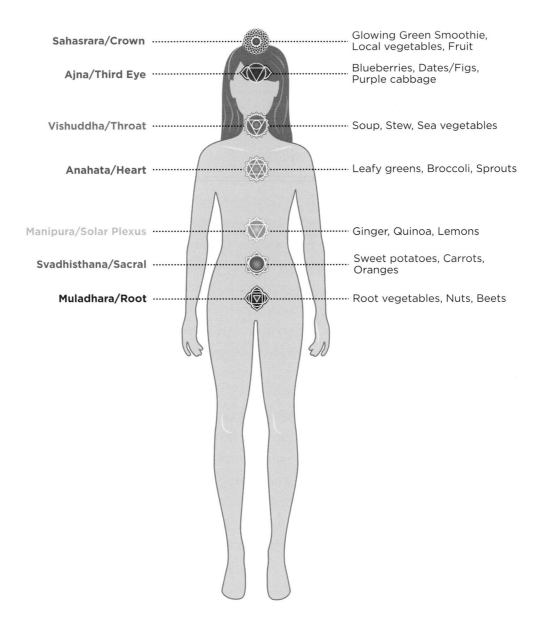

Sahasrara/Crown ········· Glowing Green Smoothie, Local vegetables, Fruit

Ajna/Third Eye ········· Blueberries, Dates/Figs, Purple cabbage

Vishuddha/Throat ········· Soup, Stew, Sea vegetables

Anahata/Heart ········· Leafy greens, Broccoli, Sprouts

Manipura/Solar Plexus ········· Ginger, Quinoa, Lemons

Svadhisthana/Sacral ········· Sweet potatoes, Carrots, Oranges

Muladhara/Root ········· Root vegetables, Nuts, Beets

emotional and mental issues associated with that particular chakra, that is, to understand the root cause of the imbalance.

It took a combination of chakra work, dietary changes, and the ongoing cleansing techniques I discuss in *The Beauty Detox Solution,* such as incorporating probiotics, taking a magnesium-oxygen product, and having enemas and gravity colonics, for me to boost my sluggish "fire" of digestion and reach new levels of health and energy. Finally, I had clear skin, and I shed the excess weight I had been carrying around. As I repeat so often, balance from within creates outer beauty.

Understanding the chakras and all the energies at various levels in your life will help you create the body and the beauty you want—in a deep and enduring way.

Chakras in Alternative Medicine

The Scientific Basis of Integrative Medicine (2005), coauthored by Lucy Anderson and Leonard A. Wisneski, MD, a fellow in the American College of Physicians and a clinical professor of medicine at George Washington University Medical Center, is one of the first books to detail the mind-body connection and to bridge Western medicine and the knowledge of ancient energy systems. According to an overview of their research published in 2005 in the journal *Evidence-Based Complementary Alternative Medicine*,[2] the authors assert that "subtle energy both informs and transcends the faculties of the five senses. It is taken into the body via openings, called chakras, and translated into a form of energy that the body can use, literally use, at the cellular level. Just as the pineal is the energy transducer for environmental information, the chakras are the energy transducers for subtle energy. Subtle energy is a healing energy that anyone can learn to perceive and utilize. It is a crucial, but often missing, component in health care."[3]

The chakras are connected to *marmas,* a foundational cornerstone of Ayurvedic medicine,[4] one of the world's oldest medical systems.[5] Ayurvedic medicine originated in India thousands of years ago and involves energy movement, much like acupuncture. Both the chakra system and acupuncture involve vibration, movement and the removal of blockages to allow vital energy to flow through the body. This flow of energy is what creates optimal health and well-being. Both systems are based on five elements: earth, water, fire, air and ether/space in the chakra system, and earth, water, fire, wood and metal in the acupuncture system. These chakra elements exist in the world around us, as well as in our bodies. Though these elements are everywhere in our bodies, it is believed that our energies "coil" into the central spinal column, and it is in the chakras, which are areas along the spine, where we can really work with them.

Prana, the universal energy that flows through the chakras, is similar to chi in Chinese medicine.[6] Acupuncture involves penetrating the skin with needles to stimulate certain points on the body and thus allow for the free movement of Qi or chi. Acupuncture has been studied in a formal context and is now widely accepted as a beneficial healing technique. Modern research provides evidence of a sympathetic nervous response when acupuncture points are stimulated.[7] A meta-analysis of randomized controlled trials of acupuncture for pain relief published in 2012 in *JAMA Internal Medicine* concluded that "[a]cupuncture is effective for the treatment of chronic pain and is therefore a reasonable referral option."(8)

While there has been less structured study of chakras, researchers have found that chakras can "alter the activity in the central nervous system" and that "the physical base of a chakra" can have an influence over the "activities of the CNS, ANS, and endocrine system."[9] Dr. John Nelson, a neurologist and psychiatrist, believes that "the chakras line up with Western stages of biological growth and psychological development."[10] We've established how psychology influences weight. Psychological distress can lead to emotional eating, and it can also create energetic patterns that can contribute to a tendency to "hold on" to weight.

Reiki, which was first developed in Japan, is an energy-based healing modality that involves balancing the energies of the chakras. According to the American Hospital Association, as of 2007 over eight hundred American hospitals offered Reiki as part of their hospital services.[11] That is roughly 15 percent of hospitals nationwide. Among the hospitals that offer Reiki are the Cleveland Clinic, Children's Hospital in Boston, and Johns Hopkins Hospital in Baltimore.[12]

A peer-reviewed study of Reiki published in 2010 in the *Journal of Alternative and Complementary Medicine* found that "heart rate and diastolic blood pressure decreased significantly in the Reiki group compared to both placebo and control groups."[13] Balancing the energies of the chakras doesn't just benefit your heart rate and your blood pressure; it can also have a beneficial effect on other parts of your body that are influenced by energy. Therefore, it is vital to your health, beauty and weight.

Professor Brian D. Josephson of Cambridge University, a recipient of the Nobel Prize, said of the ancient Hindu system of philosophy, which includes the chakra system, "Vedanta and Sankhya hold the key to the laws of the mind and thought process, which are correlated to the quantum field, i.e., the operation and distribution of particles at atomic and molecular levels."[14] It is at these subtle levels that outer form is created, including the health of your organs, the appearance and structure of your body, and your beauty.

Isabel's Story

Isabel was in a car accident some years ago, and she described it as "scary traumatic." While driving home from a movie, she was hit nearly head-on by a teenage driver. Luckily, she suffered only bruises, some broken ribs and a broken leg. Even after her wounds healed, Isabel walked with an inexplicable limp, which her doctors did not understand. She also gained a lot of weight specifically in her hips and some in her thighs while her tummy and the rest of her body stayed thin.

It wasn't just Isabel's ribs and leg that were injured during the accident. The experience threw off her sense of security and her feelings of safety, which are all related to the *Muladhara* chakra (the first chakra, or root chakra), located around the hip area. In order to rebalance her first chakra, she had to reestablish the routines of eating and working and go about her daily life. During this time, Isabel's dog was a huge comfort to her. She embraced a Beauty Detox plant-based diet packed with vitality-enhancing vitamins and minerals, as she was determined to recover fully and slim down.

Her doctor actually suggested she try doing Reiki, the healing method that aims to balance chakra energies, since other patients he had worked with had reported positive results, and it was offered in the hospital in which he was treating her. She tried it and stuck with it after her hospital release, finding a Reiki practitioner close to her home. After her accident, Isabel reduced her crazy work hours, dialed back her intense career focus and directed more energy toward taking care of herself, thus making it possible for her to attend Reiki sessions two or three times a week.

After about nine months of her improved diet, a quieter life and her regular Reiki treatments, Isabel told me that during one Reiki session she felt this incredibly deep "pop" in her hip, which she characterized as energetic rather than physical. She described it as coming from deep inside. After that "pop," or release of energy, she no longer had a limp. Energy releases can come in all forms. Sometimes they are subtle and gradual mental or emotional shifts, and other times they occur in a more defined physical moment, as in Isabel's case.

Chakra Qualities

There are seven chakras in all, and five are associated with the five elements of the universe—earth, water, fire, air and ether/space. These five elements are contained in our bodies, which are microcosms of the entire universe. We all exhibit the denseness of earth, as well as the qualities of air and space. The remaining two chakras are composed of very subtle energy and are not associated with any element of the universe.

The different elements associated with the chakras also correspond to specific emotions. For instance, the earth element, which is associated with the earth or root chakra, also known as the *Muladhara* chakra, corresponds to fear, particularly fear related to one's safety. Love is an all-pervasive emotion felt in the air-based element of your heart, and fire-based anxiety can be felt in your stomach as a bellyache or that butterfly feeling you get before a job interview or a work presentation, or before a first date.

Each chakra is also associated with a specific color. Color is pure energy, and light is simply the vibration of radiant energy that is visible to our eyes. Color is created by the interaction of photons of light with electrons. The seven colors of the rainbow all have varying wavelengths and frequencies. Red is at the lower end of the spectrum and has a lower frequency, while violet is at the top end of the spectrum and has a higher frequency.[15] Adding more of a particular color to your life—especially by ingesting foods of that color—can have a positive balancing effect and can give a specific vibrational energy boost to the corresponding chakra and the emotions associated with it.

Eating for Your Chakras

Food can help balance your chakras. What you eat doesn't affect only your physical body. It can influence your energy in multiple ways based on the different vibrations of color, elements and nutrients that comprise it, its nourishing or congestive qualities, and where and how it was grown.

We discussed the mind-body fusion earlier. Let's look at the *Anahata* chakra (the heart chakra) in this context. Eating too much of the wrong kinds of fats can compromise your cardiovascular function, partially or fully closing channels of energy around the heart (clogged or blocked arteries) and leading to an energy blockage in the area, which can contribute to feeling more emotionally "closed" to giving and receiving love. On the other hand, fiber-filled green vegetables are nourishing for the heart, as they contain vitamins and nutrients and have a cleansing and blood-purifying effect, all of which support heart health. As energy physically opens around your heart, it can help open the emotional energies that center around love.

In general, whole foods—such as the blended whole vegetables and fruit in the Glowing Green Smoothie or unrefined grains, which contain the endosperm and the outer bran— promote the wholeness and balance that we want to foster. If we are what we eat and digest, we want to eat and digest whole, natural foods. Fragmented, processed foods, on the other hand, are imbalancing, as they contain unnatural substances that have the potential to create dissonance in our systems, such as artificial spikes in energy, digestive distress, high blood pressure and reduced circulation.

The more balanced you become and the more energy can flow freely, the less weight and other energy you tend to hold on to. Excess toxins are easier to eliminate, and weight drops off easier. Often, when people commit to making a life shift, they begin with food, which may appear physical, because it can be seen and held, but you may be startled to experience energetic changes and new discoveries about yourself on a deeper level.

POWER TIPS

1. **Take some time to let this chakra information sink in.** This is especially important if it is new to you. Remember that new is good and can be very helpful to you on your path to weight loss and true joy. So take your time with it. Feel free to read this chapter again at your own pace.

2. **Consider your own chakras.** Where in your body do you feel distress or

imbalance? What particular emotions are problematic in your life? Anger? Jealousy? Anxiety? Keep these in mind as we head into the next chapter, where we will discuss the individual chakras.

3. **Give up processed foods and embrace whole foods.** You can't really "trick" your body with low-calorie, synthetic foods, packaged meal replacements or processed foods. Choose whole foods, which nourish you on all energetic levels and support a whole, balanced you.

I am a whole being that is nourished on all levels.

Energy flows freely through me.

I now achieve balance physically, emotionally, mentally and spiritually.

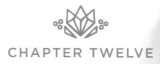

CHAPTER TWELVE

FOODS AND PRACTICES TO BALANCE THE INDIVIDUAL CHAKRAS FOR YOUR HEALTH AND IDEAL WEIGHT

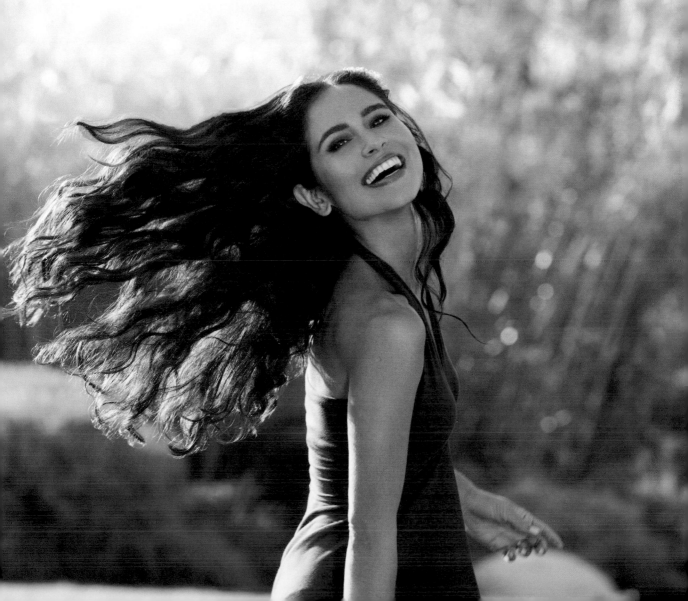

MULADHARA (ROOT/FIRST CHAKRA)

The energy of this chakra lays the foundation for all your energy systems. It governs safety and security, as it relates to your most basic survival needs and sense of belonging. Physically, it is centered around your hip area and the base of your spine.

Element: **Earth**   Color: **Red**

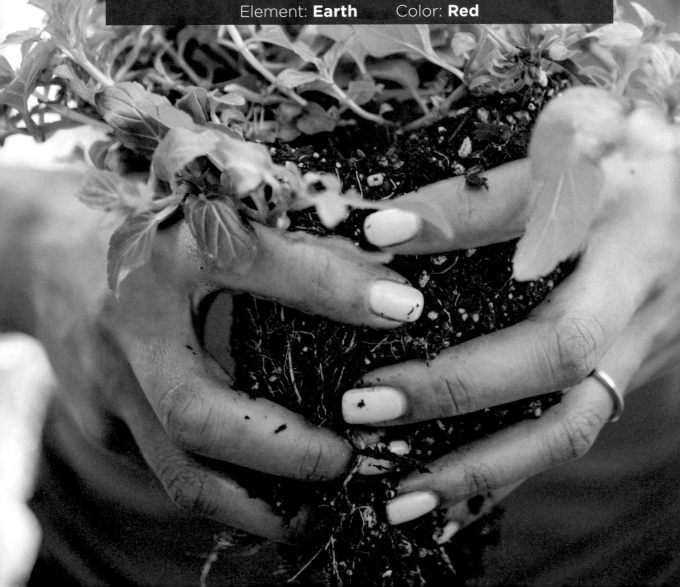

Balanced:

➤ Feeling secure and safe in all areas of life

➤ Feeling grounded

➤ Believing there is abundance for all and trusting you will always be provided for

➤ Cultivating prosperity

➤ Feeling connected to the earth and nature

➤ Having a strong sense of your life purpose

➤ Maintaining healthy boundaries in personal relationships

Imbalanced:

➤ Not feeling safe emotionally, financially or otherwise (extra weight may provide padding and protection)

➤ Feeling fearful about moving forward in life

➤ Overachieving, overworking or overeating to compensate for something that is missing in life

➤ Experiencing rifts in your family or in the groups you are from or are tied to (workplace, clubs, school, church/temple/synagogue, etc.)

➤ Feeling like you can't connect to those around you, like you are "separate" from others

➤ Feeling that parts of your body regularly break down

➤ Having difficulty functioning or seeing yourself as a contributing member of society

Physical Manifestations of Imbalance:

The root chakra is located at the very base of the spine. Any type of hip issue is related to this chakra. This energy can extend down to the lower part of your body, including the legs and feet, and can involve the adrenals, bones and immune system. Weight held in the lower part of the body, as well as inflammatory or autoimmune conditions, are associated with this chakra. Anorexia and bulimia are also linked to energy imbalances in this chakra.

Healing Eating Disorders:

Eating disorders must be treated with extreme compassion and sensitivity. Healing such disorders often requires extensive effort and courage, and entails rebalancing emotions and changing habitual patterns and beliefs, especially about oneself. Eating disorders must be taken seriously and should never be dismissed offhandedly or brushed aside.

A lack of a sense of safety or a strong identity, as well as a sense of powerlessness, can lead to deep insecurities and energy blocks in the root chakra, and eating disorders may be a physical manifestation. Eating disorders can also reflect imbalances in the solar plexus chakra (the *Manipura* chakra). Starving oneself, as in anorexia, may have to do with not feeling truly secure in oneself and one's "right to exist," as well as increased self-criticism.[1] Research has found that self-imposed starvation often represents a deep desire to decrease self-consciousness by controlling one's physical appearance,[2] which is indicative of not feeling rooted in a strong, secure sense of self.

Bulimia can also stem from feeling shame, repressed rage or anger; from perhaps feeling that you are living a life that is not a true reflection of who you are; and from not knowing who you really are. The Power Tips and Affirmations throughout this book can help foster your awareness of the truly beautiful being that you are and of your unique contribution to this planet, but as eating disorders are extremely complex issues, professional help may also be needed for you to deal adequately with an eating disorder.

Discussion:

By establishing balance in this root chakra, you create a strong foundation, which is essential to reaching your full potential in your body, beauty and life. This chakra has everything to do with safety, security and survival. If you don't feel safe, then your body and emotions may try to establish security through imbalanced means, such as building extra layers of fat for protection and insulation.

Anything you can do to feel grounded on a regular basis is important. If you feel run-down from too many activities or events or from being surrounded by too many people, set aside time to rest. Give yourself the space to nest at home, quietly reading or writing. Touch the earth and connect with it directly whenever you can, whether it's through gardening or walking barefoot on a beach, in the park or in your backyard.

Fears about life, including fear about sickness, accidents, travel and the unknown, can arise when there's an imbalance in this chakra. The more you are able to go within and feel your essential connection to the whole universe, the more you will trust the path of life and live without fear.

You are safe to be you and to live a full life. And you will always ultimately be okay. Trust and believe in yourself and life.

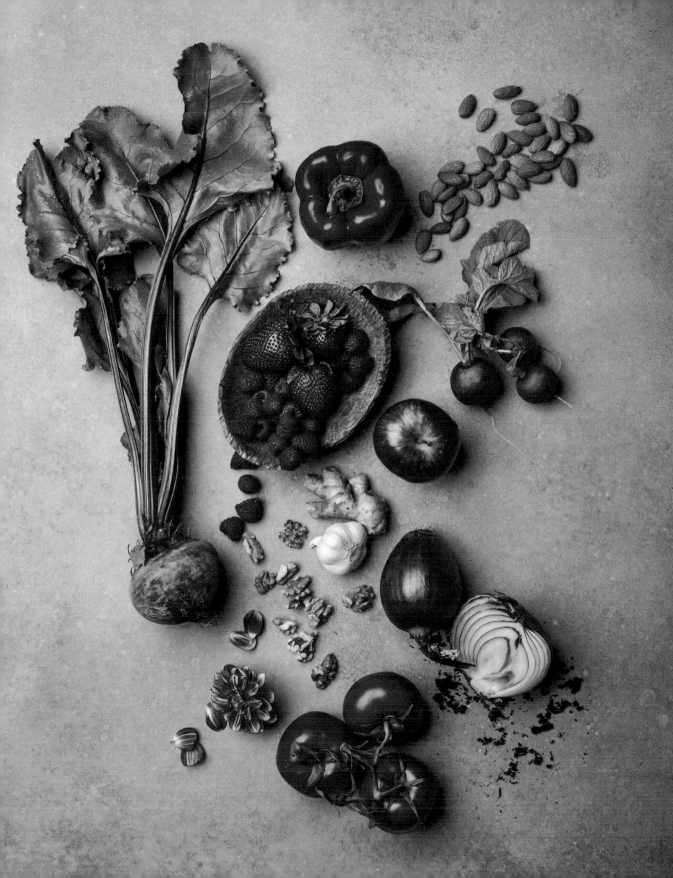

Specific Foods:

➤ Foods that are grown right in the earth are the most balancing for this chakra. Root vegetables are a primary example of solid, sturdy foods that will feel stabilizing, and they include sweet potatoes, red-skinned potatoes and other potatoes, carrots, yams, all types of squash, ginger, onions, shallots, parsnips and radishes. Hearty vegetable soups featuring these root vegetables will feel particularly grounding and are a great option to make you feel more rooted. Connecting to where your food comes from can be very healing, so make it a point to go to the local farmers' market and meet the people who grow your food.

➤ Dense, high-protein foods, such as seeds, nuts and legumes (which include lentils), are grounding in moderate quantities, so be sure not to consume too much of these foods at one time or you will feel heavy. Mushrooms are another great choice, and their texture can be appealing to those transitioning off meat. Calcium is an important mineral for this chakra, as it supports structure and shape, especially in the dense hip bones. Calcium-rich almonds and sesame seeds are exceptional choices.

➤ Since red is the color of this chakra, all red foods help boost and balance its vibration, including red apples, red pears, red cherries, strawberries, red tomatoes, radishes, red-skinned potatoes, red beets, red onions and red bell peppers. The lycopene found in tomatoes is a protective antioxidant. Beets assist in healthy red blood cell formation, which is critical to the distribution of oxygen throughout the body.

➤ Vitamin C, found in fresh fruits and vegetables, is important for supporting your collagen, including in your bones, teeth and skin, for maintaining structure all over your body.

POWER TIPS FOR *MULADHARA* (ROOT/FIRST CHAKRA)

▸ Release your fear of not having enough. Recognize that you will be able to eat when you want and you will have access to food when you need it. If you grew up in less fortunate circumstances, in a family where you had to fight to get your share at the table, or with parents for whom food was scarce at one time, you may now have to overcome this mentality of lack.

▸ If you do choose to eat some animal protein, make it a small amount and consume it, ideally, only a few times a week or month, maximum. If that sounds like a huge adjustment, then start with not eating meat more than once a day. Too much meat will make the body acidic and rigid. As I discuss at length in *The Beauty Detox Solution,* animal protein of all types takes a lot of energy, effort and time for your body to digest. If you aren't ready to become a full-fledged vegetarian, that's okay. Merely reducing your meat intake is a big improvement from a digestive and energetic standpoint. Remember, progress, not perfection!

▸ Choose organic, grass-fed and antibiotic-free animal proteins if and when you do choose to eat them. Your body also takes in the vibration of what you are eating. Meat from a factory farm contains the energy of animals that have lived a fearful life filled with pain and mistreatment. When you ingest meat from a factory farm, you ingest these energies along with it, and that can have negative energetic consequences for your root chakra. This is partly why many yoga masters stress to their students the importance of being vegetarian, especially at the beginning of their spiritual journey. And if you constantly ingest foods that are physically clogging, it can make it more difficult to transcend the material-based ego and live from higher energies.

*I am safe and secure, and I trust
that I will always be provided for.*

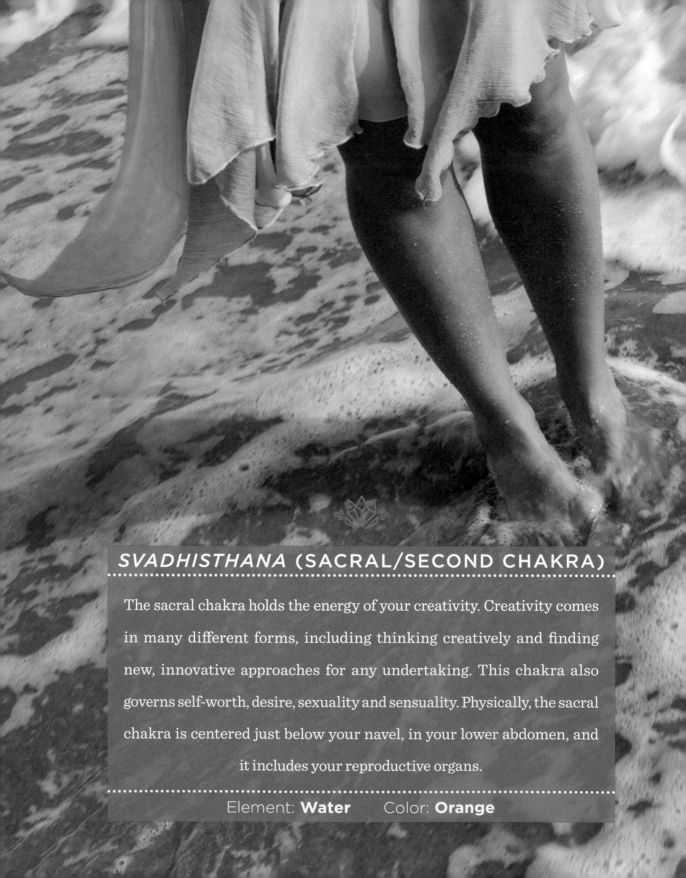

SVADHISTHANA (SACRAL/SECOND CHAKRA)

The sacral chakra holds the energy of your creativity. Creativity comes in many different forms, including thinking creatively and finding new, innovative approaches for any undertaking. This chakra also governs self-worth, desire, sexuality and sensuality. Physically, the sacral chakra is centered just below your navel, in your lower abdomen, and it includes your reproductive organs.

Element: **Water**   Color: **Orange**

Balanced:

➤   Feeling empowered to express yourself creatively

➤   Having a strong sense of self

➤   Establishing and maintaining healthy, balanced relationships based on good communication and respect

➤   Being tuned in to your emotions and your dreams

➤   Feeling liberated and fluid as you move through life, and not feeling "stuck" in any way

Imbalanced:

➤   Having difficulty expressing yourself in a direct manner and/or processing emotions

➤   Avoiding others because of a fear of not being able to relate fully to them

➤   Having repeated random, meaningless sexual encounters

➤   Fixating on the idea that you have to have something to "show" for your life

➤   Feeling powerless to achieve your dreams

➤   Engaging in self-criticism and feeling a sense of extreme guilt

➤   Deriving your self-worth from pleasing others

➤   Feeling you have to flaunt your sexuality to be liked

➤   Having relationships that are largely based on looks or on sex

➤   Feeling blocked in your creativity or feeling that you don't get to express your creativity in your life

Physical Manifestations of Imbalance:

Issues around the sacral chakra are fairly common. When creative energies are not expressed, physical issues can manifest in the most creative of organs, the reproductive system. Chronic yeast infections, infertility, endometriosis, urinary tract infections, repeated or multiple sexually transmitted diseases, issues related to the ovaries or other sexual organs in women and men, and kidney and adrenal issues are some of the physical ailments that can arise when there is an energy imbalance in this chakra.

Discussion:

Our bodies are 57 to 75 percent water,[3] which is the element associated with the sacral chakra. The very nature of water is fluid movement. At the cellular level, we exhibit the dynamic qualities of flowing motion.

This chakra has to do with the ability to manifest desires, express creativity and evolve personally. Ego can play into the energy here, such as in deriving self-worth from outer validation. Imbalanced energy in this chakra can manifest in obsessive thoughts about food and sex.

Emotions are forms of moving energy. You must allow space for emotions to flow freely like water. In fact, the word *emotion* is partially derived from the Latin verb *movēre*, meaning "to move."[4][5] Allowing yourself to be fully present and to authentically express your emotions in healthy ways, rather than bottling them up, is key to balancing this energy. Affirmations, journaling and creative outlets are all balancing tools.

Relationships created with imbalanced sacral chakra energy are often characterized by lust, dependency, control and attachment to an idealized perception of the other person. Seduction and jealousy can arise, and these tend to go hand in hand with a deeper feeling of emptiness. The relationships in your life are reflections of how you feel about yourself and the world. Are your relationships healthy and balanced? In other words, do both sides in the relationship give and receive inspiration and support? If not, how can you adjust the dynamic to create health and balance in your relationships?

Your relationship with yourself is the most important one, as it influences all others. Believing that your self-worth resides largely in how physically attractive you are to the opposite sex reflects an imbalance in this second chakra. So many of us just want to be loved. And because of that, many women give themselves to men who just pay attention to them. You are so much more powerful than your sexuality. You are beautiful because you are you.

Specific Foods:

➤ Because the element associated with this chakra is water, hydration is key to keeping movement at an optimal level in your body. Fluids are essential for flushing out old waste and toxins through your kidneys and bowels.

➤ Juicy fruits are particularly hydrating, and tropical fruits often grow in places near the mother of all bodies of water: the ocean. Pineapples, papayas, pomelos, mangoes, oranges and coconuts are some of my favorite tropical fruits. Aim to consume fruits with seeds whenever possible, as these fruits contain reproductive and creative power within, and are in their natural form, instead of hybridized, seedless fruit.

➤ Orange is the color vibration of this chakra, and orange foods include carrots, sweet potatoes, yams, butternut squash, orange bell peppers, oranges, papayas, apricots and peaches. The orange color in foods is present in part because of beta-carotene and other plant carotenoids, which help to protect your cells and keep you vibrant and fluid.

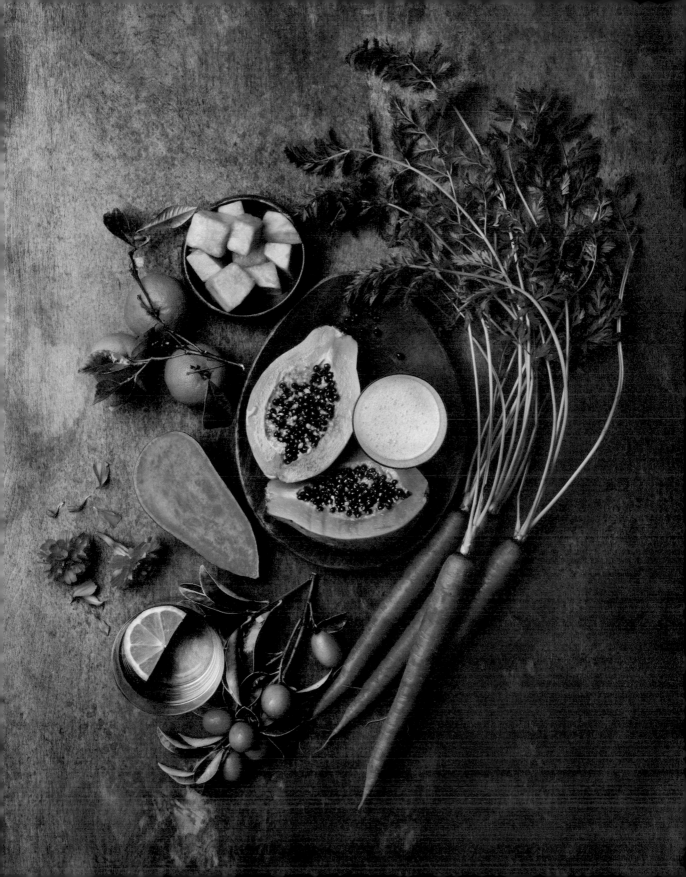

POWER TIPS FOR *SVADHISTHANA* (SACRAL/SECOND CHAKRA)

▸ Prepare your own meals as much as possible to reinforce the notion that you are worthy of proper nourishment. Tune in to which specific foods and dishes are calling to you on any given day. Prepare your food lovingly and in a relaxed way. Simple is totally fine. Whipping up Guacamole Pizza (page 299) in just a few minutes is infinitely better than buying a submarine sandwich.

▸ The next best thing to preparing your own food is having someone who loves you cook for you. Love can be transmitted in the energy of the food. I truly believe that this is the reason my clients have so much passion for the food I make them. They can sense my love for them in their food! That cannot be bought at fancy restaurants, where the kitchens are hectic. Have family members, friends or roommates take turns cooking so there are always healthy meals available. If you're expecting a crowd, try making Vegan Beauty Ranch Dressing (page 289) and serving it with veggie sticks. Meditation is the essential activity for reconnecting with your whole being and your self-worth. Please refer to Power Alignment Shift 5 for a more thorough explanation of a beginner's practice.

I am a creative, fluid being with
unlimited power to create what I want.

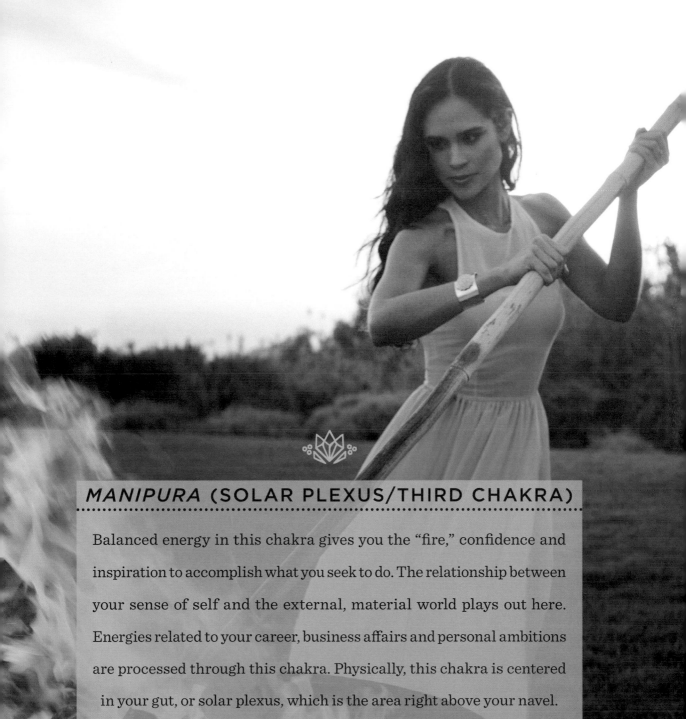

MANIPURA (SOLAR PLEXUS/THIRD CHAKRA)

Balanced energy in this chakra gives you the "fire," confidence and inspiration to accomplish what you seek to do. The relationship between your sense of self and the external, material world plays out here. Energies related to your career, business affairs and personal ambitions are processed through this chakra. Physically, this chakra is centered in your gut, or solar plexus, which is the area right above your navel.

Element: **Fire**   Color: **Yellow**

Balanced:

➤ Radiating motivation and inspiration

➤ Feeling dynamic and empowered to follow through and realize goals and dreams

➤ Being comfortable with who you are, living without judgment, and not seeking constant validation from others

➤ Not taking criticism too personally, learning from it and moving on

➤ Having healthy self-esteem and self-worth

➤ Feeling balanced in life, rather than feeling overwhelmed

➤ Having an energy of sharing and cooperation

Imbalanced:

➤ Overthinking or overanalyzing situations, to the point of exhausting and confusing yourself (and those around you)

➤ Being easily angered or irritated, being overly "fiery"

➤ Fixating on external accomplishments and competition

➤ Using manipulation and control tactics

➤ Possessing a strong attachment and/or desire for material objects and status symbols

➤ Voicing strong opinions and not being open to others' views

➤ Overcompensating in social settings due to a lack of self-esteem

➤ Lacking self-confidence and self-worth

➤ Feeling powerless to create change in your life

➤ Feeling uninspired and believing that you don't make a difference

Physical Manifestations of Imbalance:

The fire element largely has to do with digestion, and this chakra is physically centered around your midsection and digestive tract, so digestive issues, such as heartburn, ulcers, irritable bowel syndrome, diarrhea and constipation can arise with energy imbalances. Issues with the liver, pancreas, stomach, upper intestines, gallbladder, spleen and middle spine (lower thoracic region) may also be related to this third chakra. If you've ever experienced a "gut feeling" about a situation or felt butterflies in your stomach before a work interview or a speaking engagement, you've connected with your energy here.

Discussion:

A false, ego-based perception of power creates imbalances in this chakra's energy. Possessing money, material objects, status symbols, fame or externally measurable accomplishments such as educational degrees, wealth, or job titles do not in any way indicate true power. Though the media and widespread societal beliefs often reinforce the idea that external accomplishments are of the highest importance, you won't be truly happy if you believe that is where your power comes from. All these things can, of course, be enjoyed, but they should never be central to your self-worth.

True power emanates from within, feeling secure in your wholeness and inherent connection to universal energy without relying on outer things to try to make you feel or look better. The more you inspire and help to uplift others so that they discover their true light, the stronger your true connection to universal energy becomes and the more power you gain. When you approach life with this understanding of power, as well as with the mentality that there is enough for everyone, it eliminates the need to feel competitive and fixated on external accomplishments, such as your educational degree, finances, or job title, which ultimately have nothing to do with what you are. So relax and exhale, because you are awesome as you are and you don't have to prove anything to anyone!

This chakra is like a filter between you and the external world. At any given time there is a lot of information and energy passing through your being from the external world. You need to ensure there is enough energy moving within this chakra to prevent stagnation and buildup on any level, including emotional (such as anger), and physical (in the form of waste and toxins).

Eva's Story

Eva had recently landed her dream job as a high-end stylist. She always dressed like she just stepped off a fashion shoot, with her perfectly tailored clothes, her unique and perfectly put together accessories, and shoes you only see in *Vogue*. Yet her whole life was about external recognition. Naturally, Eva was one of those people who fished for compliments. She craved the validation she received all day from people telling her she had amazing style and was brilliant at what she did. But she would tell me how fierce the competition was for booking shoots, sourcing the right outfits from designers and keeping clients.

It was clear that the constant stress she was under was having an effect on Eva's health, and along those lines I could not help but notice her foul breath. I'm sure it was related to her long-term constipation issues. (By the way, I'm pretty sure my breath wasn't so great, either, when I was backed up, so I'm not one to judge.) Eva was throwing herself out of balance by holding all that frenetic fashion world energy right in her gut. She was so busy running from appointment to appointment every day that she wasn't taking time for her own wellness. Ultimately, Eva reached a breaking point of utter exhaustion and unhappiness about her low energy, her puffy belly and her dependence on caffeine surges to pep her up.

I got Eva to carve out more time in the mornings so that she would slow down and set up her day properly. She started drinking hot water with lemon as her regular morning ritual. I also urged her to take time to reflect and meditate, to find some stillness, before commencing the constant moving around that filled her days. This was not the easiest thing for her, but we found some instrumental music that really helped to settle her mind, as well as a silky eye mask, which, she said, helped calm her down when she strapped it over her eyes.

The great news is that Eva now goes to the bathroom regularly as a result of her dietary changes and a magnesium-oxygen product (such as Detoxy, which I've recommended for years and which is helpful to all of us in getting things moving!), and she is making an effort to be still and to consciously relax on a consistent basis. She also makes the time to go to the bathroom in the morning, a lifestyle change she made as a result of my explaining to her how critical giving time to her body was for loving and taking care of herself. She goes jogging in her neighborhood to let off steam on the weekends, and she tries to get to Pilates class as often as possible. Her life is still fast-paced, but she handles that pace with much more ease and balance now.

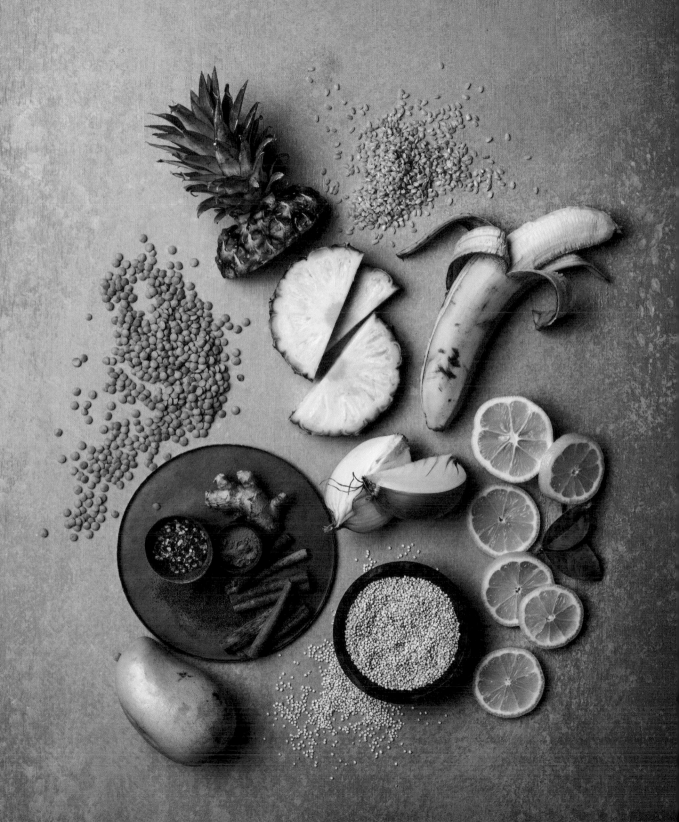

Remember that nothing and no one can add to or take away from your self-worth. You are worthy, wonderful and whole just as you are.

Specific Foods:

➤ You need enough "digestive" fire to ensure that you are absorbing nutrients and breaking down food to the maximum extent possible. Include foods with warming properties, such as ginger, cayenne, turmeric and cinnamon, in your diet regularly.

➤ Fiber is one of the most important nutrients for a healthy *Manipura* chakra, because it keeps energies moving throughout the entire system. Fiber also has a stabilizing energy to help maintain blood sugar levels. Fiber-filled foods include fruits and vegetables, such as squash, as well as complex, whole carbohydrates, such as quinoa and legumes, which release fuel into your system in a controlled way.

➤ Yellow is the color of the *Manipura* chakra, and yellow foods that can help balance the energy vibration in this area include lemons, yellow summer squash, spaghetti squash, yellow bell peppers, pineapples, grains such as quinoa and millet, bananas (one of my personal all-time faves), yellow pears and yellow apples.

POWER TIPS FOR *MANIPURA* (SOLAR PLEXUS/THIRD CHAKRA)

▸ This chakra's element is fire, and it is responsible for the transformative processes involved in digestion. Efficient digestion is a big topic in the Beauty Detox lifestyle. Be sure to eat raw plant foods at the beginning of each meal, such as green salads and veggie sticks, as these are filled with enzymes, water and fiber, and improve digestion all around.

▸ One of the most important ways to balance this chakra is to avoid stagnation. Slow-digesting, fiberless foods, such as dairy (which is difficult for many to digest), stay in your gut for long periods, contributing to a feeling of heaviness, lethargy, and feeling "blocked." Work to reduce your dairy intake, or give up dairy products completely, as I personally have. Instead of dairy, reach for oranges, almonds, greens and sesame seeds, which are just a few examples of great calcium-rich plant foods.

▸ Keep things in perspective. It's fantastic to enjoy nice things, but be aware of how these things make you feel or trying to purposely "show" what you've done or what you have. Remember that you don't have to prove anything to anyone.

▸ Doing twists, a physical practice whereby you physically "wring out" your liver and kidneys, helps work out energy in your "fire center" and helps push out toxins and stagnant energy. Keep your pelvis rooted as you stand or sit, or even lay on your back on your yoga mat, then twist your torso in both directions. You can even do this in your office chair. Do twists often (ideally daily, or at least 3-5 times a week).

True power comes from within me
and empowers me in all that I focus on.

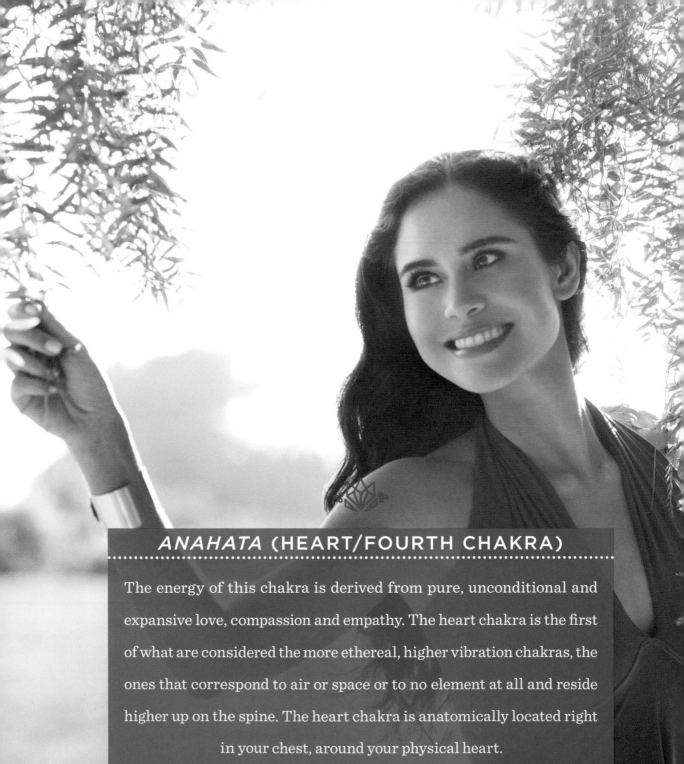

ANAHATA (HEART/FOURTH CHAKRA)

The energy of this chakra is derived from pure, unconditional and expansive love, compassion and empathy. The heart chakra is the first of what are considered the more ethereal, higher vibration chakras, the ones that correspond to air or space or to no element at all and reside higher up on the spine. The heart chakra is anatomically located right in your chest, around your physical heart.

Element: **Air**   Color: **Green**

Balanced:

➤ Feeling universal love for all, versus limiting love to individual circles, such as "my" family and friends

➤ Feeling compassionate and empathetic toward others

➤ Possessing healthy self-love

➤ Being open to giving and receiving love

➤ Committing to goals that serve the higher good and are beyond materialistic achievements and self-aggrandizement

➤ Seeing the world as a place of abundance rather than of constant competition

➤ Feeling joy from within

➤ Forgiving others with ease

➤ Feeling a higher degree of emotional wisdom, and not reacting to or being overly attached to materialistic endeavors and competition

Imbalanced:

➤ Having difficulty giving and receiving love

➤ Having difficulty expressing or being in touch with feelings and emotions, especially love

➤ Experiencing discomfort with being touched

➤ Having a cynical or overly analytical perspective on all parts of life

➤ Finding it challenging to feel grateful for yourself, others, life and/or a greater power

➤ Putting up boundaries to hide feelings

➤ Having a hard time forgiving others or yourself

➤ Holding on long term to hurt feelings and perceived rejection, and feeling that you are not loved by another in the way that you want to be loved

➤ Experiencing a loss of joy and feeling unmotivated or depressed about life in general

Physical Manifestations of Imbalance:

On a physical level, your heart, lungs and chest are in the energetic field of this chakra. Your hands and arms are considered extensions of the heart chakra, and therefore touching others is a physical extension of this chakra. Any physical conditions related to the center of your chest, including chest pains, heart attacks, other heart issues, breast issues and breathing difficulties, as well as arm and upper back issues, can be related to this chakra.

Discussion:

The joy and unconditional love that a heart-centered person emanates are so powerful that everyone around her or him can feel it. Living from your heart makes you highly magnetic to others, makes everything you do more powerful and aligns your actions with the higher good. Love is true power.

Dr. Rollin McCraty of the Institute of HeartMath reported that the magnetic field of the heart is around five thousand times stronger than the magnetic field of the brain and can be "measured several feet from the body."[6] Just as you can feel the tremendous strength of a heart-centered person, you can also sense when someone is being led more by their analytical thoughts than their heart. A healthy heart chakra is also discerning. It rises above lower energies, such as petty jealousy and cattiness. Instead, its energy reflects joy, contentment, gratitude, awe in the face of beauty, and humility. When your heart is balanced, it is easy to be grateful for the daily miracles in life. The more you let gratitude flow from your heart, the more life unfolds fluidly and without a struggle. No, all problems don't automatically go away, but your approach to them can shift so that you are in touch with the joy in your heart.

What are you grateful for? Seek out opportunities to say thank you, even for the smallest things. Smile at people you pass on the sidewalk or in the market—even if they don't smile back or give you an odd look. What you put out, you get back, so put out beauty and love and get it right back, sometimes in unexpected ways.

A robust heart chakra energy can also make it easy to forgive. After moving to Los Angeles from New York City and having to drive again, I learned how quickly the white-hot anger of road rage can rise. Avoiding it requires consciously and simply letting things go (even if the other person is so very wrong). The deeper pain of deception or hurtful words or actions on the part of family members, colleagues or friends can feel more upsetting. And in those cases, it's even more important to exercise radical forgiveness, as doing so prevents negative energy from getting lodged in your life or your body.

I know I talk about it a lot, but I strongly believe that meditation is the key to overall life improvement. (We'll talk more about this in Power Alignment Shift 5.) Meditation is also one of the most powerful ways to become truly heart centered, as it expands your consciousness and allows you to feel that your true essence is unlimited love. The more you tune in and feel your true nature, the stronger love will be in all areas of your life. It is true that you have to give love to receive it, and this most certainly starts with loving yourself.

Mary Anne's Story

Living from your heart can be difficult at first. It's natural to feel more vulnerable initially if you're used to living pragmatically. Mary Anne was almost robot-like when we started working together. I asked her questions about how she was feeling and doing, and every answer was, "Fine. I'm fine," or a high-pitched "I'm good!" When I posed these questions, I tried to hold her gaze for as long as possible to get her to connect and tell me what was really going on, but she would give me a blank, inauthentic smile and would look away often while talking. I admit that sometimes I was tempted to (gently) push her out of her chair, just to see what she would do, and to see what a genuine reaction from her would be like!

Softening a "hardened" heart can take time and effort. With Mary Anne, I worked from the root up, first addressing any energetic imbalances with the first three chakras, as these often need to be handled first in order to open up the energy of the heart, which is higher up the spine. (This doesn't necessarily mean that one chakra is more "important" than the others, as they are all important. But as you ascend the spine, the energies become more subtle to work with.)

First, I introduced grounding whole foods into her diet, such as almonds, beets, yams and pinto beans, and I talked extensively about the concept of healthy self-worth. I'll admit it was like talking to a statue of Athena for a while, because she would just sit there, stone-faced, during most of our conversations. Still, we continued our work, and I continued to do most of the talking during our sessions and our phone calls, though I was always trying to dig for more. I wanted to know what was really going on with her, what was making it so hard for her to eat regular meals in front of others, and what was causing her to binge on treats in seclusion.

Mary Anne was more open in emails and texts, where there was no opportunity for her nervous, fake laughter to glide over my questions. Since writing seemed to be easier for her, I encouraged her to note her emotions and feelings regularly in a journal, which she shared with me during our consultations. She came from an emotionally unexpressive family, one in which no one really talked about their feelings or hugged. We added loads of greens to her diet, and I encouraged her to have large salad-based meals. I had her start a *pranayama* practice, which involves breathing techniques, to help her move beyond the analytical, outer world. It was hard for her to sit still, but she could focus her mind on the proper counts for the breathing practices, and that helped open up some space between her racing thoughts.

I've been working with Mary Anne for over four years now. I can say that she now smiles—and laughs—more authentically. She is more "real." She's no longer that plastic Mary Anne I first met, and I'm not tempted to push her gently out of her chair anymore. She has largely improved her digestion, and she eats more regular meals. She looks so much younger as a result of our increased detoxification and, I believe, as a result of living more joyfully from her heart and allowing more all-around nourishing love to flow into her daily life and, in doing so, into herself. Love is at the core of being centered and authentic and of tapping into your true power.

Specific Foods:

➤ Since green is the main color vibration of the heart chakra, you can guess which foods are most important for this chakra! Green foods vibrate with the frequency of nature and cultivate healing. Leafy greens, including spinach, kale, chard, romaine, mustard greens, arugula, mâche, mixed greens, collard greens and others, will help open up the heart chakra. Other beneficial green foods include broccoli, brussels sprouts, chlorella, spirulina, green cabbage, sprouts, bok choy, green peppers, green beans, scallions, zucchini, green apples and various herbs, such as parsley and cilantro.

➤ If you are experiencing an *Anahata* chakra imbalance, then you may have a very strong aversion to green vegetables. Over time this can change, as I've seen so many times. Greens are amongst the most balancing of all foods, as they support your entire body, and especially your heart area. Chlorophyll is anti-inflammatory and high in anti-oxidants; it helps to build healthy blood, and it promotes circulation. Fresh greens are alive and ignite love energy. Have you noticed how much more alive and more connected you feel when drinking the Glowing Green Smoothie? This is due to the mind-boggling amount of nutrients you ingest, and to the fact that green is harmonizing and recharges the vibration of the heart chakra.

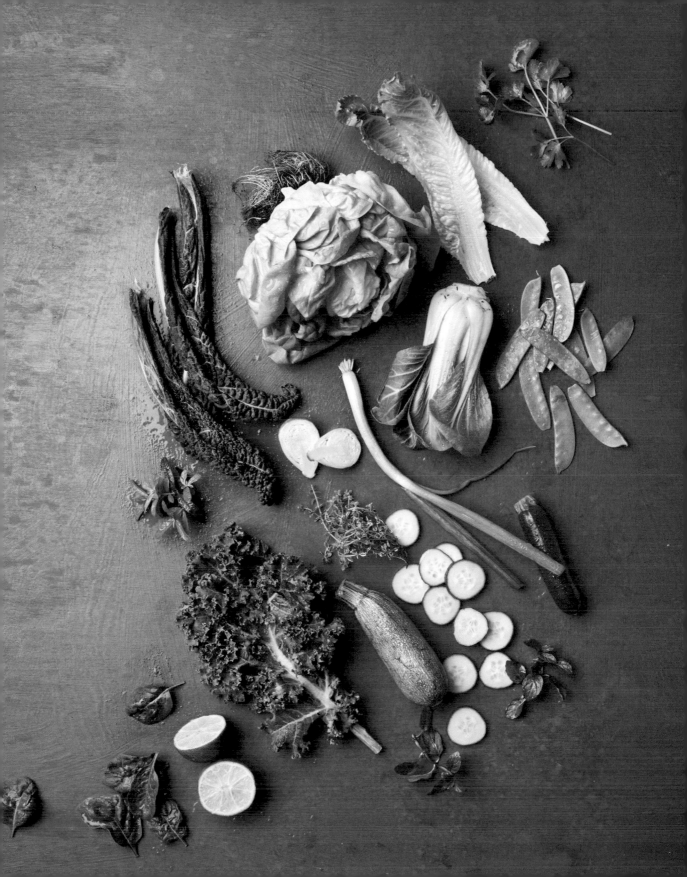

➤ Raw greens are considered to have a cooling (yin) effect, which is positive because the heart is tender. The heart chakra is associated with the air element, so light foods, like raw greens, are supportive of this energy.

POWER TIPS FOR *ANAHATA* (HEART/FOURTH CHAKRA)

▸ My beautiful mother, Sally, always used to say that the state of your refrigerator—how empty or how full it is—is a gauge of the love in your life. Keep your fridge stocked to cultivate love in your life.

▸ When you eat in a loving, compassionate, relaxed and open atmosphere, you actually digest your food better. Share your meal with your loved ones, or if you are eating alone, enjoy your food in a non-rushed, peaceful way. Avoid talking about politics or stressful work or family issues while eating. Treat your meals, even when brief, as sacred time.

▸ Take a moment before eating to express gratitude and usher in the energy of grace and love. Your expression of gratitude can be simple, so long as it means something to you. Sound is a powerful vibration: I often recite yoga mantras and sing song lyrics while I cook. Here's a super-simple one for you to invoke your connection to higher love and gratitude: *Om Namah Shivaya,* which translates as "I bow down to the light within."

I am pure love, and unlimited love
flows through me and surrounds me.

VISHUDDHA (THROAT/FIFTH CHAKRA)

This chakra governs self-expression, self-knowledge and communication. It enables us to gain wisdom from our inner truth and experiences, rather than relying on analytical sources alone. Through the throat chakra we allow our authentic expression to flow through us and into the world. Physically, this chakra is centered in our throat area.

Element: **Ether/Space**   Color: **Blue**

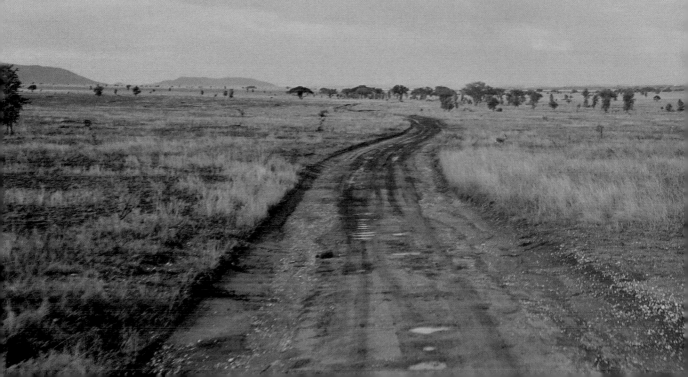

Balanced:

➤ Always speaking honestly to yourself and others

➤ Living with alignment between what you believe, what you say and your actions

➤ Expressing inner creativity

➤ Teaching and learning effectively

➤ Seeking truth in every situation and thus going beyond analytical data, which has limits

➤ Taking responsible action and speaking up for your own needs

➤ Feeling empowered to voice your needs and beliefs

Imbalanced:

➤ Feeling "blocked," or choked up, when trying to express emotions, feelings or thoughts

➤ Lying

➤ Speaking from fear or doubt instead of from truth

➤ Lacking conviction behind your words

➤ Directing critical or hurtful words at others or the world

➤ Being overly talkative and not listening to others

➤ Experiencing difficulty in really hearing others

➤ Expressing your feelings, emotions or ideas in an overly aggressive way

Physical Manifestations of Imbalance:

The throat or neck region is related to the energy of the *Vishuddha* chakra. Common dysfunctions of this chakra include laryngitis and other voice or vocal cord issues, sore throat, TMJ, mouth ulcers and swollen glands. Issues with the neck vertebrae, trachea, gums, teeth, esophagus, thyroid, parathyroid, hypothalamus and ears are also governed by this chakra.

Discussion:

When you are in alignment within your *Vishuddha* chakra, you speak in truth. What you see is what you get. Isn't that such a refreshing and attractive quality? We've all been around phony people who smile and give compliments while mentally criticizing others. In contrast, those with balanced energy in this chakra possess a calm wisdom, tend to have a broader perspective on any given situation, and consider the good of others, rather than just themselves, when making decisions.

The element of this chakra is space, which does not signify "emptiness" in any way, but rather vibrating potential energy that can be consciously shaped with the power of your voice and your expression. As you start to align more with the love and the wisdom within you, you are honest with yourself and others, and you express yourself through your words. There's a real power in that. Paramahansa Yogananda taught that "[t]here is incredible creative power behind the words of one who always speaks truth."[7]

Ellen's Story

When I started working with Ellen, a restaurant manager, she used to lie to me all the time. She would lie about how much alcohol she drank, about what she ate and about other details of her life, though it really did her no good to lie to me at all. I was not a Supreme Court judge sitting in judgment; I was her teacher and nutritionist and was trying to help her!

The problem was that I could see things in her face and her body that simply did not equate with what she was telling me. For instance, she told me once that the only thing she had put in her body was "salad and some mushrooms" the day before, but I could tell from the way she looked that she had chased them down with something. Everyone else in Ellen's life was a yes-person, but not me. I would challenge her, which she didn't like at first. One time she sent me a super nasty email, then later apologized profusely (after I didn't reply). I knew not to take it personally, because I know resistance can rise up in communication channels when you are pushing through energy blocks.

I worked on making her feel safe to tell me the truth, and I expressed disapproval only when I sensed she was lying so that she looked like a "perfect" student to me. One time, she had a little outburst in public and hissed at me, "Okay, fine. I ate the freaking pizza, okay? I'm a cheese whore. Are you happy now?" I just sat silently, being present with her. After a minute or two, I could see her hunched shoulders relax, and a softness appear in her eyes. She apologized, but witnessing her peaceful energetic transformation, her shift from stressful posing to just surrendering and being herself, was far more gratifying to me.

The more Ellen opened up to me honestly, the more we closed the gap between what she said and what truly was, and the more powerful she became. We found replacements for some of her old go-to foods, ones that didn't serve her anymore, while she transitioned. Over time, she even gave up some of her favorite processed foods, switching, for instance, from packaged protein bars to almonds or oranges as a snack. Her honesty enabled her to gain strength, and in turn it was easier for her to stick to a balanced, healthy lifestyle program. Even with her occasional hiccups, when she would revisit her favorite junk foods, Ellen was still able to progress. She lost over fifteen pounds in six months and kept it off, which was her goal, and she did it without the struggle and hunger she had experienced with other diets in the past.

Examine areas or relationships in your life where there is less than completely honest expression. When you live in truth, everything becomes aligned and, therefore, stronger. Feel your power to shape your world, be authentic, and nothing can hold you back.

Specific Foods:

➤ There aren't too many foods that correspond to this chakra's color, which is blue, but not dark shades of blue (darker blues, such as the blue of blueberries, belong to the sixth chakra). Foods that are balancing for the energy of this chakra often combine different elements, like water and earth, from the other chakras.[8] Soups, stews, fruits with a high water content, and sea vegetables are examples of such foods.[9]

➤ Consuming sea vegetables, including dulse and nori (the seaweed wrapping for sushi), is an excellent way to incorporate into your diet the wide variety of trace minerals from the sea, and sea vegetables are a great complement to land vegetables. They are high in iodine and can help balance your thyroid and your metabolism. Sea vegetables are also a superb source of B vitamins, iron, and vitamins A and E. Sea vegetables have been consumed by the peoples of Asia and Northern Europe, including Ireland, for centuries. You can purchase them online, in the Asian section of your local market and in Asian markets. Once you stock up on nori, be sure to give the Sprouted Quinoa and Veggie Sushi recipe (page 284) a go!

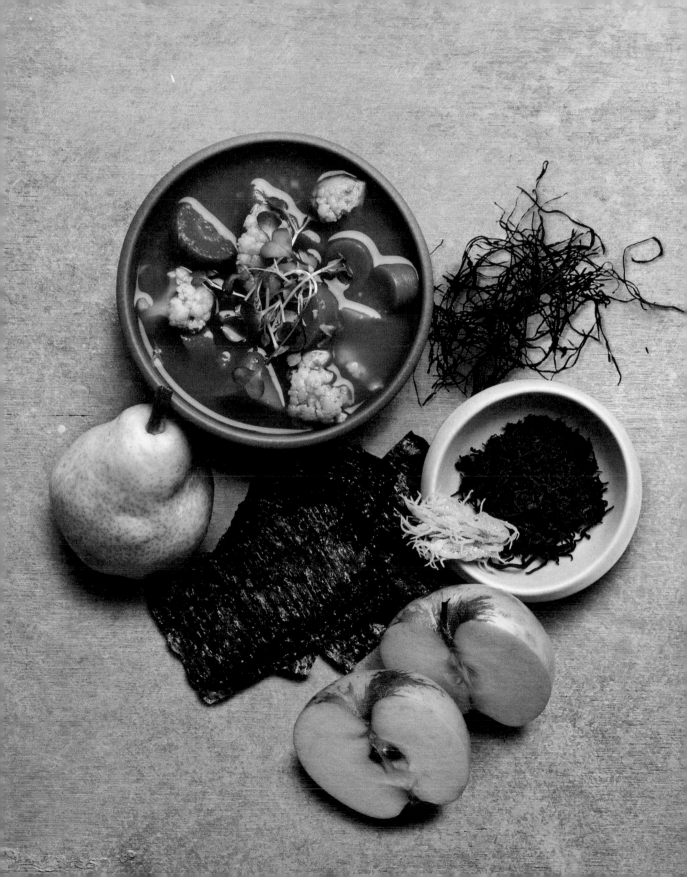

➤ Pureed or chunky vegetable-based soups, eaten mindfully one spoonful at a time, are soft and easy to digest, and they are soothing to your throat and jaw, too.

POWER TIPS FOR *VISHUDDHA* (THROAT/FIFTH CHAKRA)

▸ Physically connect with your foods the minute you start to smell them and put them in your mouth. Chewing thoroughly is key, not only for the assimilation of nutrients, but also for a truthful connection to what you are doing at that exact moment.

▸ Eat openly. If you find yourself trying to "hide" when you eat certain foods, it may indicate deeper, disempowering feelings of shame that stem from overeating or "cheating." Remember, no one expects you to eat the ideal diet all the time. If you are going to eat something less than ideal, own up to it and be candid about it!

▸ Examine areas or relationships in your life where there is less than completely honest expression. This was a hard area for me in the past, as I would stay in relationships that I knew were not right for far longer than I should have, instead of using my power to express that and walk away sooner. Breakups and other relationship and friendship shifts can be hard at first, but being authentic is so tremendously empowering that you will feel a force supporting your genuine expression, one that perhaps you did not even know you had.

I am empowered to express myself fully.

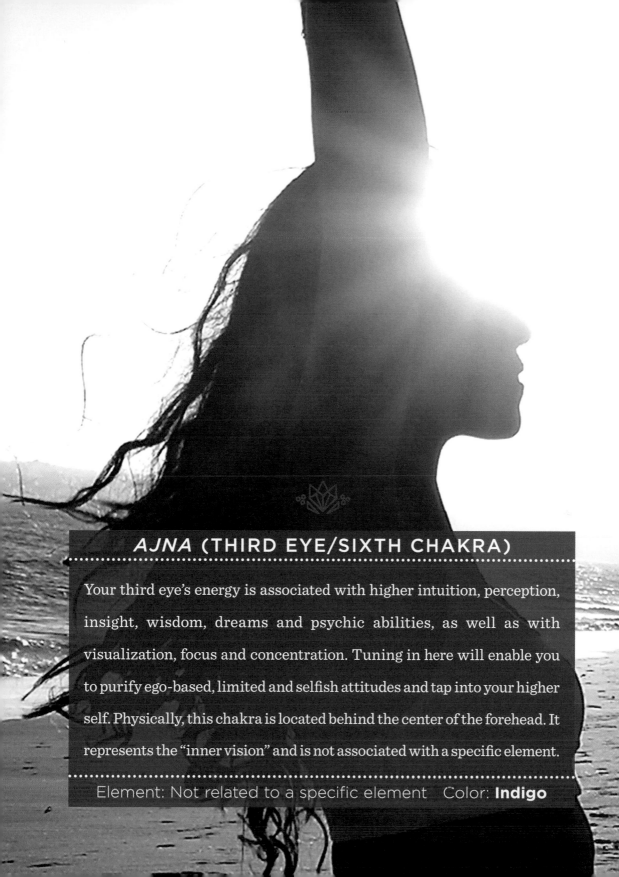

AJNA (THIRD EYE/SIXTH CHAKRA)

Your third eye's energy is associated with higher intuition, perception, insight, wisdom, dreams and psychic abilities, as well as with visualization, focus and concentration. Tuning in here will enable you to purify ego-based, limited and selfish attitudes and tap into your higher self. Physically, this chakra is located behind the center of the forehead. It represents the "inner vision" and is not associated with a specific element.

Element: Not related to a specific element   Color: **Indigo**

Balanced:

➤ Trusting yourself and your intuition when making decisions, and having awareness of the motivations behind all your actions

➤ "Seeing" the truth that you and everything else are part of a larger whole

➤ Living in a fearless (rather than a reckless), courageous way

➤ Feeling in control of your life and following your dreams

➤ Not being attached to material things and situations

➤ Having psychic or higher-intuition experiences

➤ Being confident in yourself and not looking to others or outside means to feel whole or complete

➤ Observing the "outer theater" of life from a calm inner point of view

➤ Feeling inspired by your vision of your purpose

➤ Regularly practicing meditation or another technique to feel aligned to divine guidance or higher truth

Imbalanced:

➤ Not being able to stand up for yourself

➤ Fearing success on a deep level

➤ Being ego-based, that is, stuck in "my," "mine" and "I"

➤ Experiencing confusion, indecision and a lack of clarity, despite overanalyzing

➤ Exhibiting an inability to concentrate or focus on the task at hand

➤ Suffering from depression or extreme moodiness

➤ Possessing obsessive-compulsive characteristics

➤ Feeling cut off from your life purpose

Physical Manifestations of Imbalance:

This chakra is located in the middle of the forehead, in the area between the eyebrows and slightly higher, and so the physical issues that can arise from imbalance in this chakra concern the face, the forehead, the central nervous system, the brain and pituitary gland, and the nose. Such physical issues include headaches, reoccurring nightmares, sinus problems, memory issues, blurred vision, blindness and other eye problems.

Discussion:

Balanced energy from your third eye is what some refer to as your "sixth sense." The energy of this chakra enables you to have a deeper perception in all situations, a penetrating vision that "sees" beyond the limitations of the physical and is more sensitive to picking up nonverbal communication, which is where true communication largely takes place. For example, I'm sure you can think of a time when a friend insisted she was happy and then smiled, but you had an inner knowing that something was off.

Healthy *Ajna* energy enables you to focus and think more clearly. You'll feel more intuitive about the decisions you make and the steps to take in your career and relationships, as well as in everyday life, including when it comes to what to feed yourself. There is such a joy in this. You feel like you're flowing along in the sea of life, rather than thrashing around, trying to keep your head above the waves. You naturally seek less validation from other people, because your confidence and your trust in yourself has expanded.

Have you ever wondered why Hindus traditionally place the *bindi,* or red dot, on their forehead? It's because the *bindi* represents the third eye and reminds Hindus to cultivate their spiritual vision. Regardless of your spiritual beliefs, this energy center is present, and its balance is extremely beneficial. In many forms of meditation, including Kriya yoga meditation, which I practice, you focus your energy upon the third eye, right above the middle of your eyebrows. This area is said to be the seat of spiritual sight, where you can perceive what the two physical eyes cannot see.

My Story

Before and during college and for some time afterward, though I put up a good front, deep down I was actually totally confused as to my purpose and direction. I tried to find a sense of belonging through constantly going to parties and seeking out activities with friends and groups of people. Back then I did have periods of regularly consuming vodka and beer... and I am *so* grateful that our livers repair themselves!

I always felt compelled to find out what others were "up to" that night and join in. I sought validation and depended on input from others to make my decisions: where to go, what to do, what to wear, what activities to participate in, even what to eat. At the time it was hard for me to imagine that I could ever get sick of going out. So I understand that we all are on a personal journey, and some of us are not at the point yet to go out less, to spend more time eating at home and not in restaurants, or to be alone more and meditate, because I was very much there myself.

But a shift happened, gradually. I read the books *Scientific Healing Affirmations* and *Autobiography of a Yogi,* both by Paramahansa Yogananda, and they changed the direction of my life. I was inspired to seek the inner joy that Yogananda spoke of, the joy that was possible from spending time being still and meditating. It was a foreign, but thrilling prospect to me.

I started to transition into eating the Beauty Detox way, and I naturally got to the point where I didn't want to put alcohol in my body regularly (though I'll still have a glass of wine from time to time, if I really feel like it) and I wanted to get up earlier to meditate with a clear mind, rather than a groggy one. I gradually started becoming conscious that I was happier spending time with friends in smaller groups and spending more time alone instead of going out several times a week. I still enjoy social events, but not as often.

Perhaps the biggest leap into healthy *Ajna* energy for me is living with a clear vision of my purpose, which is creating a lifestyle that enables me to evolve and live my best possible life, and inspiring and teaching others to do the same through this lifestyle. I now focus my energies on whatever supports this purpose, and I have eliminated in my life those things that do not. It's as clear as that. What truly nourishes me is meditation, learning in all forms, travel, writing, creating in the kitchen, practicing yoga and connecting on a deeper level, through authentic communication, with my husband, friends and family, not just my biological one but an expanded one that includes you and all others in our Beauty Detox community.

Balancing my *Ajna* chakra also really changed the way I interact with people. I really "see" more than hear what people are saying when I'm with them. I work from a place of much deeper intuition with clients and with whomever I'm talking to, feeling what they need to be nourished holistically. Learning and prescribing textbook knowledge are important in some instances, but it takes subtle awareness to work with people from this place of deeper vision. We all

> have the ability to develop this sensitivity, but it takes working to balance *Ajna* and the other chakras in our own selves first. There is no right or wrong path to living life. No matter where you may be, look inward and try to listen to yourself more and more. If you create more space, you will live more from your "inner vision."

Specific Foods:

➤ To create balanced perception, it's important to avoid excessive amounts of caffeine and sugar, which alter your mood and can overstimulate your system, creating anxiety.

➤ Certain spices, herbs and spice blends, such as ginger, turmeric and curry, have stimulating qualities, but they are also protective. They help balance blood sugar levels and have anti-inflammatory properties.

➤ Purple/indigo foods resonate with the vibration of this chakra. These foods include purple grapes, purple cabbage, blackberries, blueberries, purple kale, purple potatoes, dates, purple plums, figs and black raisins.

➤ Dark purple foods contain an antioxidant known as anthocyanin, which protects your brain and nervous system.

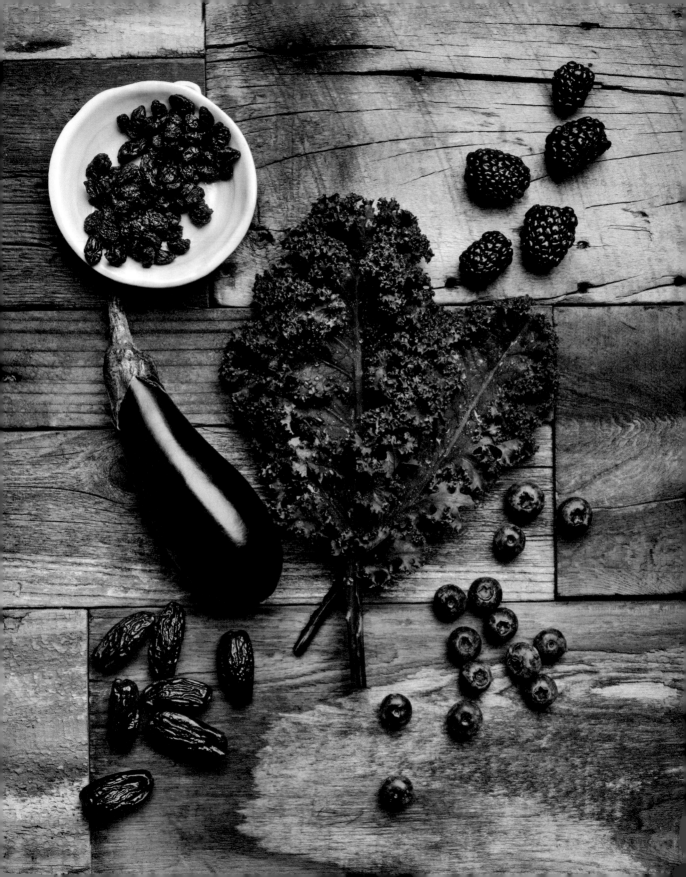

POWER TIPS FOR *AJNA* (THIRD EYE/SIXTH CHAKRA)

▸ Use your intuition when making everyday food decisions. When you go to the market, stand in the produce section for a moment. Try to feel which vegetables and fruits are calling out to you, as this may signal which ones are most nourishing to you right now. You might feel lost at first by not sticking to a set shopping list, but the more you try it, the more confident you'll feel when making your decisions. Do the same when eating at a restaurant. Does your body need something more grounding, such as a bean dish, dense protein, such as a tempeh dish or brown rice, or do you need something lighter, like a big salad? Don't just order what your friends have chosen. Listen to yourself.

▸ When you talk to people, try to tune in to more than their words. Notice their body language, the expression in their eyes. Determine their emotional or mental state based on more than what they say. Don't judge them in any way, but just focus on being more present and "seeing" more with your inner vision. As you practice this, it will foster more powerful and effective communication with your friends, family and coworkers.

▸ Excessive alcohol and drugs must be avoided, as they act as clouds over the third eye and can muddy its perception. They are drains of your true power and can lead to depression and sluggishness. Chemical-laden artificial foods and beverages, including ones in circus-like neon colors, are also congestive to your body and energy, so please avoid them.

I have access to infinite inspiration and power, because I am one with the whole.

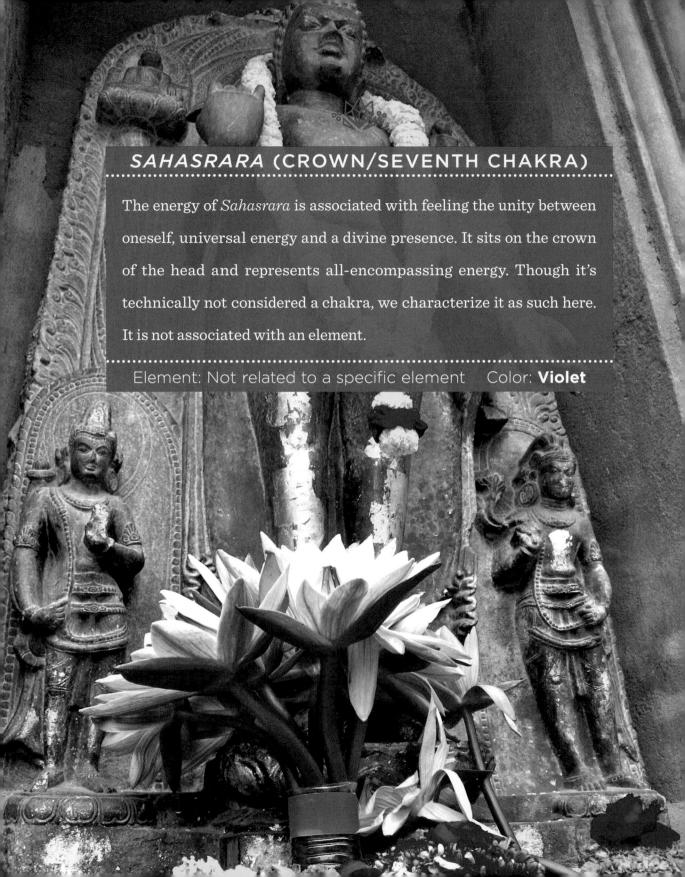

SAHASRARA (CROWN/SEVENTH CHAKRA)

The energy of *Sahasrara* is associated with feeling the unity between oneself, universal energy and a divine presence. It sits on the crown of the head and represents all-encompassing energy. Though it's technically not considered a chakra, we characterize it as such here. It is not associated with an element.

Element: Not related to a specific element   Color: **Violet**

Balanced:

➤ Believing there is a power greater than yourself (this can be based on spiritual practices or on a reverence for nature/the universe) and trusting that you are part of this greater universal power

➤ Going beyond materialistic pursuits alone and feeling abundant joy, a sense of purpose and curiosity about life

➤ Surrendering to the present moment

➤ Feeling animated and connected to your purpose for existence

➤ Practicing any form of devotion that feels authentic to you, including meditation, prayer, the chanting of hymns or mantras, a yoga practice approached with bhakti (devotion), or spending time in nature if you are an agnostic

➤ Being an agent for universal peace

➤ Feeling liberated from material labels

➤ Feeling connected and feeling that you are never truly alone

➤ Having a strong interest in humanitarian efforts and service to others

Imbalanced:

➤ Feeling the need to always debate or defend your beliefs with others

➤ Feeling confused about what you believe

➤ Being overly materialistic, rational, skeptical or cynical

➤ Having strong religious or spiritual viewpoints, to the extent that you are not open to others' beliefs

➤ Lacking purpose or inspiration

➤ Having difficulty learning new information

➤ Lacking sensitivity to the greater good or to the needs of others, animals and/or the environment

➤ Feeling limited and not expansive beyond your limited being

➤ Feeling bored with life

➤ Feeling chronically tired and worn down

Physical Manifestations:

There is less of a physical essence to this chakra than to the others. It can be likened to the aliveness of your vibration as a total being. Since it is more broad-spectrum, it oversees hormonal and nervous system function, and an imbalance can lead to a deterioration of the central nervous system or depression. An imbalance in this chakra can also lead to general accelerated aging.

Discussion:

When your crown chakra energy is balanced, you feel centered and capable of reaching your full potential. It is easy for you to tap into your connection to the ocean of universal energy. The electrical activity of your central nervous system and the firing of neurons and synapses throughout your body are part of this etheric energy.

In some Eastern traditions *Sahasrara* is described as a gradually blooming lotus flower, which represents a life increasingly rooted in spirituality. The lotus rises out of the mud into the sunlight and sheds debris as it fulfills its potential as a radiant, pure blossom. Some have theorized that the halo depicted in religious imagery of Jesus Christ and other Christian saints is representative of the seventh chakra.[10] It's pretty interesting whether you are Christian or not. But in a broader sense, you can simply focus on the imagery of overall balance and feeling your limitless energy and potential.

Greg's Story

I've had so many clients who are intensely attached to their coffee, but one of the most extreme cases was my client Greg. He had a high-powered technology career, but many facets of his job were far from glamorous. Dealing with constant office politics and red tape, conference calls, meetings and endless emails led to chronic stress. Coffee was definitely one of Greg's daily treats, and he was very strongly protective of it. He drank seven or more cups of joe on an average day. Eating less dairy and more veggies? That he could handle with no problem.

But there was no way he was giving up his coffee!

I noticed that Greg's days were bookended by coffee drinking in the morning and staying up late at night. He told me he consistently went to bed at around one in the morning or later. His whole lifestyle was imbalanced. I couldn't control his job, but I knew that it was important for him to cut back on his extreme coffee drinking, which was acid forming in his body (especially given the creamer he added to his cup) and contributed to the imbalance of his nervous system and adrenals. The key would be to help him experience feeling better without coffee. In this case, we had to tackle not only Greg's morning routine but also his late nights.

We reached an agreement that he would get into bed by eleven o'clock for at least two weeks. Since he would often get sucked into watching a TV show (and then the one after that) and would end up staying up late, I asked him to commit to leaving the television off when he got home and not even browsing the web. I told him he could read magazines or books instead. He didn't really want to do that (he was not a big reader, apparently), so he just naturally ended up going to sleep earlier. Though he got more sleep, he still drank coffee in the morning, but it was now easier to improve his diet. I instructed him to consume larger amounts of vegetables, to keep easy-to-stock fruit, such as blueberries, to snack on in his work fridge, to give up dairy, and to stock the necessary ingredients to whip up super-easy and energizing natural energy drinks.

Greg now feels a lot more balanced and has energy throughout the day. These days he usually goes to bed before midnight. He still drinks coffee . . . but only one or two cups a day and sans creamer. A huge improvement!

Specific Foods:

> Practicing nonattachment to particular foods is a great way to balance energy. People always ask me what I eat when I travel. The answer is that I do my best but remain flexible. It's hard to find big salads when I'm in Rwanda, but I eat a lot of cooked greens and tons of yams and potatoes. In South Korea I get a lot of great sea vegetables and kimchi, but I have to forgo some of my favorite fruits, like fresh figs, which I can get readily in California. In Greece I missed making smoothies, but I was incredibly grateful to be able to enjoy salads and *fava,* a dish made of yellow split peas. Try to practice this openness no matter which restaurant you visit or which place you travel to.

> Simplicity goes hand in hand with nonattachment. The Glowing Green Smoothie in the morning, instead of an elaborate breakfast, fuses the glory of the earth's perfectly crafted fruits and vegetables, which radiate with the brilliant harmony of the crown chakra. Edible flowers are another way to ingest the essence of beauty embodied in nature.

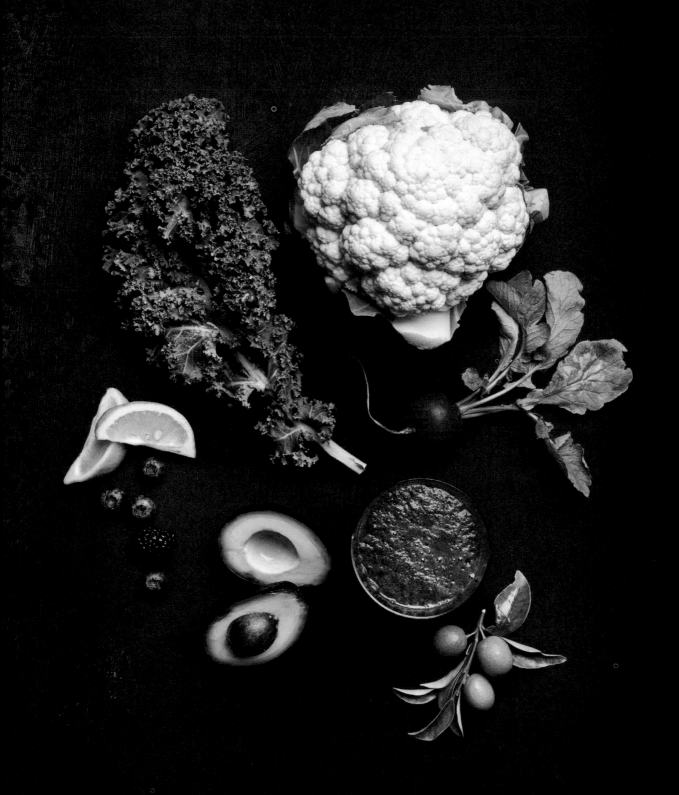

➤ Adhering to *The Beauty Detox Solution* principle of eating 80 percent alkaline-forming foods, which increases the oxygen circulating in the body, is of utmost importance. Eating this way also fosters greater detoxification, the removal of heavy old matter, and this makes more room for lightness and space to circulate through the body.

POWER TIPS FOR *SAHASRARA* (CROWN/SEVENTH CHAKRA)

▸ Find moments to listen to the universe around you, of which you are part. Listen to the birds, the wind rustling the tree branches, and the sounds of human life if you live in a city. Experience your connection, rather than isolation, to everything around you that you can hear, feel and see.

▸ Stay curious to cultivating new knowledge and experiences, as this keeps energy flowing freely. To help open new pathways and neurons in your brain, take up crossword puzzles and/or brain games, or take a class in a subject that interests you.

▸ To balance the crown chakra, it is also important to spend more time in the limitless elements of nature, and especially in the sunlight (exercise moderation), and to swim in the ocean or in lakes or ponds. Opening up space in your body can help you feel more expansive, so enemas or gravity colonics, which are water-based tools for cleansing waste from your digestive system, can be very helpful.

*I fulfill my unique purpose
and reach my full potential.*

Practical Power Practices

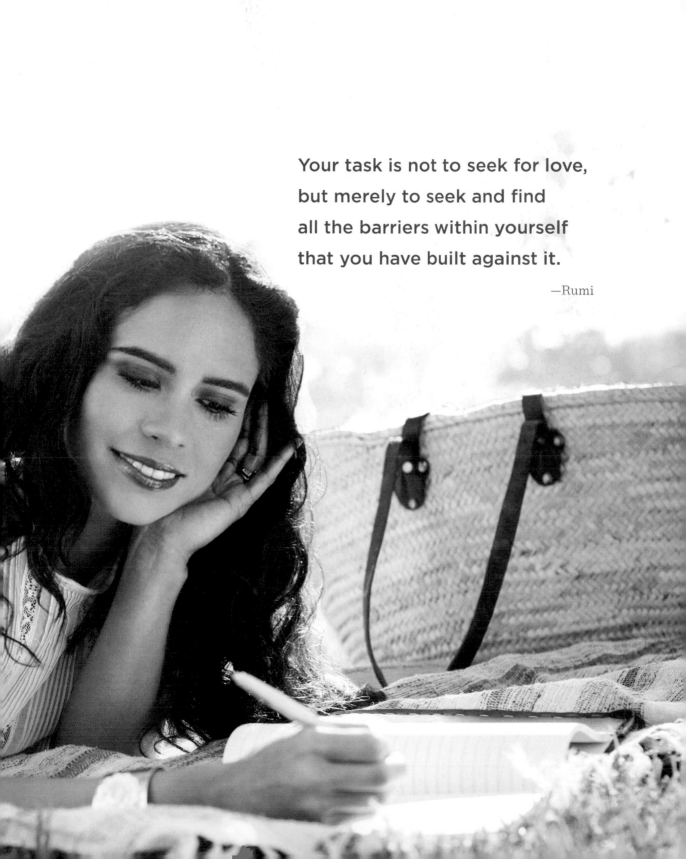

Your task is not to seek for love,
but merely to seek and find
all the barriers within yourself
that you have built against it.

—Rumi

Relationships are important to address, because the people you surround yourself with—and *their* thoughts, emotions and perspectives—can affect your overall well-being and weight-loss efforts.

While you are working on integrating the deep, perspective-shifting information found in the earlier chapters, I want to provide you with some practical power practices that you can start implementing right away. Remember, it's not just what is on your plate that influences your weight long term, but all aspects of your life, which are all interconnected.

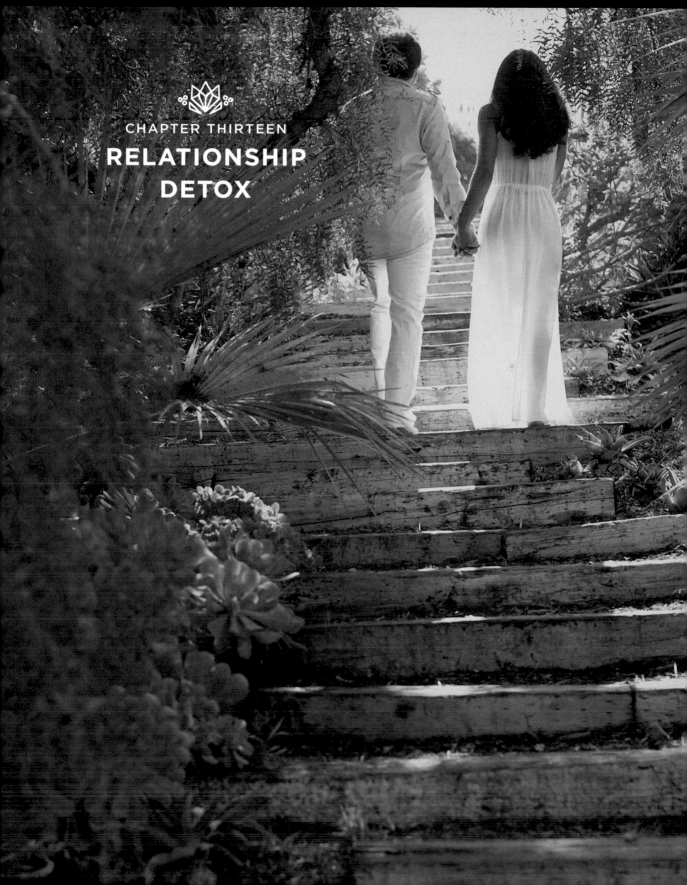

CHAPTER THIRTEEN

RELATIONSHIP
DETOX

A large epidemiological study carried out in the United Kingdom examined the level of conflict the study participants experienced in their closest relationship and found that those unhappy in their current closest relationship were more likely to gain weight.[1] In her comments on the study's findings, Susan Krauss Whitbourne, PhD, a professor of psychology at the University of Massachusetts Amherst, observed, "If you're gaining weight but don't know why... you might want to take the pulse on your relationship. It's not a matter of love or even sex that causes the need to let out your belt when things aren't going well. Instead, it's being able to confide in your partner, feel that your partner will help you with what you need done and, perhaps most important, to feel that your partner can help you alleviate your stress."[2]

But you're not off the hook if you are single. Your relationships with your close friends and family members can also have a powerful effect on your emotions, thoughts and beliefs, which, as we've established, all have an impact on your weight. Patterns of weight gain can be connected to your social networks, with some research revealing a shocking 171 percent increase in the weight of one person in a friendship when the other becomes obese.[3]

According to research conducted at North Carolina State University and the University of Texas at Austin,[4] when significant others resisted healthy changes and were not supportive of their partner's weight loss, the relationship suffered. I would infer from this study that making improvements in your lifestyle has the potential to create friction with friends, family members and colleagues who are resistant to such changes, and not just with significant others.

If your best friend, boyfriend, girlfriend, partner, spouse or favorite coworker scoffs at your GGS or about your journaling or starting a meditation practice, or is simply disapproving or pessimistic in general, it can pull you down emotionally, reinforce limiting thoughts, or create more stress in your life. You love that person, but you might feel deep down that this information is benefiting you and is now important to you and you don't appreciate their negativity.

On every energetic level, sharing takes place between people who are closely entangled. A study conducted by researchers at the University of California, Davis, and published in *Emotion*[5] in 2012, and a study completed at the University of Arizona and published in the *International Journal of Psychophysiology*[6] the same year found that romantic partners, even when seated several feet apart, synchronize their heart rates and breathing. The two studies also found that women tend to adjust their heart rate and respiration to their partners more than the other way around.[7] Such synchronization also occurs with close friends and family members. A study conducted at Aarhus University in Denmark and published in the *Proceedings of the National Academy of Sciences* showed that when an observer watched a friend or a relative walk across hot coals, the observer's heart beat sped up at the exact same moment as the friend's or relative's.[8] So be aware of those you choose to surround yourself with and the impact your actions and emotions have on each other.

I mentioned a prior relationship of mine in the Chocolate section of Chapter 10 (Overcome Your Specific Food Cravings). I was starting to binge on huge amounts of chocolate toward the end of our relationship, when I was subconsciously looking for love and intimacy from chocolate rather than from my partner. Definitely not a good sign! What finally ended things was when he got upset one day because I made a batch of the Glowing Green Smoothie from the greens and celery he happened to have purchased that time. We both took turns buying groceries, and I hadn't had time to restock the fridge. He was upset that I had used up "his" produce. In his anger, he made a very strange comment. "This car only has one seat in it, and that belongs to me," he said.

In that moment, I heard him loud and clear. He ultimately only wanted to take care of himself. It dawned on me that other comments he had made in passing about my goals and dreams were actually negatively affecting my self-esteem, even if that was not his conscious intention. His bizarre car analogy was the impetus I needed to say finally, "I'm out of here." I knew I had to end the relationship immediately. And I did. It was very difficult, because I had to deal with many repercussions from that decision, such as working out a new living arrangement, ending my relationship with his mother, whom I loved, and handling awkward social situations, since we had many mutual friends. I knew that as hard as those particulars would be to figure out, I would get through them, because of utmost importance was getting out of a relationship that was not good for me or my well-being.

At that time, I was looking a bit softer and rounder than usual, and my skin had started to break out again. Perhaps I was filling out in a quest for emotional protection (and because of so much chocolate!). But after I ended that relationship and healed from the breakup, my body became more toned and my skin cleared up nicely. It was as if the strong decision I had made, which was difficult but vital, had been translated into a visible strength in my body and across my face. Also, following the breakup, my energy shifted and opportunities around my passions for nutrition, wellness, writing, yoga and travel accelerated exponentially.

Don't worry! You don't have to get divorced or go through a breakup, ditch all your friends and disown your family to move forward in your life. But I do think it's important to take stock of all your relationships. In this chapter, we'll cover the different types of close relationships, as well as tips and strategies for navigating them in a way that infuses the most positivity into your life to support your weight loss, health and goals within those very relationships.

Your Significant Other and Family Members

Emotional ties run incredibly deep between you and your husband, wife, boyfriend, girlfriend, or partner and other family members. There are things you can do to maximize harmonious and positive energy within these relationships, which may be the closest ones in your life.

When you make dietary or health changes, or work to make any type of improvement in your life, it can sometimes be perceived as threatening by your significant other and those in your family. Perhaps it may bring up challenging feelings for them that they are doing something "wrong," and it makes them feel uncomfortable. When something new is uncomfortable and intimidating, there is some type of fear involved. So proceed with sensitivity and kindness. Food is a particularly charged topic, because so many people and families have emotional connections intertwined with food.

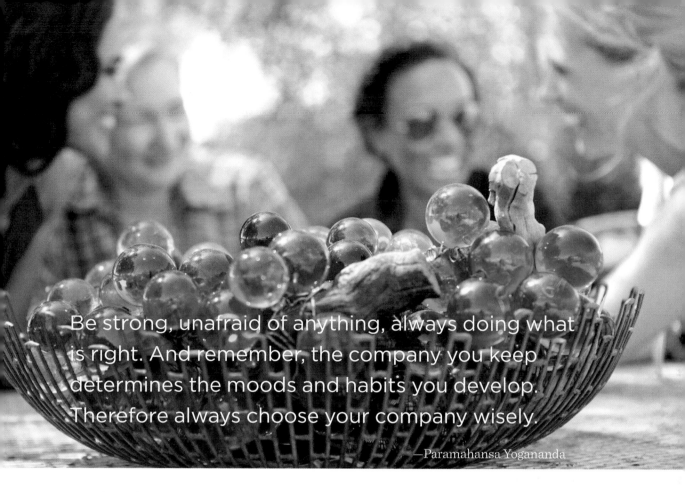

Be strong, unafraid of anything, always doing what is right. And remember, the company you keep determines the moods and habits you develop. Therefore always choose your company wisely.

—Paramahansa Yogananda

I have found that the best way to quell this fear is to make your relatives or significant other feel safe and to show them that you are not trying to prove them wrong. Focus on what you are doing as it pertains to yourself. For instance, if you start preparing Vegan Beauty Ranch Dressing (page 289), instead of reaching for the old family fave, regular ranch, and your mom or your brother or your husband questions you about it, you can always stick to, "I just feel better having this." Making the change about you takes the pressure off of them and keeps them from feeling that they are doing something wrong. Also, making the change about your feelings makes it harder to argue with, because it's not going to spark a fact-based discussion, such as you trying to mentally dig up all the exact information about why consuming dairy is not helpful to your weight loss.

There is no need to try to prove others wrong or to convince others to eat a certain way or follow a regimen if they are not ready for it. People come to discover things in their own time. Forcing them never works. But love does. Commit to remaining loving, open and nonjudgmental as you focus on your own goals and the steps you are taking to realize them. That is how you can be your most powerful. As you focus on your own goals, your energy will increase and you will become so magnetic that others won't even need any convincing to join you in your new pursuit in the future. They may start to ask you about what you are doing, and they may become interested in learning more. If they seem threatened in some way by the changes you are making, you can take steps to show them that you love them and that your new perspective on eating and being a whole being in no way compromises your relationship or your love for them. Go out for a walk, a hike, a tea, a movie, or find creative other ways to spend time together with your loved ones that doesn't always involve food.

If members of your family continue to be negative, all you can do is choose to be happy and keep your space and focus on your upward improvement. Shining with happiness and joy and focusing on realizing your best life is the best you can do.

Dana's Story

I've heard many stories from friends, readers and clients about their husbands being difficult and resistant to changes they were trying to make for their health and long-term weight loss. Some wives, too, but more often husbands. Sorry, guys, but it's true from my experience! A lot of the time it has to do with resistance at the dinner table, when they don't want to eat quinoa instead of chicken.

The stress Dana felt from her husband not wanting to improve his eating habits became overwhelming. He refused to sample the Glowing Green Smoothie, calling it sludge (how dare he!). He complained about not having anything to eat when she made vegetarian dinners, even if they contained hearty ingredients, such as beans and lentils. I reminded her that if she was feeling chronic stress building, it was because she was trying to use force. Force is the opposite of flow. You can't force things to be just the way you want them to be when you want. You have to find a way to flow with the situation while maintaining your personal power.

I suggested that she make her Beauty Detox dish and a separate portion of chicken or meat, simply prepared, which he could add to his plate if he chose. That way everyone would be happy, and she didn't have to cook two entirely different meals. For instance, when she made the Gluten-Free Spaghetti and Lentil Meatballs (thankfully, he couldn't tell that the pasta was gluten-free!), she prepared a side dish of chicken, which he could add to his meal. (It was not a Beauty Food–Paired combination, but for him it was still an improvement). This practice reduced her daily stress immensely.

Dana kept going with her Beauty Detox regime and lost over twenty-five pounds. After about a year of Dana receiving compliments on how she looked a decade younger and on how her energy was soaring, her husband, the former meat/food snob and Glowing Green Smoothie offender, decided he, too, needed to lose some weight, and he started drinking the GGS. He actually grew to love it! Dana was so surprised and happy that she texted me that she cried the day he started drinking the GGS. He now eats a few vegetarian dinners a week with Dana, and he has lost over twenty pounds. He has more to go, but he is on his way, because he chose to change himself. So, ladies, be patient, because this is definitely not the only time I've seen a very reluctant husband come over to the green side when he was ready and it was on his own terms.

Your Friendships

It is simpler to be selective and discerning with your friends, to whom you don't have a biological, legal or professional attachment. As your awareness expands, you may realize that some of your friendships are not serving you anymore. Make sure to spend the most time with friends who are positive and supportive, and who leave you feeling *good* after you see them.

Beware of negative friends, the ones who consistently make negative comments, such as complaining about their job or other people, or about how hard it is to lose weight, and even judgmental comments about the changes you are making in your own life. This includes those "energy drain" friends, the ones who take more and more of your energy and, you may now notice, infect your space with little tidbits of negativity, which can add up. Deep down you might feel that it isn't helpful to your well-being to be around people like this, at least not in large doses. This may be the case even if you have been friends with them for a long time.

Negative friends can make it harder for you to implement the energetic and life changes needed to clear out old emotions and drop weight. They can also make it more difficult to "lighten" up and make better choices and thus visibly become more healthy and beautiful. Though you don't want to hurt anyone, it is best to minimize your exposure to negativity. You can handle things delicately. You don't have to have dramatic confrontations with friends (unless you think facing the issue head-on is the right thing to do). Instead, you can intelligently and carefully avoid those individuals and reduce the number of occasions when you have to be with them for an extended period of time.

I know this isn't always easy, because I've been through it myself. Over the years, I have had to distance myself from some friends, including some with whom I had long relationships. But I felt we had grown apart and the friendship wasn't supporting my growth and evolution. This was especially true when I came back from my around-the-world trip. I suddenly had a very different outlook on life, including on how I wanted to spend my time and what I wanted to put in my body. It was awkward at first, especially at social gatherings. I was the one with a glass of water instead of a fancy cocktail. But more importantly than drinking alcohol or not, I found that I couldn't really talk about the things I was interested in with those groups of people. I knew they wouldn't understand what I was talking about, and I knew deep down that while I could love those friends from afar, I wasn't going to be spending a whole lot of time with them in the future.

Remember that you deserve the best in life, including being supported and surrounded with love and positivity. If you handle your friendships with love, kindness and honesty, you will be able to focus on building only uplifting friendships. Don't see distancing yourself from a certain friend as being selfish. By doing so and creating a stronger support system in your life, you will grow in power, and this will enable you to create more positivity in the world and inspire more people around you. It's not necessarily good or bad; it is just the way it is.

Anna's Story

Anna had a close friend, and they had gone on many vacations together. They were both single, and besides traveling together, they often enjoyed going to dinners, lounges and parties together and with other friends.

Anna was trying to improve her skin and digestion. She suffered from acne and IBS. She started to eat more whole plant foods, and she cut out dairy (though she still enjoyed goat cheese) and greatly reduced her meat intake. Her friend did not like that one bit. She was on a high animal protein diet, which she staunchly believed was the "right way" to eat. She didn't like that Anna no longer wanted to go to some of the same restaurants they had gone to in the past and that she was trying to do something different. She often made demoralizing comments. She told Anna that her new "hippie" way of eating didn't have enough protein and wasn't good for her. Deep down, her friend's reaction was fear based: Anna's new diet made her friend feel threatened because she misinterpreted it as an accusation that she was doing something "wrong."

I could see that Anna was having a really hard time with this. This girl had been her friend for over six years and was a big part of her social world. I advised Anna to just keep taking care of herself and to refrain from sharing so much about her dietary choices or goals with her friend. Anna kept progressing. All the fiber and greens in her diet had a profound effect on her. Anna's eyes brightened, her energy increased and she started to become much more conscious and to make better choices. For the first time in her life, she made time for regular grocery shopping and got up earlier to have time in the morning to make hot water with lemon and to spend some quiet moments grounding herself before her day started. She cut back a good deal on her alcohol intake, though she still enjoys wine or a cocktail sometimes. She told me that she could now see plainly that her friend was actually really negative about life in general. She complained all the time about her job, insisted that there were no "good" guys left and constantly lamented being single and "fat."

Soon after making all those positive changes, Anna met a really great guy online and they started dating. She took her time, but eventually she grew close to him. Her diet is now fantastic, her skin has largely cleared up and her digestion has improved immensely (thanks not only to eating more plant

foods, but also to giving up gluten and
taking probiotics). She and her friend
still maintain a friendship, but she sees
her far less regularly and they haven't
been on a vacation together in over

a year. The situation worked itself out
in more ways than one. When Anna
put herself and her needs first, her
relationships played out peacefully.

Your Job and Your Relationships with Coworkers

Oftentimes, you spend more time with your coworkers than with your friends and family. You may not be able to quit your job, but you can still create healthy work relationships. You can also establish certain boundaries, such as not bringing up or engaging in conversations about dietary habits, complaints or gossip.

For some people, their job or career creates a lot of fear in their life. The fear can be centered on the potential of job loss, structural work changes and a lack of control over projects. Such work-related fears can elevate your stress levels, which in turn can affect your weight and overall health. Worrying is a form of fear, and it takes you out of the present moment. It also doesn't serve a useful function, such as making things better. Realize that you don't have to figure out the whole future. Sometimes the best way to handle your job-related fears is simply to revamp your perspective and your interactions with your coworkers. But if you feel that your job is stagnant and there is no way to shift or grow within it, explore other options. Follow your heart and do not let fear get in the way.

If your now heightened start of awareness makes you notice that your colleagues are pessimistic or negative, start creating other places and ways to spend lunch breaks and don't share too much about your personal life, including about your weight and health goals. By the way, if you are a mom or dad this can translate into your relationship with other parents at your child's school or sporting events. Other parents are sort of "coworkers" in working to raise your children in shared group environments. You can be polite and have a great working relationship, but still be carefully selective with sharing information to maintain the most positive environment around you for your weight and health goals.

POWER TIPS

1. **Engage in authentic conversations with your loved ones.** Show them that you love them and that your changes are for yourself and do not threaten them. If you make an effort to hold a space of love, hopefully, they will be more loving and supportive of you, as well.

2. **Avoid debates.** If questions come up about your new way of eating or your new activities or daily practices, always make it about you and your personal feelings. For instance, if you are questioned about your food choices, simply answer, "Eating this way makes me feel good."

3. **Consider how your friends make you feel.** If you notice that some friends are negative and are not supporting your efforts to improve your health and well-being and to achieve weight loss, or if you realize that you don't feel as uplifted or as joyful when you are around them, take steps to reduce the amount of time you spend with them. If you feel it is necessary, have an honest talk with them to see if they have a desire to evolve. A clean break in the relationship may be healthier for both of you.

4. **Seek out some positive, like-minded friends in healthy environments.** There could be a new friend just around the corner at your local yoga studio, art studio, dance class or moms' group or even at the farmers' market. You may be surprised by how you start to attract more positive friends as you become aware that optimism and joy are important to you. The positive side of consciously chosen technology and social media is that you can tune in to inspiring communities online at any hour of the day, whenever you need a boost. I'm thrilled to constantly witness Beauty Detox community members interacting, sharing and supporting one another on our Instagram, Facebook and Twitter pages. Please check out our social media channels (@_kimberlysnyder, Facebook.com/KimberlySnyderCN) to align with like-minded people along this path.

5. **Remember that you are not what you do.** Start to become conscious of any ego-based identities you have created for yourself around your job. The more you realize that you are just you, the more you will lessen the fear, anxiety and stress that accompany attachments to outcomes in your work and too much emphasis on the future.

All my relationships are healthy,
and I give unlimited love to all.

All my friendships are uplifting and positive
and supportive of my growth and goals.

I am passionate about living my best life.

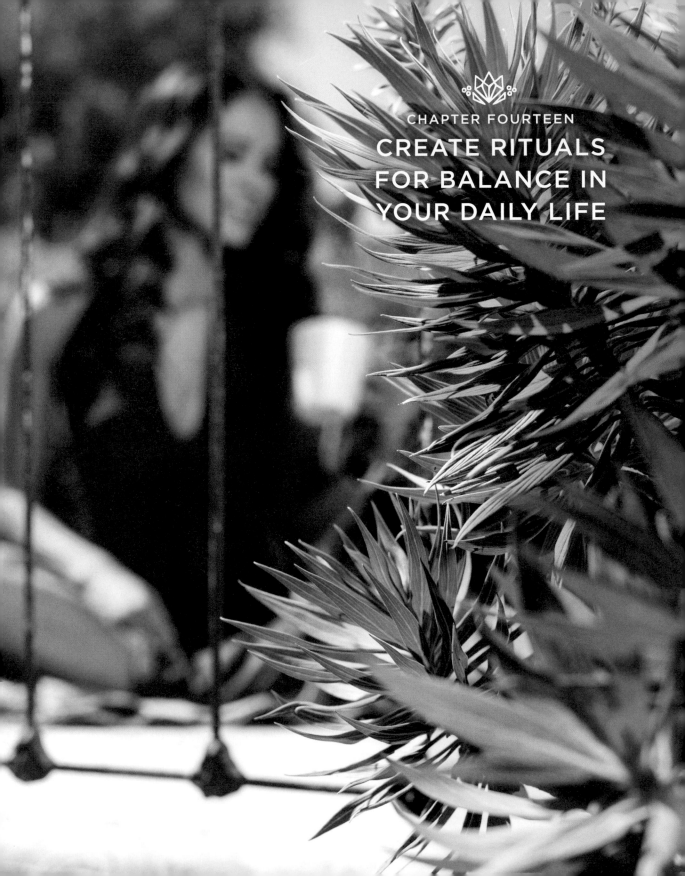

CHAPTER FOURTEEN

CREATE RITUALS
FOR BALANCE IN
YOUR DAILY LIFE

You can consciously create rhythms in your day to foster greater awareness. Let's focus on the everyday activities, which add up. I hope that the practices I share with you in this chapter will inspire you to make them your own. They are all rooted in mindfulness, which is a gateway to weight loss and joy.

Sadhana means "practice" in Sanskrit. These are the regular rituals you create in your life to work toward a given purpose. Some of the most powerful rituals, in terms of creating balance in your life and supporting your weight and well-being goals, are the ones with which you start and end each day.

Morning Practices

How you start the day is critical to improving your health and beauty, and to empowering you so that you have a great day ahead of you. It's easier to continue on the path of making great food choices when that path is paved with good morning habits. Here are some of the most important ones to make part of your life.

➤ Keep your phone in airplane mode while sleeping. Not only will you have less radiation in your midst, but you won't wake up and immediately be pulled in different directions by emails and text messages that have come in during the night.

➤ Start the day by planting your feet firmly on the ground for at least three minutes and simply tuning in to your breath as you breathe in deeply and slowly through your nose. This will help you get grounded. Do this *before* you turn your phone back on. I call this "the 3 minutes" with my clients. This is a simple beginning to fostering a regular meditation practice. (See Introduction to a Simple Meditation Practice on page 210.) Or, if you have a different or longer personal practice that you adhere to in the morning, honor it and create the time for it.

➤ Fresh water and hot water with lemon should be the first things that enter your body each morning. They reinforce the fact that you are doing something good for yourself, as well as ensure that you start your day off from the powerful place of being hydrated.

➤ Nourish your whole being every morning with the Glowing Green Smoothie (GGS). It infuses your body with a powerful blend of minerals, vitamins, enzymes, fiber and many other phytonutrients from whole plant foods grown in the earth. Consuming the GGS (page 255) is the most beautifying, health-promoting and weight-balancing daily gift you can give yourself.

➤ Say your Power Affirmations or listen to them while you're getting ready in the morning. Choose the affirmations that resonate the most with you. Select any of the affirmations in this book, or focus on the ones in the chapters that correspond to areas in your life you are working on. Feel free to customize these affirmations so they are specific to you.

Evening Practices

How you wind down each day is just as important as how you start it. Your preparation for sleep greatly affects your body, the quality of your rest and your health. Here are some of the foundational practices to incorporate into your evening routine.

➤ At bedtime, always create space between the busy day and nighttime. Turn off the TV at least (at least!) half an hour before bed. That way you have some time to clear your mind of external chatter and messages and turn inward, where your true power resides, before bedtime.

➤ As a relaxation ritual after a stressful or full day, try sipping the Nourish Your Nervous System Elixir (page 335) in the evenings.

➤ In the evening have your three minutes of quiet mindfulness once again or practice a full meditation. See the tips in the Morning Practices section on the preceding page. Allowing for relaxed stillness at the end of the day is an important ongoing practice, as it enhances deep beauty sleep and provides the opportunity daily to let go of anything that doesn't serve you emotionally, mentally or on any level anymore. This is essential for optimal health and weight control.

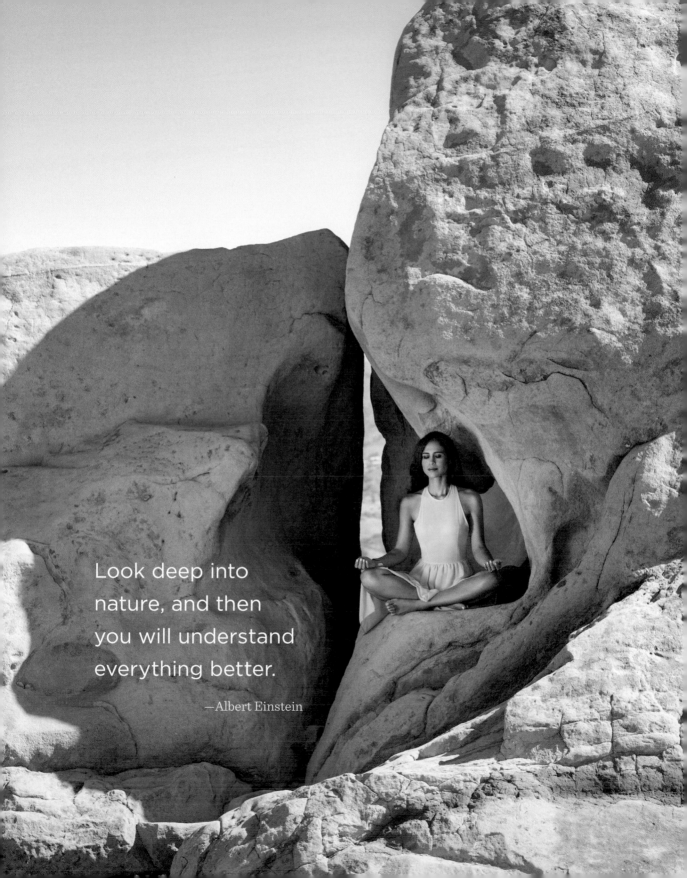

Look deep into
nature, and then
you will understand
everything better.

—Albert Einstein

Introduction to a Simple Meditation Practice

Developing a meditation practice is the key to increased joyfulness, regardless of outer circumstances, and the attainment of your highest potential in all areas of your life. When you meditate regularly and increasingly deeply, you reunite your consciousness as a limited being with the unlimited whole. This infuses unlimited power into all that you do. And you will experience the realization that happiness comes from within, and does not depend on outer things.

➤   Choose a way to sit that allows your spine to be straight and is comfortable for you to be in for some time. If you sit cross-legged, it can help to elevate your hips with a pillow. If your legs consistently go to "sleep," it may be better for you to sit in a chair with both feet planted on the floor, as I personally do for longer meditations. It is also helpful to designate a meditation space, whether it be a small corner in your bedroom or in another room, and to have a pillow or chair that is only for meditation. This reinforces in your mind that it's time to drop into your meditation practice.

➤   Once you're settled, close your eyes completely or soften your gaze and close your eyes halfway, if you prefer. Do a quick body scan and notice if you're holding tension in any area of your body, especially in your shoulders and jaw. Relax your entire mouth and prevent your tongue from pressing against the roof of your mouth. Take a deep inhale in through your nose and exhale out your mouth, consciously releasing stress and tension.

➤   You can start with an intention such as a simple "I offer up gratitude and peace"; a silent or audible "Om," the vibrational sound of Oneness; or a brief prayer of any kind that is meaningful for you. Now start a simple *pranayama* breath exercise, one with a 4-4-4 breath count. Breathe in through your nose for a count of four, retain the breath (with a sense of ease rather than strain) for a count of four* and then breathe out through your nose for a count of four. Keep the breaths smooth and deep. Remember to relax completely to keep the pathways open for fuller breaths. Avoid hunching your shoulders or constricting the muscles in your neck. Your breaths can be silent—there is no need to strain to produce a loud noise for this practice.

➤   Keep going with your 4-4-4 breath count practice for several cycles. If you find yourself being pulled toward different thoughts, just keep mindfully bringing your attention

*If you are pregnant or you have a health issue that precludes holding your breath, just omit this middle step of retaining your breath and practice the inhales and exhales only.

back to your deep, slow breaths. When you feel ready—there is no set time—lift your internal gaze, or your attention, to the space between your eyebrows, that is, to your *Ajna* chakra.

➤ Rest here for as long as it feels right to you, observing feelings as they arise but trying not to follow thought chains. You can say a simple mantra, such as *"Shanti, shanti,"* or "Peace, peace," if it helps to have something to repeat. If your mind wanders (as it does at times for everyone), keep bringing it back peacefully to the lifted inner gaze. You can also use this space to offer another personal prayer. Sit for at least three minutes, or longer, perhaps for ten, twenty or thirty-plus minutes. When you feel complete, bring your hands together in *anjali mudra*, a position created by pressing both of your palms together in front of your chest, and close with another silent or audible "Om," if you choose, or offer another intention of gratitude or peace, such as "I am thankful for everything. May my thoughts and actions contribute to peace and positivity for the greater whole."

➤ It takes practice to create inner and outer stillness, and constant effort is required to keep bringing your attention back to the inner lifted gaze and away from the different thoughts that may arise. Be incredibly patient with yourself. Don't judge yourself or get frustrated. The fact that you are attempting a meditation practice at all is a huge step, and it means you are progressing amazingly well. Even if you are restless or fidgety, remember that it is a practice, and it will get easier to sit still. So keep consistently carving out these precious, highly beneficial moments in your life for your practice. With continued practice, over time your meditations will leave you feeling increasingly joyful—I promise. This is sacred time for your well-being in immeasurable ways, so bravo and infinite love to you!

➤ If you are interested in learning a highly effective meditation system that will enable you to go much deeper in your practice, I highly recommend the Kriya yoga methods taught by Paramahansa Yogananda, which I personally practice. You can learn more at www.yogananda-srf.org.

Go in Nature

Nature is a constant reminder that we are all equally part of a much larger cosmos. It has tremendous healing power. Nature mirrors the perfection of the universe. It doesn't have an ego, and it doesn't try to project a certain image of itself. It just is. There is a micro-macro relationship between nature and us, as the universal five elements of earth, water, fire, air and ether/space are present in both.

When I was going through the most difficult parts of adolescence and was stressing out about fitting in and about my body and my acne, I would go hiking in the woods very often, sometimes daily. There were numerous hiking trails in the Northeast town in which I grew up, and one was within walking distance, and so the forest became my sanctuary. After breathing in the fresh air and being with the trees for so long, and often walking next to free-flowing creeks, I would always feel calmer, revived and stronger.

Creativity is at play in all areas of your life, and thus you have the ability to create the body and life you desire. Creative power is the very essence of the universe and all of nature, which you are a part of. You can create a beautifully fit, strong body. Why not? When you connect with consciousness, there are no limitations to this power.

I firmly believe that the best way to connect with your creative power is to spend more time in nature. We are all a part of nature, so if you are disconnected from your natural surroundings, you will fall out of alignment with the very essence of who you are. Many of us have lost touch with it, but our creative capacity is embodied in our cells, and by reconnecting with nature, we also reconnect with its boundless creative power. The connection is intrinsic and integral to our very being.

My Story

Between my junior and senior years of high school, I took a monthlong Outward Bound course in Colorado and Utah. I had always been attracted to the forest, and I enjoyed hiking along the trails surrounding my town. But I had never been out West, and the prospect of being in the wilderness for a month was thrilling. I begged my parents to let me go, and they finally relented.

This Outward Bound adventure had me hiking up many different mountain peaks on loose scree (loose stones and rock fragments), rappelling into desert canyons, using a compass to navigate the way to food drops or water and finding the best places to put our mats down for shelter at night. The course culminated with a solo expedition, where I had to survive in the woods completely by myself for a few days and nights.

When I look back on my life, I credit that extended time in nature as the early burgeoning of my creative power. Had I not gone on that adventure, I do not think I would have had the courage to undertake my three-year world journey and all it entailed. In turn, the world journey involved spending a lot of time in nature, which indelibly shaped my perspective and opened my mind and heart to nature's inspiration.

Today, no matter where I may be, I recognize and embrace the fact that the pulse of creativity from nature inspires me in all my ventures. I walk barefoot on grass or sand as often as possible, and especially before writing sessions or work on a new creative project. I eat outside as much as I can, I hike, I go for walks and I watch the sunset as often as possible. Nature is a master teacher for all of us.

POWER TOOLS FOR CONNECTING WITH NATURE

▸ Spend as much time in nature as possible. Nature is there to remind us silently but strongly that we are part of a much bigger whole, and we can always draw energy from this universal connection. If you live in a city, spend more time in parks and take excursions into the surrounding countryside as often as you can. Choose vacations where you are in nature at least part of the time. Hike, walk, look at trees and local plants and flowers, or enjoy any outdoor activity that resonates with you as often as you can, whether it's swimming, planting flowers, letting yourself drift on your back in the ocean or stargazing.

▸ Eat fresh foods from a farmers' market or grow your own food. Keeping a Beauty Detox diet of mostly plant foods will also connect you with nature, especially if you prepare at least some of the simple dishes yourself. Having a lot of plants in your home so there are living things all around is also something I encourage. You can cultivate a simple herb garden or sprouts on your windowsill to remind you of your connection to living things and the whole of nature.

▸ Select outdoor activities over indoor ones whenever possible to take advantage of breathing fresh air and moving in a natural way over uneven terrain. For instance, choose hiking or walking outside when the weather allows over going to the gym. Even sedentary activities, like lunches and meetings, are opportunities to get some fresh air and sunshine. You need only find a picnic table or a bench in a nice garden or a park.

Practice Healing Touch

Skin is special and unique in that it is a visible line of demarcation, the divide between the limits of your physical body and the energy beyond. Physical touch has been shown to promote healing[1] and to foster growth (it helps newborns develop).[2] Abhyanga, a highly recommended practice in Ayurveda that involves massage oils for the body, is said to have a therapeutic effect, helping to calm the mind and the nervous system.

Since touch, a form of nourishment, increases overall well-being and helps reduce stress and worry,[3] it can help prevent overeating and weight gain. Unfortunately, in the Western world there is a lack of touch. It's as if everyone lives in their own little bubble and is very uncomfortable with the prospect of someone else touching them. I even see it in yoga class, when people make a concerted effort to avoid touching someone else's yoga mat or (gasp!) brushing against somebody's shoulder or hand. But touching is natural and healthy, and so you should make it a regular healing practice in your own life.

POWER TOOLS FOR PRACTICING HEALING TOUCH

▸ Practice self-massage daily. At bedtime, take a few minutes to massage coconut or another healing plant-based oil into your feet, your calves, your elbows and your hands. I keep a jar of coconut oil next to my bed, and I do this for myself nightly. It's something I look forward to at the end of the day. Healing self-touch fosters self-love.

▸ Get yourself a luxurious-feeling body scrub or make your own (see below). Take a few minutes to scrub your limbs, back and belly lovingly with it while you shower. As you do, imagine you are scrubbing any lingering stress or negative energy off your being that you may have picked up from others during the day.

▸ Take turns giving and receiving massages of any length with your significant other, roommate or friends. It can be an amazing way to connect in a deeply nourishing way.

BEAUTY DETOX BODY SCRUB

½ cup coconut oil
½ cup organic sugar
15 drops lavender essential oil

Mix all the ingredients together in a small bowl until well combined. Pour the mixture into a waterproof, BPA-free container and keep it in your shower.

Begin or Deepen a Yoga Practice

Yoga is infinitely more than just a form of exercise. Though many associate *asanas* (poses) with yoga, in reality they are actually only a very tiny part of what yoga truly is. Regularly and properly practiced, yoga creates a union or alignment with all parts of your being—your mind, body and spirit—and with the infinite or greater power (however you personally define that). It makes you aware of your breath—one of the most powerful and instrumental ways to reclaim your power in the present moment.

How "advanced" your yoga practice is does not hinge on the level of complicated poses you can do. Nor are you "bad at yoga" if you are not flexible. Those are really not the important parts! The Western approach is often so focused on success, according to external measures, and thus it reinforces the ego, instead of addressing the internal, formless benefits derived, which cannot be seen with the eye. In yoga these include a deepening awareness of breath and an alignment of all parts of your being. The poses are fun to try to create with your body, and I have a lot of fun with them myself, but do not become attached to them or think they are the be-all and end-all of yoga. They are not.

Yoga also promotes the release of old energy, energy that is stored in various parts of the body, in the hips, spine or hamstrings. Releasing patterns are a tool to release the "old," stored emotions and to move on without holding on to them. Due to its innate intelligence, *prana,* or energy, moves automatically to the places in the body and mind where there are blockages preventing the free flow of energy. In your yoga practice, you will bend your spine and twist your body in ways that you usually do not in other forms of movement.

Learning how to hold a *drishti* (focused gaze) and balance poses for long periods of time facilitates the development and sharpening of higher levels of focus in other areas of your life, such as your dietary choices. (In other words, yoga enhances your ability to follow through with making the most nourishing food choices for yourself and to stick with them.) When you develop higher levels of focus through yoga, you are able to hold the gaze of others, to look right in their eyes, as you are talking to them. I see so many women looking away or looking down when they are engaged in conversation. Holding the gaze of others means that you are confident about holding space and being in the world, and that you value what you have to say and contribute.

Svadhyaya means "self-observation" and is a tool for becoming truly aware of who you are and what your true needs are. This starts with simply observing your breath. It is

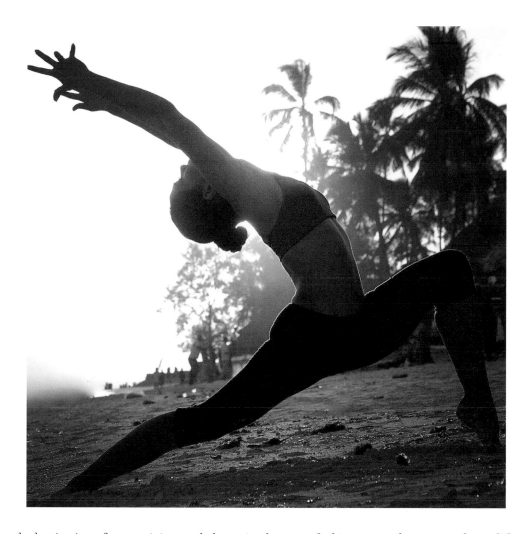

the beginning of recognizing and observing how you feel in many other parts of your life, such as when you eat certain foods versus others, and how you feel being around certain people and their energy.

POWER TOOLS FOR OFFERING UP A POSE

▸ If you prefer a home yoga practice all or at least some of the time (as I do), or if yoga classes are inconvenient or out of your budget, try using DVDs or online yoga programs. There are many good ones. You can also check out my online yoga course and videos, if you're interested.

▸ Check out local yoga studios and the different types of classes they offer to find ones that work for you. Remember that there are many types of yoga (Hatha, Vinyasa, Iyengar, Ashtanga, Kundalini, Anusara, Heated/Power Yoga and others), so if you are not connecting with one type in particular, explore others.

Reduce the Noise

The mass media is a part of all our lives. It's good to be in the know of what's going on, to an extent, but it's important to put your energy into living your own life fully and making your own decisions based on what is truly nourishing and supportive for *you*. There's a lot of noise out there, in the form of other people's messages, beliefs and values, and it is being pushed on us. When you tune in to what's on TV or surf the internet, you give up your consciousness for that period of time. So always choose whatever media you tune in to consciously and carefully, rather than casually.

You want to avoid becoming passive and being drained of energy from watching too much TV or spending excessive amounts of time browsing the internet, as this can have a negative effect on your overall balance and your ability to focus your energy positively on long-term healthy weight loss.

POWER TOOLS FOR REDUCING YOUR MEDIA INTAKE

▸ Selectively choose the television programs you want to watch. Be strict with yourself and do not watch any others. Choose programming that is positive or that you can learn from (such as documentary programming). Avoid drama and negativity, as you want to keep those energies completely out of your life.

▸ Record TV shows so you can fast-forward and skip the ads and commercials, which feed the ego and create a desire for excess.

▸ After watching TV and before going to bed, be sure to have a space, ideally to meditate, to clear out those thoughts and become centered on your own.

▸ Be vigilant about not getting sucked into excessive internet surfing, especially if you frequent sites that are heavy on gossip and negativity. And no matter what, be sure never to leave negative comments on sites or social media channels, as these will ultimately boomerang on you, bringing negativity back to you.

I create balance in my environment,
which fully supports my growth and goals.

I live an authentic life.

I have all the power I need to
create the body and the life I want.

Beauty Detox Power Recipes

Your soul is a beacon of infinite power. You can expand that power from within and give light and health and understanding to others.

—Paramahansa Yogananda

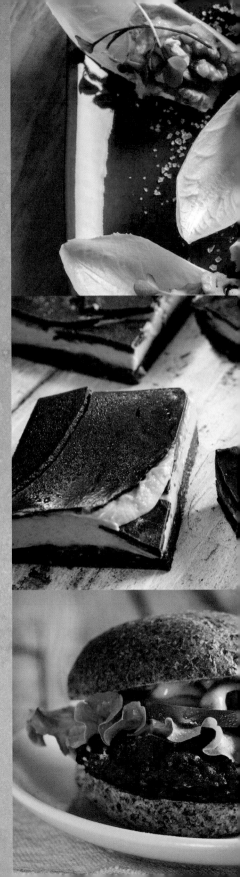

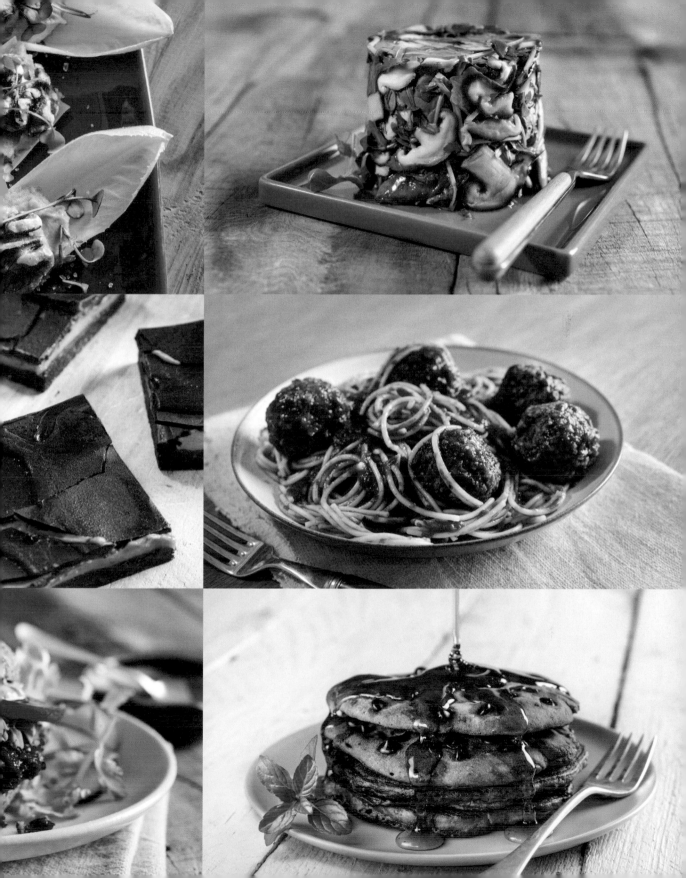

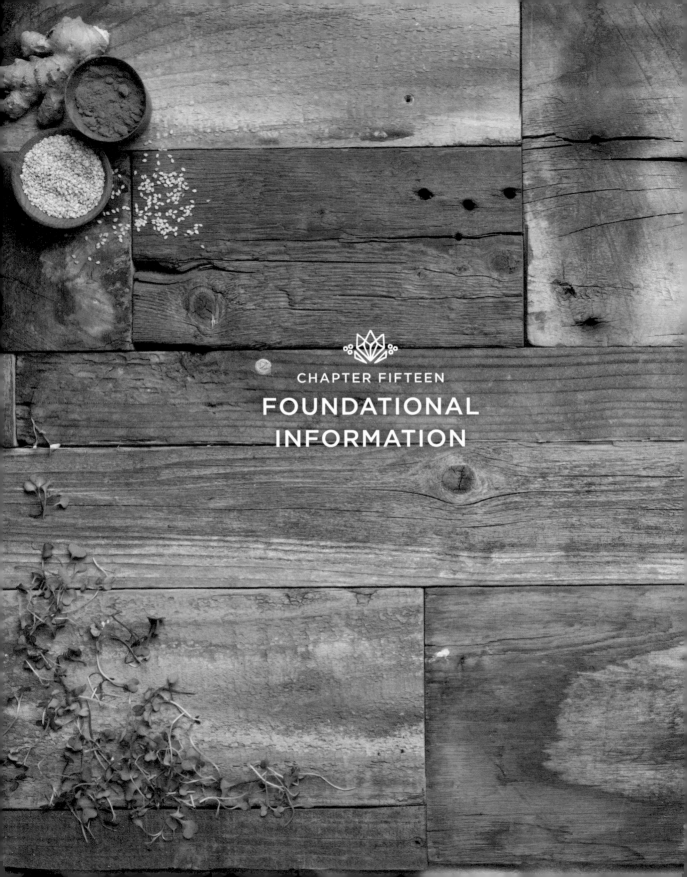

CHAPTER FIFTEEN

FOUNDATIONAL
INFORMATION

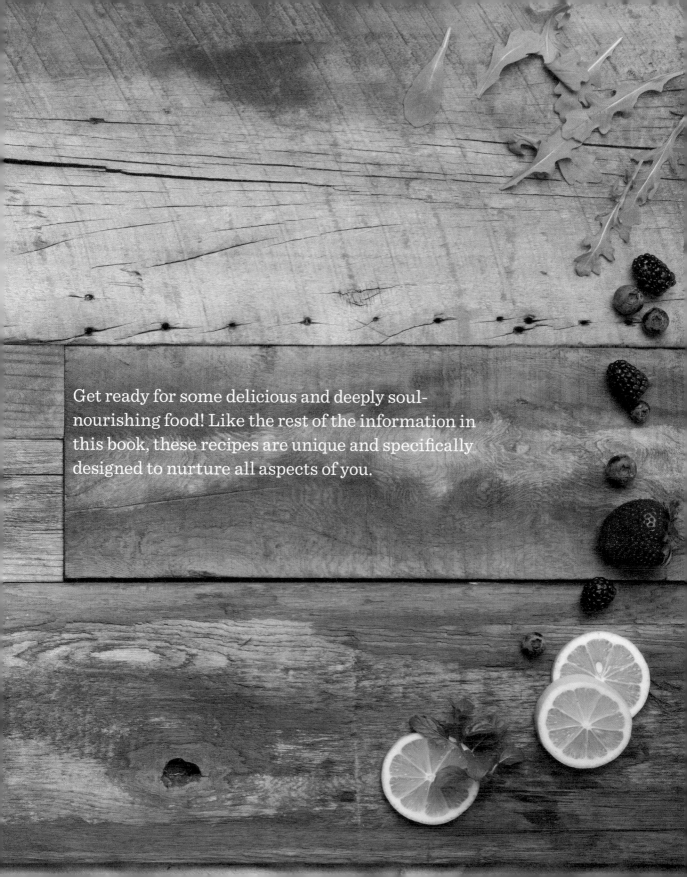

Get ready for some delicious and deeply soul-nourishing food! Like the rest of the information in this book, these recipes are unique and specifically designed to nurture all aspects of you.

The recipes in this book are organized according to the chakras and cravings, rather than by course (soup, salad, entrée, dessert and so on). The textures, colors, tastes and element-based qualities that we discussed in Power Alignment Shifts 3 and 4 dictated the order of the recipes. This way, when you are working to remedy a particular chakra imbalance or craving, you can turn to specific whole food–based, healthy recipes geared to that specific chakra or craving, knowing that you are nourishing yourself on multiple levels. Even if you are craving such things as fatty foods, sweets or chocolate, you can enjoy these recipes confidently, as they are much healthier alternatives. You might make a few recipes from one chakra or craving section or mix and match.

Each time you return to this book, you may receive the information here differently, because you are an ever-changing, dynamic being. And you may discover recipes that were right in front of you before but that you weren't called to make until a later time.

UNIQUE RECIPES TO BALANCE YOUR ENTIRE BEING

Here are some of the reasons these recipes are particularly special and powerful:

➤ As with all Beauty Detox recipes, these are based on Beauty Foods and are 100 percent plant based* and gluten-free.

---

* There are a few recipes in this book that call for honey and there is one with bee pollen. Both of these products are produced by bees. I encourage you to source these products from an ethical beekeeper. If you prefer to avoid honey for whatever reason, you can replace it with the other sweeteners.

➤ All the recipes are free of:

- soy products, except for the organic fermented soy products tamari, miso and tempeh (which may be easier to digest given that the fermentation process does away with some of soy's unfavorable qualities)

- artificial sweeteners, agave nectar or syrup, and cane sugar (see more in the Sweet Heart section)

- polyunsaturated vegetable oil and vegetable oil–based products (such as vegan butters and vegan mayonnaise).

➤ Each recipe is carefully designed to adhere to the Beauty Food Pairing Principles, outlined in *The Beauty Detox Solution*. Simple, beneficial combinations of foods ensure optimal digestion and convey health and beauty benefits. Remember that having excellent digestion can help you lose weight more easily, as well as help you look and feel your most beautiful.

These recipes are easy to customize. If the Beauty Food Pairing Principles are still vague to you, just try to stick to the general categories (for instance, switching up the green vegetables, and swapping vegetables and nuts for other options in those categories) so that these dishes will still promote optimal digestion. Listen to your body. As you continue to heal and become balanced on a very deep level, you will hear what your body is telling you more clearly.

Please choose organic foods as much as possible within your budget. It's particularly important to always source organic tamari and miso, which are fermented soy products, since organic means they are non-GMO. You can find all the ingredients in these recipes in a health food market or even online. And take advantage of what's available from your local farmers' market. The food from local farmers is the freshest and tastes great, and you'll be supporting local farms.

A little goes a long way with many of these ingredients, so you won't have to buy them often. For shopping tips and more information on specific brands, please be sure to visit my website, www.kimberlysnyder.com.

Enjoy your Beauty Detox Power adventure in every way, including with these recipes to balance your entire being!

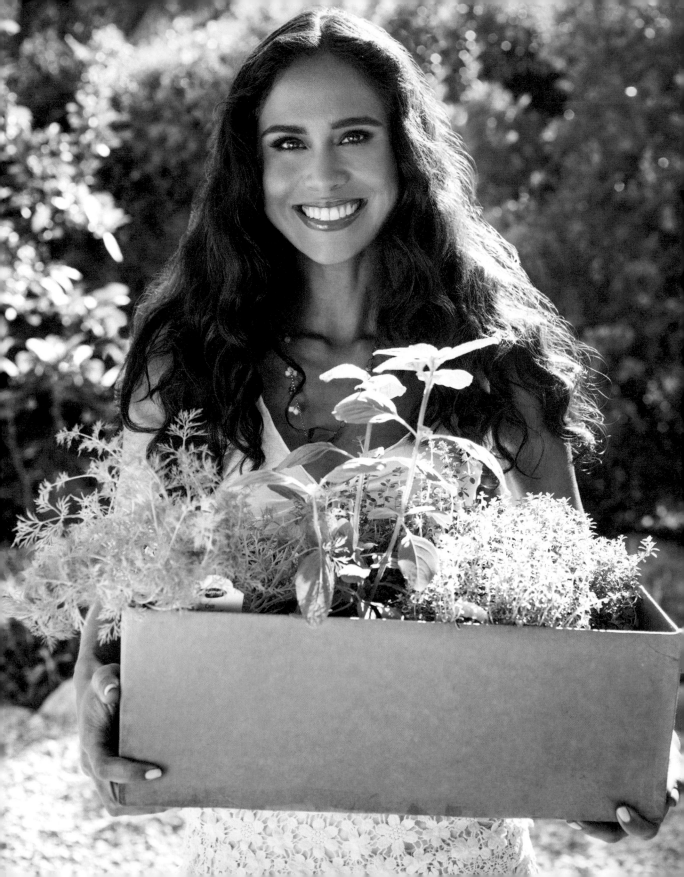

*I honor myself by nourishing
myself with the best foods.*

SWEET HEART

Sweeteners are not only for desserts. They act to balance the overall flavor profile of dressings, sauces and savory dishes. A little goes a long way when it comes to sweeteners, and over the years, I've experimented with many. In the recipes you can always swap one for another if you prefer, as I indicate. Here are my go-tos:

STEVIA:

Stevia has been used as a sweetener for centuries in South America. It's naturally derived from a plant, though forms of stevia other than the whole leaf form have undergone processing. Still, I find it to be a good choice because it is low on the glycemic index, it is calorie free, and only a small amount is needed at a time.

COCONUT NECTAR:

Coconut nectar is my go-to liquid sweetener, since it is rich in minerals and amino acids, has little impact on blood sugar levels, and is low in fructose. It does *not* have a coconut taste. It has a neutral flavor, and so it works great in a wide variety of dishes.

MAPLE SYRUP:

Maple syrup is an easy-to-source option. Its historical roots are with the indigenous peoples, including the Algonquians, who recognized that maple syrup was an excellent source of energy and nutrition and called it *sinzibukwud,* meaning "drawn from wood."[1] Naturally derived (though not raw), it contains sucrose, but for most of us, it is acceptable in small amounts. Maple syrup has an array of minerals, such as manganese and zinc, as well as other phytonutrients and antioxidants.

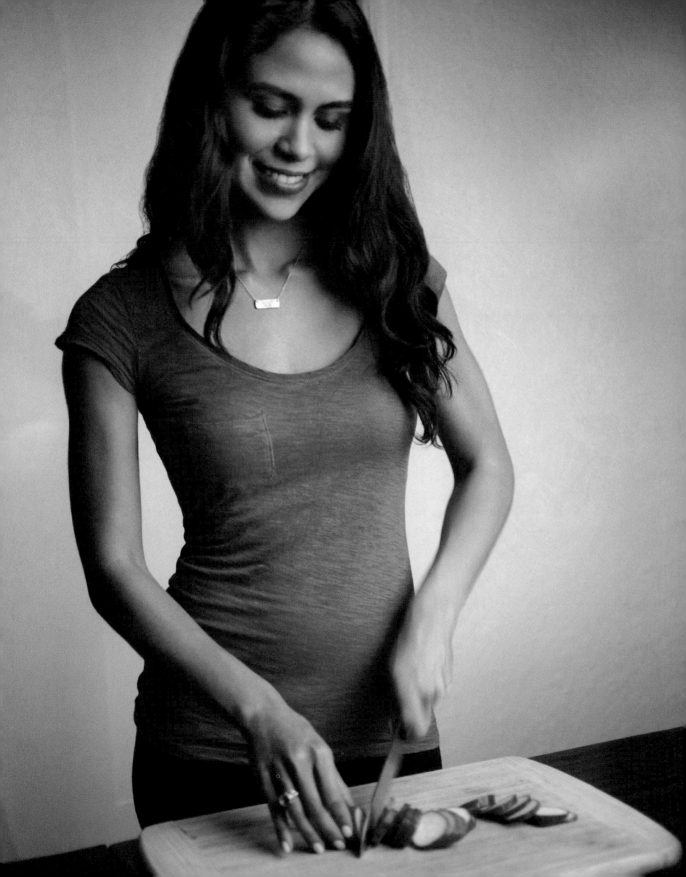

HONEY:

I am fascinated with honey's magical properties, just as I am with bee pollen. Honey has been used for thousands of years in Ayurvedic medicine, and early Roman, Greek, Islamic and Vedic texts have documented its health benefits. Honey is very concentrated and supersweet. It possesses antiseptic and antibacterial qualities, and so it may be useful in treating wounds. It may also help boost your immune system.[2] Choose raw honey, ethically sourced, from a local farmer whenever possible.

SUGAR ALCOHOLS:

Sugar alcohols, such as erythritol and xylitol, are derived from plant foods, such as fruits, and are most often available in a powdered form. I've had clients who used sugar alcohols because they didn't like the taste of stevia. If you're in that boat, be sure to use organic varieties of sugar alcohols, and be wary of using too much xylitol, which can lead to diarrhea. Sugar alcohols should not be substituted for equal amounts of stevia. Check the conversion charts on the products you buy to determine the correct amount of each to use.

VEGAN AND GLUTEN-FREE BAKING STAPLES

It took many trials to perfect recipes such as the crust for John's Crispy Crust Pumpkin Pie, Kimberly's Brownies with Raw Cacao Glaze, as well as the Chocolate Chip Galaxy Pancakes. The key to successful vegan and gluten-free baking lies in the ingredients. Here are a few I rely on and information to keep in mind with my recipes:

GLUTEN-FREE FLOURS:

You'll find brown rice flour, sorghum flour, coconut flour and millet flour in these recipes. Gluten-free flours work better in combination, and there are others beyond the ones I use regularly.

TAPIOCA FLOUR/TAPIOCA STARCH:

Yes, tapioca flour and tapioca starch are the same thing! Tapioca is derived from the South American cassava plant. It acts as a binder in our gluten-free recipes and helps to improve the texture of the baked goodies.

ARROWROOT STARCH:

This can be used as a thickener in sauces, and it is good for baking. It is extracted from the roots of the arrowroot plant, *Maranta arundinacea,* which is native to South America.

ENER-G EGG REPLACER:

Ener-G Egg Replacer mimics what eggs do in traditional baking, and I've found this product extremely helpful. Plus, it lasts for ages. It consists mostly of plant-based tapioca starch and potato starch, and unlike most of the other egg replacers out there, it is gluten-free, soy-free, dairy/casein-free, yeast-free, tree nut-free, peanut-free, and cholesterol-free, and it is low in protein.

GUAR GUM/XANTHAN GUM:

Guar gum and xanthan gum are thickeners and binders, and they need only to be used in very small amounts. Guar gum comes from the endosperm of the seeds of the guar plant, a legume cultivated in East India. Xanthan gum is a plant-based substance that is produced through the fermentation of carbohydrates by the bacterium *Xanthomonas campestris.*

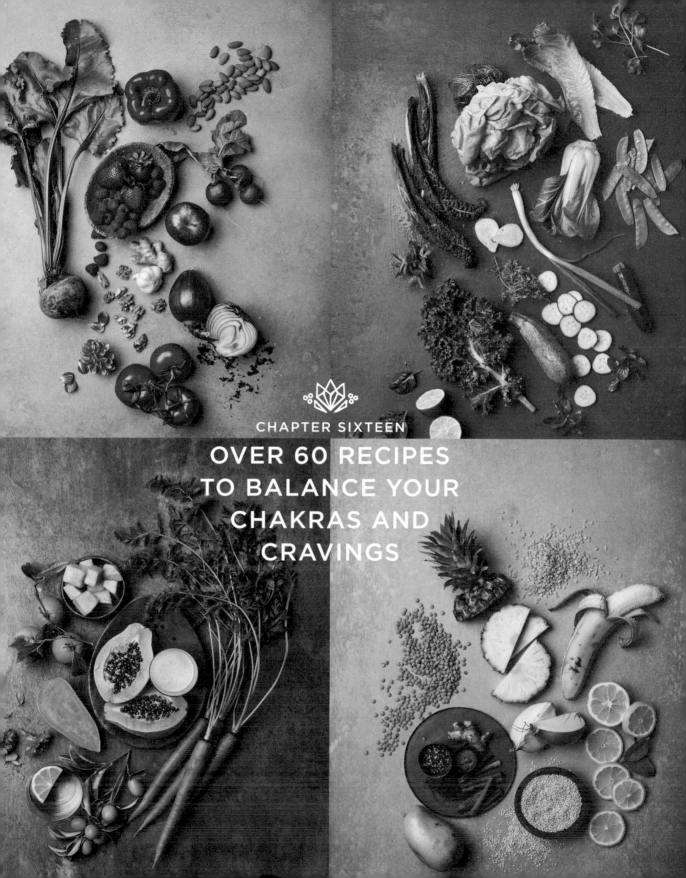

CHAPTER SIXTEEN

OVER 60 RECIPES TO BALANCE YOUR CHAKRAS AND CRAVINGS

CHAKRAS

CRAVINGS

MULADHARA

(RED, EARTH, ROOT)

....

BEET RAVIOLI WITH ROSEMARY NUT CHEESE

....

Yield: About 15 ravioli pieces

Thinly cut beet slices are so pretty. They almost look like jewels. This fun dish works as an appetizer or even as an entrée after a big salad. It's also a big hit at parties, when people discover the ravioli "dough" is actually 100 percent beets! Brilliantly colored red beets help strengthen your connection with nature and your own "roots" in the earth.

INGREDIENTS:

2 medium red beets

¾ cup pine nuts
(or substitute walnuts
or cashews)

2 tablespoons sesame seeds

1 tablespoon freshly
squeezed lemon juice

1 teaspoon minced fresh
rosemary or ⅓ teaspoon
dried rosemary

1 small clove garlic, peeled

¼ teaspoon sea salt

1 cup microgreens or
chopped greens, for
garnishing

DIRECTIONS:

▸ Rinse and peel the beets. Slice them very thinly with a knife or a mandolin and set aside. You should end up with about 30 slices.

▸ Make the Rosemary Nut Cheese by combining in a food processor all the remaining ingredients except for the microgreens and processing until smooth.

▸ Top a reserved beet slice with 2 teaspoons of the Rosemary Nut Cheese, place another beet slice on top, and arrange the ravioli on a large plate. Repeat this process until all the beet slices have been used. Garnish each ravioli with microgreens and serve. Enjoy!

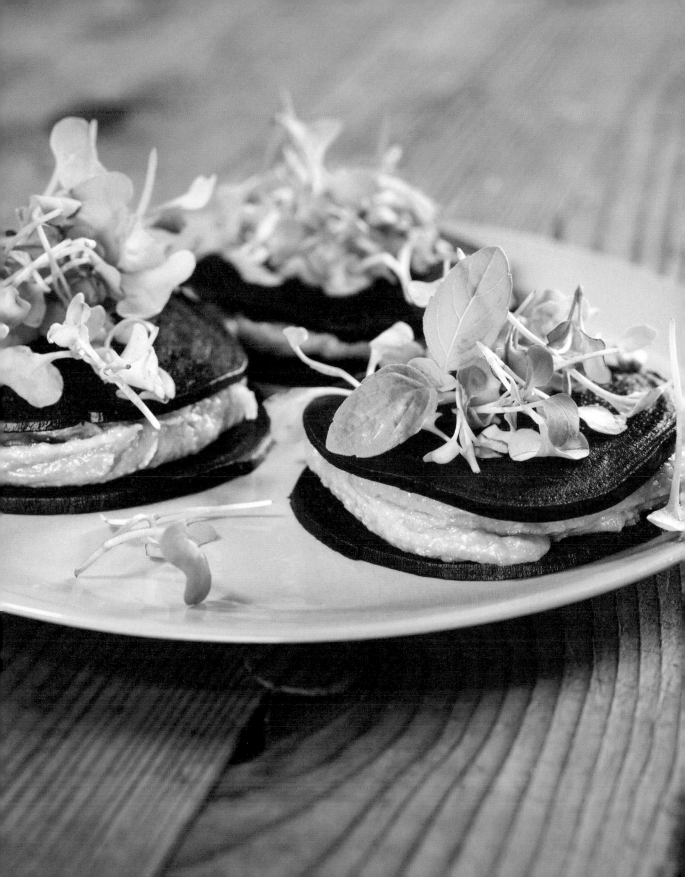

BLISSFUL BURGERS

Yield: 8 burgers

There's been a burger in each Beauty Detox book, and continuing with that tradition, here is our *Beauty Detox Power* burger. It was inspired by my dear friend Ylva, who also happens to be an awesome photographer and shot many of the pictures for this book. She loves beets and requested a veggie burger with beets recipe. So, dear Ylva, here it is!

The deep red color of the beets, grown right in the earth, are a supportive root chakra food to help you feel grounded and safe.

INGREDIENTS:

1 tablespoon coconut oil, plus more for greasing the baking dish

1½ cups filtered water

¾ cup quinoa, soaked overnight and rinsed well

¼ cup minced shallots

1 cup shredded red beets

1 cup shredded carrots

½ cup chopped spinach

1 teaspoon minced fresh thyme

¼ teaspoon red pepper flakes

1 cup shredded zucchini

Sea salt, to taste

Freshly ground pepper, to taste

1 tablespoon Ener-G Egg Replacer mixed with ¼ cup very hot filtered water

1½ cups gluten-free bread crumbs (made from about 6 pieces of toasted gluten-free bread)

DIRECTIONS:

▸ Preheat the oven to 350°F. Grease a baking sheet with coconut oil and set aside.

▸ Heat the water in a medium saucepan over medium-high heat to just under a boil. Add the quinoa, reduce the heat to medium and cook for 12 to 14 minutes, or until the quinoa is tender and no water remains. Set aside.

▸ Meanwhile, heat the 1 tablespoon coconut oil in a large skillet over medium heat. Add the shallots and cook until softened, about 2 minutes. Add the beets, carrots, spinach, thyme and red pepper flakes, and cook until the vegetables are tender, about 5 minutes. Add the zucchini and cook for another 2 minutes.

▸ Remove the skillet from the heat, stir in the cooked quinoa and season with sea salt and pepper. Allow the quinoa mixture to cool completely. Next, stir in the Ener-G Egg Replacer and water mixture and then the bread crumbs, combining well. Cover and refrigerate until the quinoa mixture is cold and firm, about 40 minutes.

▸ Shape the quinoa mixture into eight ½-inch-thick patties, pressing firmly. Arrange the patties on top of the baking sheet and bake them for 40 minutes, flipping them halfway through the baking process to ensure those babies cook evenly!

▸ Serve the Blissful Burgers between slices of gluten-free bread or in buns, for traditional burgers, wrapped in collard green leaves or romaine leaves, for natural wraps, or right on top of a big salad.

NOTE: Freeze extra Blissful Burgers to have on hand for quick meals and to use in the Comfort Chili recipe (page 239).

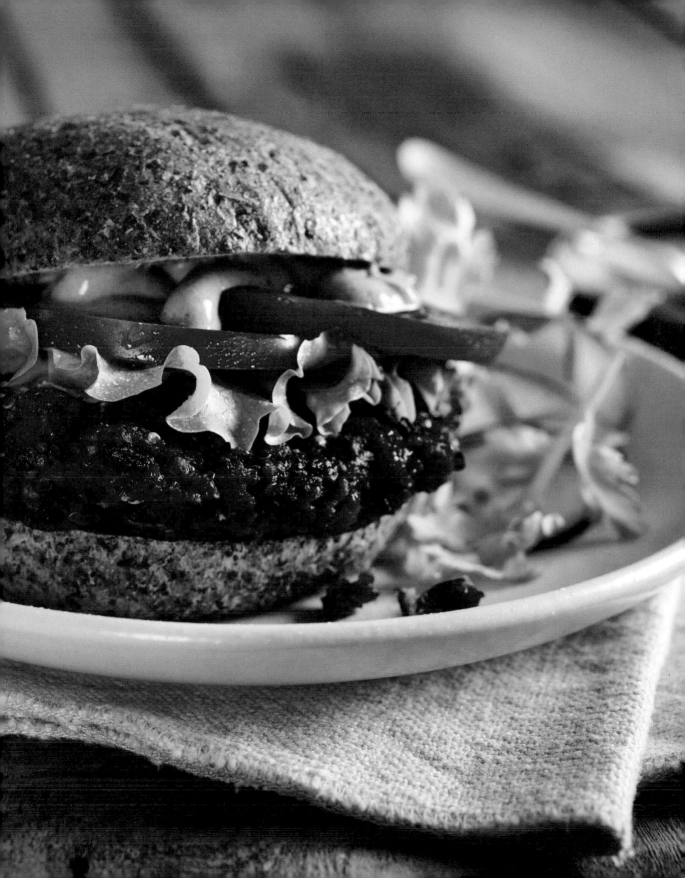

RAW BEET AND JICAMA SLAW WITH LEMON ZEST

Yield: 6 servings

Colors have an effect on your mind and body, as they are vibrations of energy, and this red slaw certainly makes a bold color statement. This salad keeps great in the refrigerator for a few days, so make a batch and enjoy it over several lunches and dinners!

INGREDIENTS:

4 cups julienned raw red beets

2 cups julienned jicama

½ cup minced fresh parsley

¼ cup thinly sliced shallots

3 tablespoons freshly squeezed lemon juice

1½ tablespoons honey (preferably raw) or coconut nectar

½ teaspoon freshly ground black pepper

½ teaspoon sea salt

1½ tablespoons olive oil

Zest of one medium lemon, for garnishing

DIRECTIONS:

▸ Toss the beets, jicama, parsley and shallots in a large mixing bowl to combine.

▸ In a small bowl, whisk together the lemon juice, honey, pepper and sea salt. Add the olive oil and whisk continuously until emulsified.

▸ Add the dressing to the vegetables and toss well. Adjust the sea salt and pepper to taste. Cover the slaw and refrigerate it, allowing it to marinate and soften into perfection, for a few hours or overnight.

▸ Before serving, garnish the slaw with lemon zest. Voilà! Red. Raw. Rooted. I want to hear you Roar!

COMFORT CHILI

Yield: 6 servings

I love a big one-bowl (or two) meal after some salad. One-pot cooking is just so simple yet satisfying. While I was cooking chili for a client, I wanted to add more gusto somehow, so I scanned the fridge and saw that I had some leftover veggie burgers. *Aha!* I chopped them up and threw them in the pot. The chili was a huge hit, and I've been doing it this way ever since. The veggie-burger bits work beautifully, adding great texture and enhancing the taste.

INGREDIENTS:

¼ cup low-sodium vegetable broth, plus 1 cup

1 cup diced white onions

2 medium cloves garlic, peeled and minced

2 cups chopped baby bella (cremini) mushrooms (about 8 ounces)

1 cup sliced carrots

1 cup sliced and halved zucchini

½ cup diced celery

3 cups packaged diced tomatoes (preferably from a carton, not a can)

1 cup diced fresh Roma tomatoes

1 cup cooked kidney beans

2 veggie burger patties (see Note), cut into 1-inch pieces (about 1 cup)

1½ tablespoons chili powder

3 bay leaves

2 teaspoons ground cumin

1½ teaspoons smoked paprika

¼ teaspoon cayenne pepper

Sea salt, to taste

Freshly ground black pepper, to taste

DIRECTIONS:

▸ Heat ¼ cup of the vegetable broth in a large heavy saucepan over medium heat. Add the onions and cook until they become translucent, about 4 to 6 minutes. Add the garlic and cook for another minute.

▸ Add the mushrooms, carrots, zucchini and celery and mix, also stirring in some love and good energy. (You have an unlimited supply, so offer it up freely to your food when you cook!) Next, stir in the remaining 1 cup vegetable broth, both kinds of tomatoes, the beans, veggie burger pieces, chili powder, bay leaves, cumin, paprika and cayenne pepper. Cover, bring the mixture to a boil, and then reduce the heat and simmer, covered, for at least 40 minutes and up to an hour, or until the chili has thickened to your liking.

▸ Season the chili with sea salt and pepper to taste and remove the bay leaves before serving.

NOTE: You can use the Blissful Burgers on page 236, or any type of gluten-free and soy-free veggie burgers in this recipe. Avoid any burgers containing seitan or textured vegetable protein. These contain gluten, are highly processed and are potentially very difficult to digest.

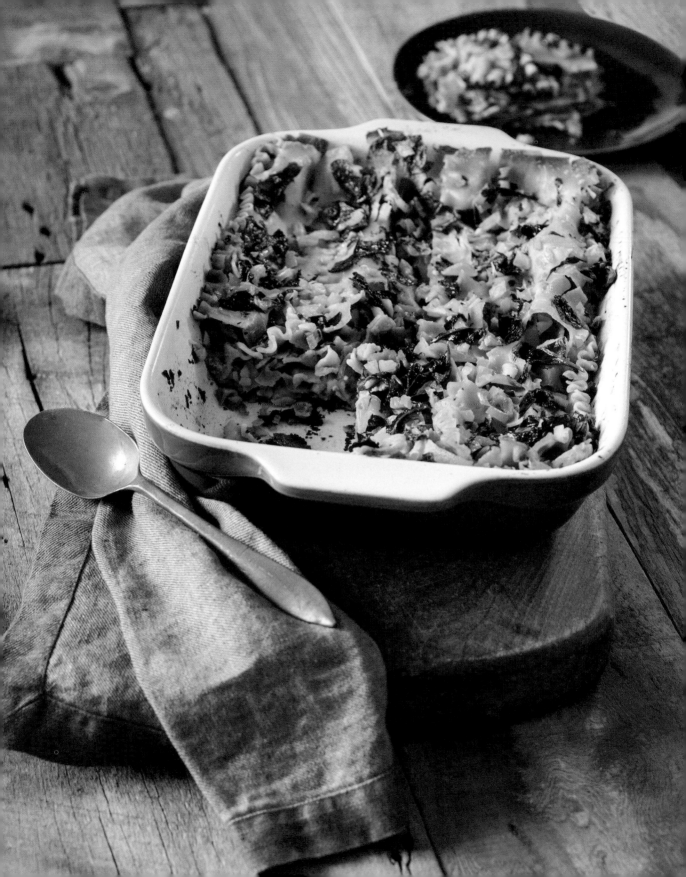

SVADHISTHANA

(ORANGE, WATER, SACRAL)

....

VEGETABLE LASAGNA WITH BUTTERNUT BÉCHAMEL

....

Yield: 6–8 servings

This truly delicious recipe requires a few steps but is well worth it. It's especially popular with my husband, my dad, and male friends because of how hearty it is, so, ladies, if you are looking for something hearty enough for a man, this is your recipe. But, on the other hand, there's definitely no man needed to love this yourself. I love it, as do many of my female friends and clients. You can easily make a batch and freeze individual portions, which you can later thaw and enjoy whenever you want a piece. The butternut squash is a wonderful, creamy base for this beauty-building sauce, which is supportive of your creative chakra.

INGREDIENTS:

Coconut oil, for greasing the baking dish

2½ pounds butternut squash, peeled, seeded and cut into 2-inch cubes (about 5 cups)

14 ounces gluten-free lasagna noodles

⅓ cup low-sodium vegetable broth, plus 1½ cups for the squash

¾ cup diced yellow onions

2 medium cloves garlic, peeled and finely minced

½ pound fresh spinach, stems removed and chopped

1 teaspoon minced fresh thyme

Sea salt, to taste

Freshly ground black pepper, to taste

2½ cups unsweetened coconut milk

⅓ cup nutritional yeast

¼ cup freshly squeezed lemon juice

DIRECTIONS:

▸ Preheat the oven to 375°F. Lightly grease a 9 x 13-inch baking dish with coconut oil. Spread the squash cubes out on the baking dish, and bake for about 45 minutes, or until soft. Remove the squash to a large plate, set it aside to cool and reduce the oven heat to 350°F.

▸ Meanwhile, bring a large pot of lightly salted water to a boil over high heat. Add the lasagna noodles, reduce the heat to medium and cook the noodles as directed on the package. Once cooked, drain the noodles and lay them out on clean kitchen towels to dry. Note that some types of gluten-free pasta do not need to be cooked. They will cook in the oven right along with the other lasagna ingredients.

▸ Heat ⅓ cup of the vegetable broth in a large heavy saucepan over medium-high heat. Add the onions and cook until they become translucent, about 4 to 6 minutes. Add the garlic and cook for another minute. Next, add the spinach and thyme, and cook until the spinach softens, about 2 minutes. Season with sea salt and pepper to taste and set aside.

▸ Transfer the reserved butternut squash to a blender, add the remaining 1½ cups vegetable broth, the coconut milk, nutritional yeast and lemon juice, and blend until smooth. (You may want to blend the ingredients in multiple batches, depending on the size of your blender.) Season the Butternut Béchamel with sea salt and pepper to taste.

▸ To assemble the lasagna, spoon some of the Butternut Béchamel into the bottom of the baking dish used to cook the squash and spread it out to thinly coat the bottom. Add an even layer of the reserved noodles to the baking dish, spoon some Butternut Béchamel on top, and then add an even layer of the reserved spinach mixture. Keep layering until you run out of noodles, sauce and spinach mixture (you should make about 3 layers of each ingredient). Be sure to arrange some of the spinach mixture on the very top to make for a beautiful presentation.

▸ Cover the baking dish with aluminum foil, but don't let it touch the lasagna directly, and bake at 350°F for 40 minutes. Remove the foil and continue to bake for 20 minutes. Remove the lasagna from the oven and let it stand, uncovered, for 10 to 15 minutes before slicing and serving.

SHAKTI POWER SALAD

Yield: 2–4 servings

I don't eat raw broccoli very often, but I love it in this salad. One of the best things about this salad is that the lemon juice "cooks" the veggies and helps them soften overnight, so the salad keeps getting better and better. Because the veggies are raw, they retain their water and are very hydrating, and thus in alignment with the fluid energy of water element–based *Svadhisthana,* or the second chakra. This salad is also packed with fiber, powerful enzymes and vitamins to support the power of Shakti, the ubiquitous cosmic energy dynamically moving through you and the entire universe. Offer this salad to yourself as a way of honoring your creative power!

SALAD INGREDIENTS:

3 cups small broccoli florets

1½ cups shredded carrots

1 cup diced cucumbers

1 tablespoon minced fresh parsley

DRESSING INGREDIENTS:

¼ cup raw tahini

2 tablespoons freshly squeezed lemon juice

1½ tablespoons organic tamari (preferably low sodium)

1 tablespoon Dijon mustard

2 teaspoons coconut nectar or ¼ teaspoon stevia

Freshly ground black pepper, to taste

Sea salt, to taste (optional)

DIRECTIONS:

▸ Toss all the salad ingredients together in a large mixing bowl.

▸ Combine all the dressing ingredients in a small bowl and mix well. Pour the dressing over the salad and toss again so all the veggies are coated.

▸ You *can* eat this salad right away, but I prefer to let the vegetables marinate and soften in the dressing for 3 to 4 hours, or overnight.

ROASTED ROSEMARY AND SCALLION SWEET POTATO WEDGES

Yield: 2–4 servings

I *really* love sweet potatoes, so if you're like me and eat large amounts of them on salads and just plain, this recipe serves two (or just one, over a day or two...maybe!). I find these wedges to be a truly satisfying replacement for French fries. The vibrational bright orange color of sweet potatoes is nourishing to your sacral chakra.

INGREDIENTS:

1½ tablespoons coconut oil, plus more for greasing the baking sheet

1½ pounds sweet potatoes (about 2 medium), peeled and cut lengthwise into ½-inch wedges

½ cup diced scallions

2 teaspoons minced fresh rosemary

1 medium clove garlic, peeled and minced

½ teaspoon sea salt

⅛ teaspoon freshly ground black pepper

DIRECTIONS:

▸ Preheat the oven to 450°F. Grease a baking sheet with coconut oil.

▸ Combine all the ingredients in a large bowl and toss the sweet potato wedges well to coat.

▸ Arrange the sweet potato wedges on the prepared baking sheet in a single layer. Bake for 15 minutes, then turn and bake for another 15 minutes, or until the wedges are soft on the inside and lightly browned on the outside. (Your kitchen is going to smell divine!) Serve at once.

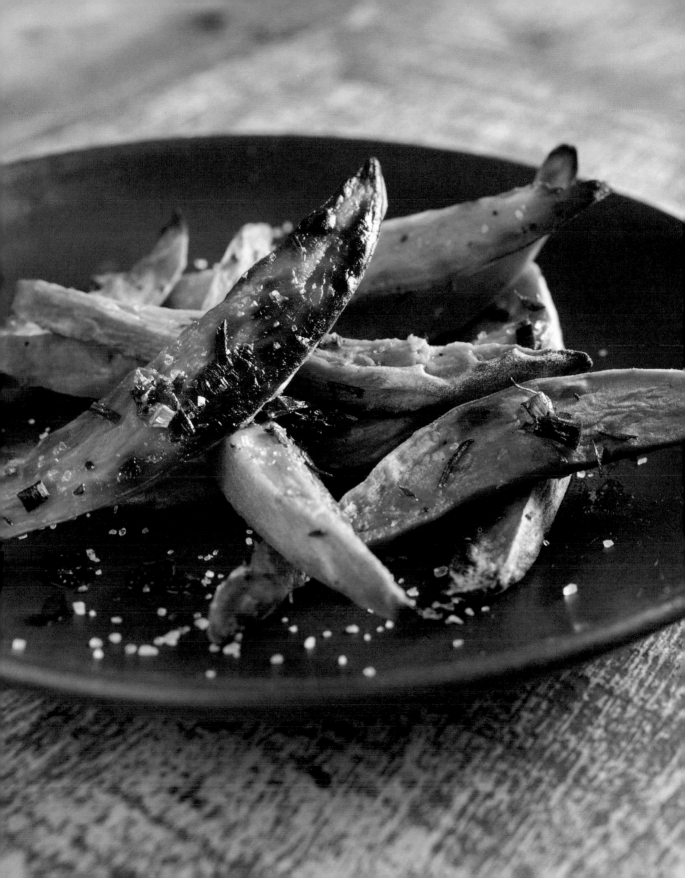

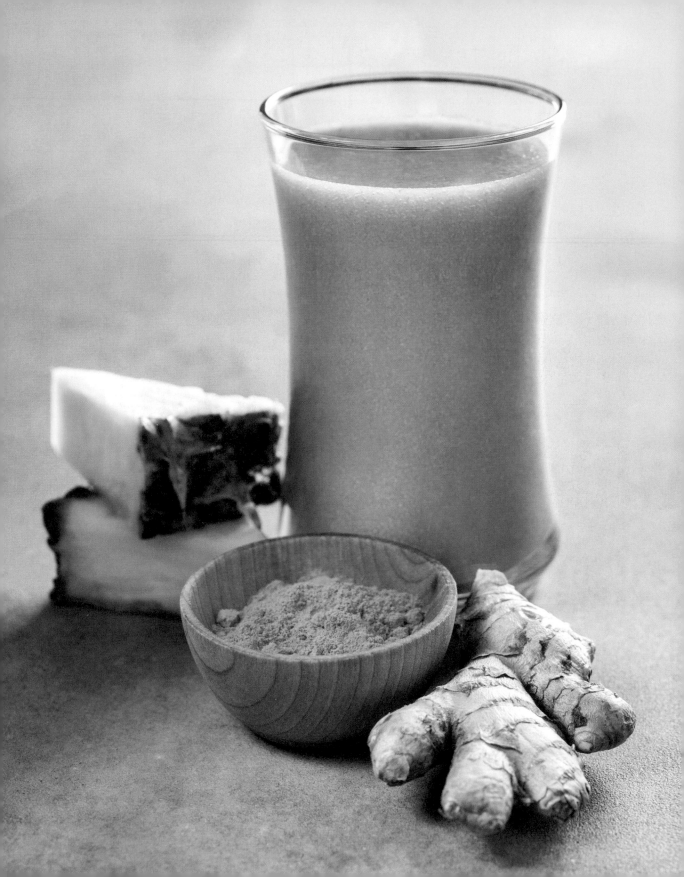

ZANZIBAR SHAKE

Yield: One 16-ounce serving

This shake was inspired by my adventures in Zanzibar, an island off the coast of Tanzania. Zanzibar is not only abundant in juicy tropical fruit, but it also has a vibrant spice market, called Stone Town, where I saw bins of fresh ginger and turmeric. Though the color of this shake is really more yellow than orange, I wanted to share it in the *Svadhisthana* chakra section because of its water-based properties.

INGREDIENTS:

1 cup chopped ripe, fresh pineapple (frozen works, too)

1 cup chopped ripe, fresh banana (frozen works, too; see Note)

1 cup cold coconut water

1 teaspoon minced fresh ginger

⅛ teaspoon ground turmeric (or a pinch of grated fresh turmeric)

DIRECTIONS:

▶ Combine all the ingredients in a blender and blend until smooth.

▶ While blending, take a deep breath in and then breathe out any tension, relaxing as you would on a tropical island, to resonate with the chilled-out energy of the locale in which these ingredients are grown and to feel the full effects. *Hakuna matata!* (No worries!)

▶ Serve the shake at once.

NOTE: Frozen bananas add even more creaminess to this shake. This is another great reason to peel and freeze your ripe bananas!

SUNSHINE PÂTÉ LETTUCE WRAPS

Yield: 8 wraps, or 1 ¼ cups pâté

You'll see why I named this recipe Sunshine Pâté Lettuce Wraps when you make it for yourself. The combination of the bright orange carrots—so nourishing to the water-based sacral chakra—perky garden mint, lemon juice and pumpkin seeds will lift your energy like early morning sunlight meeting your skin for the first time that day. This is a bright and "happy" pâté. You can wrap it in lettuce leaves, as I suggest, toss it in a salad, use it as a chunky veggie dip, or wrap it in nori wrappers.... The possibilities are endless. It's a great afternoon snack or lunch during the work week, or enjoy it whenever you need some more sunshine in your life!

INGREDIENTS:

1 cup raw pumpkin seeds

1 medium carrot, peeled and coarsely chopped (about ⅔ cup)

⅓ cup filtered water

2 medium Medjool pitted dates

¼ cup freshly squeezed lemon juice

2 tablespoons minced fresh mint

1½ tablespoons organic tamari (preferably low sodium)

¼ teaspoon sea salt

8 butter lettuce leaves or romaine leaf halves

DIRECTIONS:

▸ Combine all the ingredients except for the lettuce leaves in a food processor and pulse until smooth.

▸ Arrange a lettuce leaf on a plate. Spoon about 2½ tablespoons of the pâté on the center of the lettuce leaf and then roll up the leaf. Arrange the lettuce wrap on another plate. Repeat this process until all the lettuce leaves are rolled. Serve the lettuce wraps at once.

▸ The pâté will keep, covered, in the fridge for up to 4 days, so you can make it ahead and assemble the wraps at your convenience.

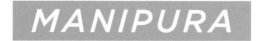

MANIPURA

(YELLOW, FIRE, SOLAR PLEXUS)

YELLOW PEPPER- AND CAPER-STUFFED PORTOBELLO MUSHROOMS

Yield: 6 stuffed portobello mushrooms

This recipe has a decent number of ingredients, but it's totally worth it, because it results in a decadent dish that is almost like a mushroom pie (with the mushrooms as the crust, that is!). The turmeric deepens the yellow color, which resonates with the vibration of your *Manipura* chakra, and its warming properties will stoke your digestive fire.

MARINADE INGREDIENTS:

½ cup organic tamari (preferably low sodium)

½ cup filtered water

¼ cup freshly squeezed lemon juice

1 tablespoon coconut nectar or maple syrup

1 teaspoon lemon pepper seasoning

1 small clove garlic, peeled and finely minced, plus 2 small cloves garlic, peeled and finely minced

MUSHROOM INGREDIENTS:

6 medium portobello mushrooms (stems removed)

1½ medium yellow bell peppers

½ cup unsweetened coconut milk

2 tablespoons nutritional yeast

½ teaspoon ground turmeric

1 tablespoon coconut oil

¼ cup diced white onions

2 tablespoons capers

2 tablespoons minced fresh parsley

1 teaspoon minced fresh rosemary

1½ cups gluten-free bread crumbs (made from about 6 pieces of lightly toasted millet or brown rice bread)

Sea salt, to taste

Freshly ground black pepper, to taste

DIRECTIONS:

▸ Prepare the marinade. Whisk together the tamari, water, lemon juice, coconut nectar, lemon pepper seasoning and 1 of the garlic cloves in a large bowl. Set the marinade aside.

▸ Arrange the portobello mushrooms in an ovenproof 9 x 13-inch baking dish, the undersurface of the caps (the gills) facing up. Spoon the reserved marinade over the mushrooms, allowing it to collect in the middle of them.

▸ Cover the baking dish and marinate the mushrooms in the refrigerator for at least an hour. I usually let them marinate for a few hours, during which time I prepare other dishes or exit the kitchen for a little while!

▸ Meanwhile, combine the yellow peppers, coconut milk, yeast and turmeric in a food processor (or blender) and blend until there are no lumps, but do not allow the mixture to become supersmooth. Set the yellow pepper mixture aside.

▸ Heat the coconut oil in a large skillet over medium heat. Add the onions and sauté for 3 or 4 minutes, stirring frequently. Next, add in 2 remaining cloves of garlic and cook for 1 more minute, then stir in the capers, parsley and rosemary. Remove the skillet from the heat and stir in the reserved yellow pepper mixture. Then add the bread crumbs, sea salt and pepper to taste, and mix well. Set the stuffing aside. (Transfer the stuffing to a medium bowl and refrigerate it if the mushrooms have not finished marinating and need more than 20 minutes.)

▸ Preheat the oven to 350°F about 10 minutes before the mushrooms finish marinating. Remove the marinated mushrooms from the refrigerator and spoon the stuffing into each. Cover the baking dish containing the stuffed mushrooms with the aluminum foil, making sure the foil does not touch the mushrooms, and bake for 30 minutes. Remove foil and bake for another 10 minutes.

▸ Serve the stuffed mushrooms fresh out of the oven with a big salad.

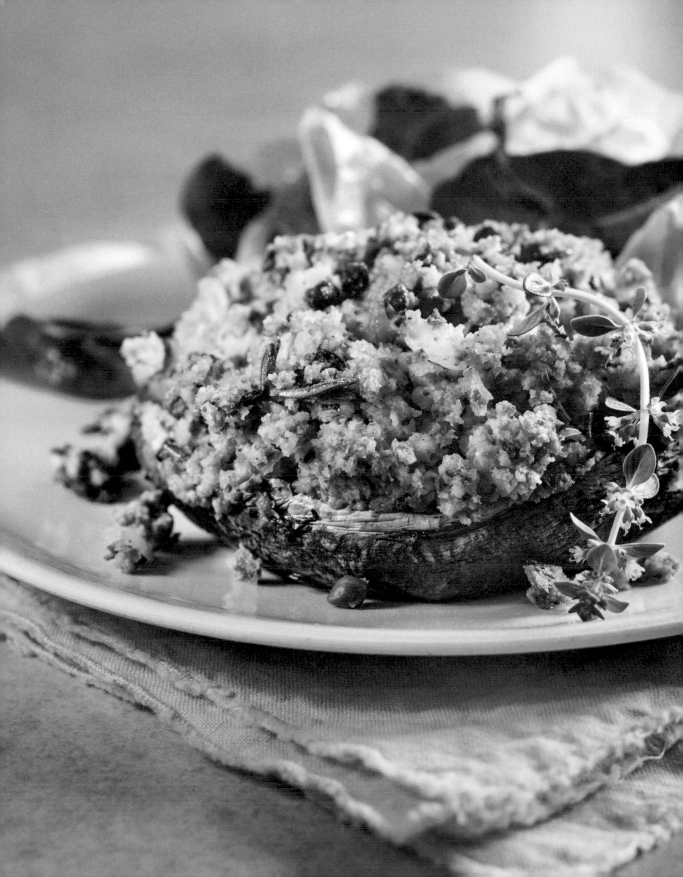

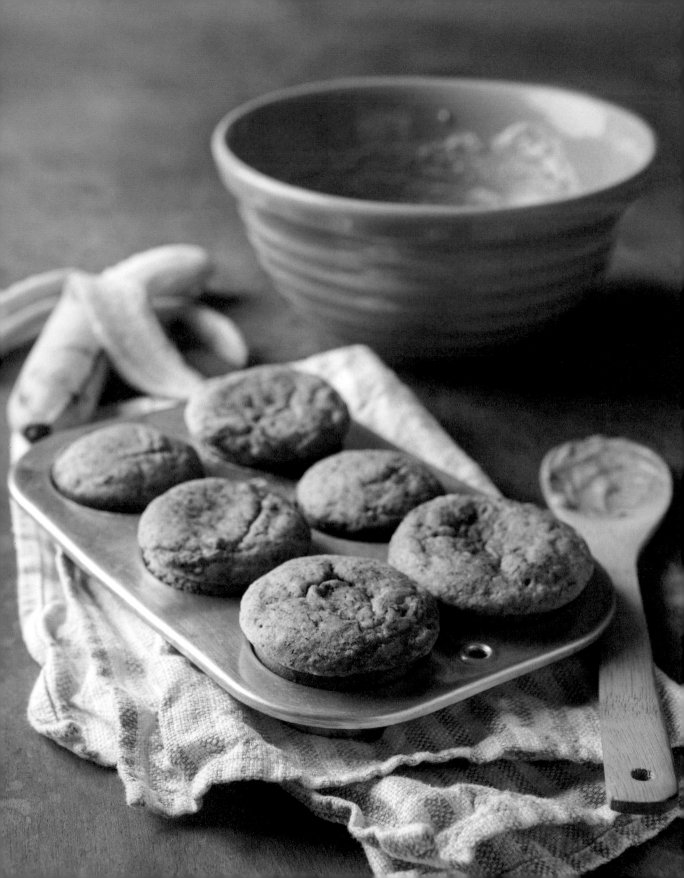

GLUTEN-FREE BANANA MUFFINS

Yield: 12 muffins

These are a moist and delicious version of the often oily, gluten-filled classic banana muffin. The flours in this muffin might be new to you, but once you try them, I don't think you'll miss any of the old ingredients. Use your arm power to mash those bananas and mix the batter. It will make that first luscious bite of muffin even more rewarding!

INGREDIENTS:

2 tablespoons coconut oil, plus more for greasing the muffin tin

¾ cup brown rice flour

½ cup sorghum flour

¼ cup tapioca flour

1 teaspoon baking powder

½ teaspoon sea salt

1 cup unsweetened coconut or almond milk

2 teaspoons vanilla extract

1 teaspoon raw apple cider vinegar

¼ cup coconut nectar or maple syrup

½ tablespoon Ener-G Egg Replacer mixed with 2 tablespoons hot filtered water

3 large ripe bananas, peeled and mashed

DIRECTIONS:

▸ Preheat the oven to 350°F. Grease the wells of a 12-cup muffin tin with coconut oil.

▸ Sift together the brown rice flour, sorghum flour, tapioca flour, baking powder and sea salt in a large mixing bowl. In a small bowl, whisk together the coconut milk, vanilla extract and the apple cider vinegar.

▸ Fold the coconut milk–vinegar mixture into the flour mixture. Next, stir in the coconut nectar, the remaining 2 tablespoons coconut oil, and the Ener-G Egg Replacer and water mixture. Then add the mashed bananas, and mix well so there are no lumps.

▸ Spoon the batter into the wells of the prepared muffin tin, filling them nearly to the top, as these gluten-free, vegan muffins aren't going to swell up like conventional muffins do. In other words, what you see is what you'll get.

▸ Bake the muffins for about 25 minutes, or until the tops are golden brown and a fork comes out dry when you prick the center of a muffin with it. After removing the muffins from the oven, allow them to set for 10 minutes before removing them from the muffin tin. Serve the muffins at once or refrigerate them for up to 3 days.

OIL-FREE RADIANCE DRESSING

Yield: About ¾ cup

There is something magical about lemons, which we may take for granted because they are so "common." But take a fresh look. Just holding them in your hands can brighten your day! They are truly a beauty gift from nature, and in this dressing we take in the lemon's radiance not only from the juice, but from the beautiful and nutritious peel, as well. Packed with vitamin C and enzymes, lemons are a brilliant yellow that vibrates with the energy of your third chakra.

INGREDIENTS:

½ cup filtered water

⅓ cup coarsely chopped Hass avocado

3 tablespoons freshly squeezed lemon juice

1 tablespoon coconut nectar or honey (preferably raw) or ¼ teaspoon stevia

1 small clove garlic, peeled

¾ teaspoon sea salt (or to taste)

½ teaspoon lemon zest

DIRECTIONS:

▸ Add all the ingredients to a blender and blend until smooth. This dressing will keep in the fridge, covered, for 2 to 3 days.

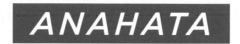

ANAHATA

(GREEN, AIR, HEART)

GLOWING GREEN SMOOTHIE (GGS)

Yield: About 60 ounces

This beloved GGS recipe is at the heart of the Beauty Detox program. I hope that you embrace it and make it part of your everyday beauty, health, energy and natural weight-control regimen for life. Greens nourish your entire body and have so many life-enhancing qualities and nutrients, and they will also help nourish your *Anahata* heart chakra.

I generally recommend starting out by consuming around sixteen ounces of the Glowing Green Smoothie daily and then working up to twenty-four ounces or more (depending on your size, appetite, metabolism and activity level). I personally drink around twenty-four to thirty-two ounces throughout the morning, along with eating some fruit. Use the best blender you can to ensure that your GGS is nice and smooth. The Vitamix is my absolute favorite blender—it is so powerful, helping you derive the most nutrition out of your food, makes the GGS in only a few minutes and is really easy to clean, which is important when you make this smoothie a part of your regular daily routine.

Making a full blender of GGS, as in this recipe, means you can share it with your family or roommates, or you can store it in the fridge and drink some in the afternoon or over the course of the next day or two. It can be stored, covered, for up to three days. Just be sure to give it a stir, shake, or reblend before serving, as it may settle. You can also freeze individual portions and thaw them out the night before.

NOTE: I encourage you to rotate your greens and fruit regularly, based on what looks good at the market. Vary this recipe by using kale, chard or arugula or other greens in place of the spinach and romaine, and pineapple, mangoes or other fruits in place of the apple, pear and banana. Just avoid melons, as they are a type of fruit that digests better on its own.

INGREDIENTS:

7 cups chopped spinach (about a medium bunch)

6 cups chopped romaine lettuce (about 1 small head)

2 cups cold filtered water

1½ cups chopped celery (about 2 medium stalks)

1 medium apple, cored and coarsely chopped

1 medium pear, cored and coarsely chopped

1 medium banana, peeled and cut in thirds

2 tablespoons freshly squeezed lemon juice

OPTIONAL INGREDIENTS:

½ cup minced fresh cilantro (stems are okay)

½ cup minced fresh parsley (stems are okay)

Ice cubes (if you prefer beverages on the colder side, but add only as many as you need)

DIRECTIONS:

▸ Combine the spinach, romaine and water in a blender and begin processing on low. Gradually move to higher speeds and blend until smooth.

▸ Next, add the celery, apple, and pear, and the cilantro and parsley (if using). Lastly, add the banana, lemon juice and ice (if using), and blend until smooth. Serve at once or refrigerate, covered, for up to 3 days.

▸ Congratulate yourself for doing something life changing and incredibly positive for yourself on all levels. Awesome for you!

NOTE: The reason I encourage blending the greens first is to ensure they have the most time to break down in the blender. The fruit is made of simple sugars and water and doesn't need to be blended as long.

GLOWING GREEN SMOOTHIE, SINGLE SERVING

Yield: About 24 ounces

If you don't want to make a whole pitcher of the Glowing Green Smoothie and just want to make enough for yourself, try this recipe! Sip this throughout the morning, or have a second serving in the afternoon.

Because I always encourage you to mix and match your veggies and fruit, you'll find that this recipe is slightly different from the single-serving version in *The Beauty Detox Foods*. This is just to give you another idea about how to switch things up.

INGREDIENTS:

2 cups chopped spinach
or kale

1 cup chopped romaine
lettuce

1 cup cold filtered water

1 small pear (or ½ large
pear), cored and coarsely
chopped

½ medium banana, peeled
and cut in thirds

1 tablespoon freshly
squeezed lemon juice

DIRECTIONS:

▸ Combine the spinach, lettuce and water in a blender
and begin processing on low. Gradually move to
higher speeds and blend until smooth.

▸ Next, add the pear, banana and lemon juice and
blend until smooth. Serve at once or refrigerate
for up to 3 days.

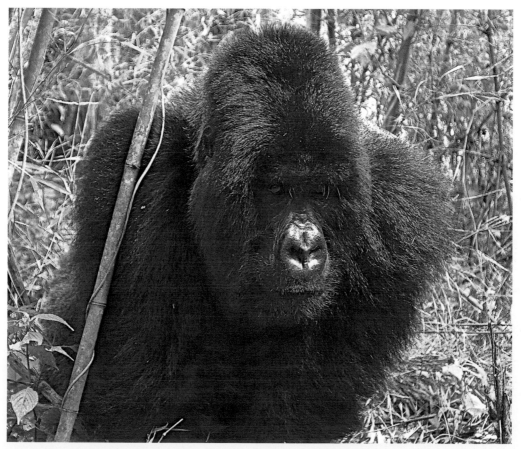

Here is one of the magnificent and strong silverbacks, who are natural plant eaters, we
encountered (in a very up close and personal way) during our gorilla trek in Rwanda. The
Glowing Green Smoothie will help make you strong, like a gorilla.

THE GORILLA BOWL

Yield: 2 servings

I've always been a gorilla fan, but after my gorilla trek on foot with a guide and a tracker in the volcanic jungles of northern Rwanda, I became a full-on gorilla lover. The wild gorilla troop we spent time with in Rwanda was so playful, and though the trackers urged us to keep a distance of some meters away, a juvenile ran up to me and mischievously tapped me on the shoulder, and a silverback charged John and playfully hit him on the back, then twisted his shirt into a ball with his very humanlike hand!

The green, heart-nourishing bok choy and the pea shoots in this recipe resemble the kinds of plants I saw the gorillas eating on that adventure. Millet is a grain grown in parts of East Africa, relatively near to where the gorillas live. Enjoy this meal gorilla-style by eating slowly and chewing very thoroughly!

INGREDIENTS:

1¼ cups filtered water

½ cup dried millet, soaked overnight and rinsed well

1 tablespoon coconut oil

⅔ cup sliced scallions (the white part, but some green is okay)

2 medium cloves garlic, peeled and minced

1 pound bok choy (1 large bunch), trimmed and cut into bite-size pieces

1 tablespoon organic tamari (preferably low sodium)

2 teaspoons raw apple cider vinegar or rice vinegar

¼ teaspoon crushed red pepper (or to taste)

¼ teaspoon sea salt (or to taste)

2 teaspoons sesame oil

2 cups pea shoots or more bok choy

DIRECTIONS:

▸ Bring the water to a boil in a large pot over medium-high heat. Add the millet, reduce the heat to medium and cook, covered, for about 15 minutes.

▸ Meanwhile, heat the coconut oil in a large skillet over medium-high heat. Add the scallions and sauté for about 1 minute. Stir in the garlic and cook for another minute.

▸ Next, add the bok choy, tamari, vinegar, crushed red pepper and sea salt, and cook, stirring, for about 2 minutes. Add the cooked millet to the skillet and stir until it is incorporated.

▸ Remove the skillet from the heat. Stir in the sesame oil, combining well, and then fold in the pea shoots. Serve at once.

NOTE: Pea shoots are available at farmers' markets and some natural-food stores.

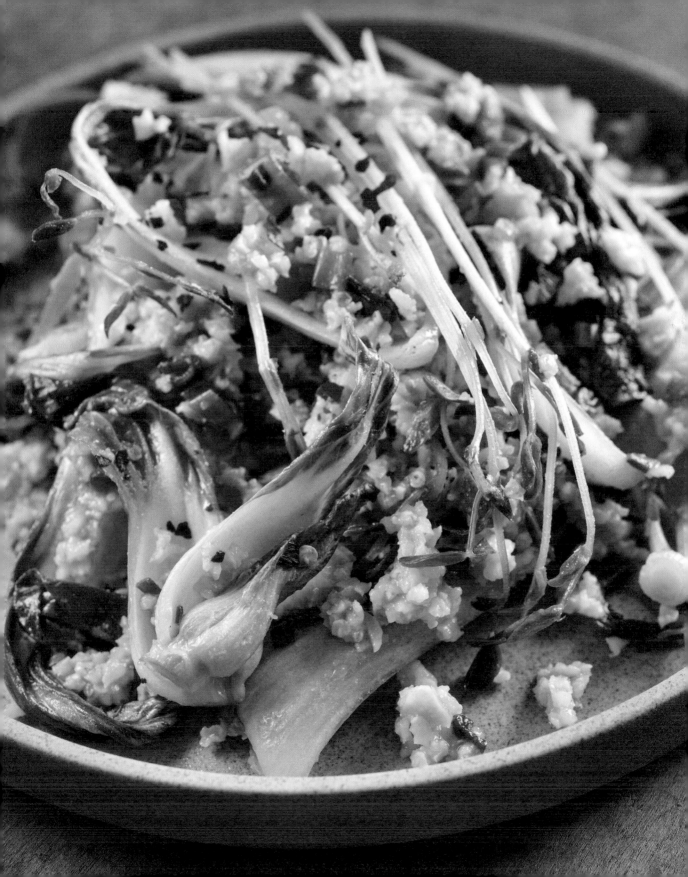

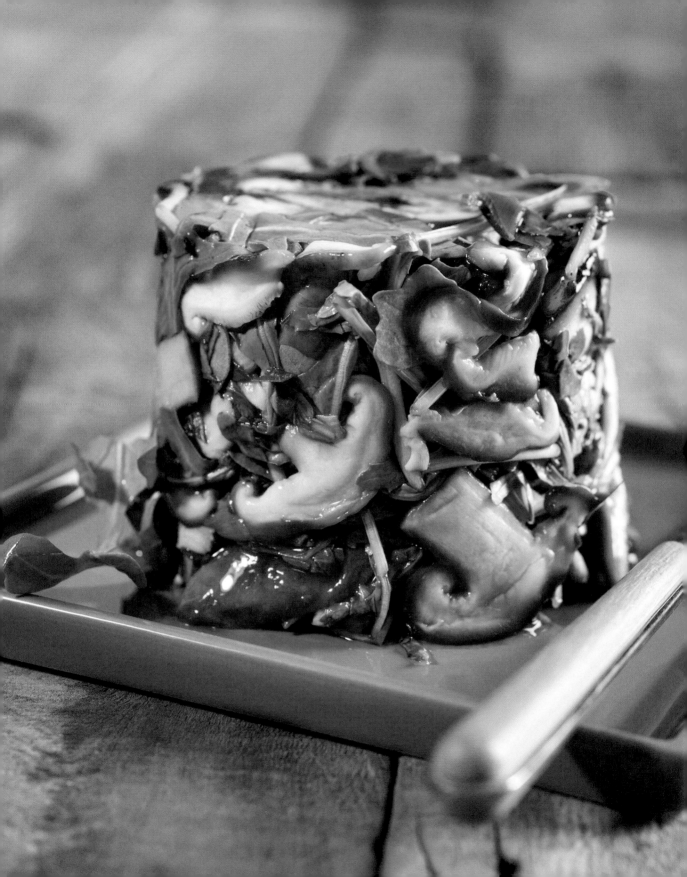

SPINACH AND SHIITAKE MUSHROOM COMPRESSED SALAD

Yield: 2–4 servings

I usually make huge green salads that are free in their leafy, wild wonderfulness. But sometimes shaped, compressed salads are also fun, as they burst open on the plate, from containment to freedom, the minute you reach in and touch them. Just like our hearts.

INGREDIENTS:

1 tablespoon coconut oil

1 cup diced scallions

6 cups sliced shiitake mushrooms (or substitute cremini)

1 cup sliced bok choy

2 tablespoons freshly squeezed lemon juice, plus 1 tablespoon for the arugula

2 tablespoons organic tamari (preferably low sodium)

6 cups arugula (preferably wild, available at farmers' markets and some natural-food stores)

Sea salt, to taste

DIRECTIONS:

▸ Heat the coconut oil in a large pot over medium-high heat. Add the scallions and sauté for 2 to 3 minutes, or until softened.

▸ Add the shiitake mushrooms, bok choy, the 2 tablespoons lemon juice, and tamari, and cook, stirring occasionally, for about 5 minutes, or until the mushrooms have softened. Drain the mushroom mixture in a colander and set aside.

▸ Place the arugula into a large bowl and toss with sea salt and the remaining 1 tablespoon lemon juice. Fold in the mushroom mixture.

▸ Next, pack the salad tightly into 2 medium bowls or 4 small bowls (or into square molds) with a spoon or your knuckles. Cover each bowl with a plate and invert each. Serve the salads at once.

NOTE: If the salads fall apart on the way to the table, it's totally okay. Think of it like a Jackson Pollock painting. Art doesn't have to be "perfect," right? And neither does food. It will be still be delicious, no matter how it looks in the end.

THE CEDRIC SMOOTHIE

Yield: One 16-ounce serving

This smoothie was named for and inspired by the sweetest little boy in Rwanda. He had been abandoned, and was malnourished before being adopted by a member of our nonprofit partner, Gardens for Health International (GHI, www.gardensforhealth.org).

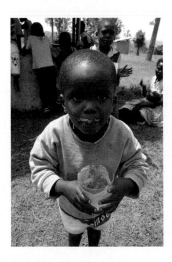

Now he is thriving! GHI has a beautiful farm where they test the best seeds to give to mothers so that they can cultivate their own vegetable gardens for their families, as well as grow vegetables and fruits to sustain a daily community lunch program that feeds over fifty people. GHI members also make a version of this smoothie every day for all the village children. Because malnourishment is a big issue in Rwanda, avocado is added to the children's smoothies for extra sustenance, as in this recipe.

The innocent love of these children, who truly adore their green smoothies, and green kale and avocado, which resonate so beautifully with your heart, make this a powerful, heart-supporting recipe. Since this smoothie has fat, it's a good one to try in the afternoon, as a snack, or when you need a quick, light lunch to keep going. I advise you to forgo this smoothie in the morning and stick with the classic Glowing Green Smoothie recipe.

Please send some love to Cedric and Rwanda, and into the world in general, as you drink this! It will make this smoothie all the more delicious.

INGREDIENTS:

1½ cups chopped, ripe mango (frozen works, too)

1 cup chopped curly or Lacinato kale

1 cup coconut water

¼ cup cubed Hass avocado

1 tablespoon freshly squeezed lime juice

DIRECTIONS:

▸ Combine all the ingredients in a blender and blend until smooth. Serve chilled.

▸ Be sure to sip the smoothie slowly (rather than chugging it), and chew a little as you do to mix the ingredients with the digestive enzymes in your mouth and thus promote better digestion.

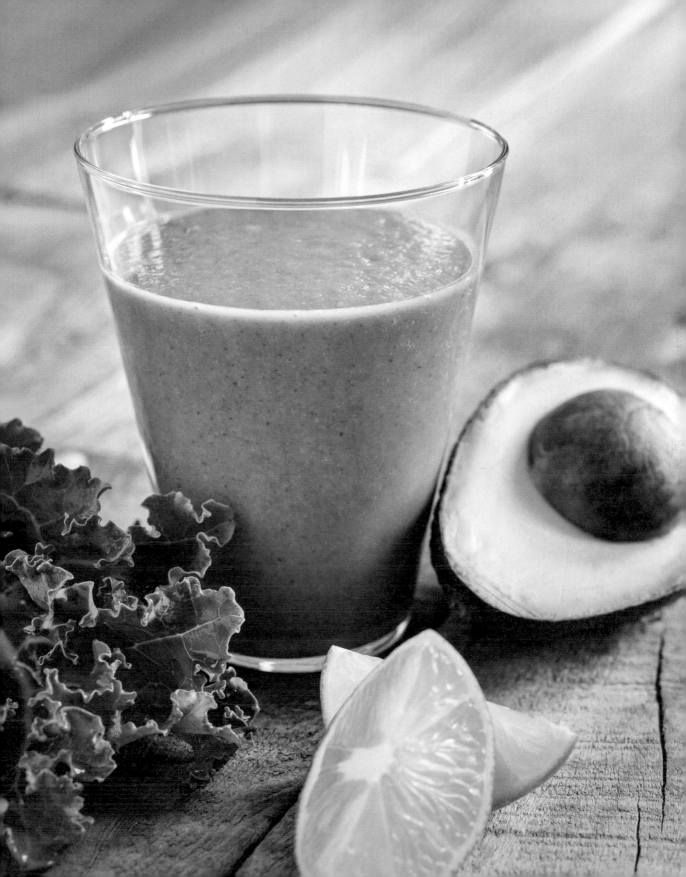

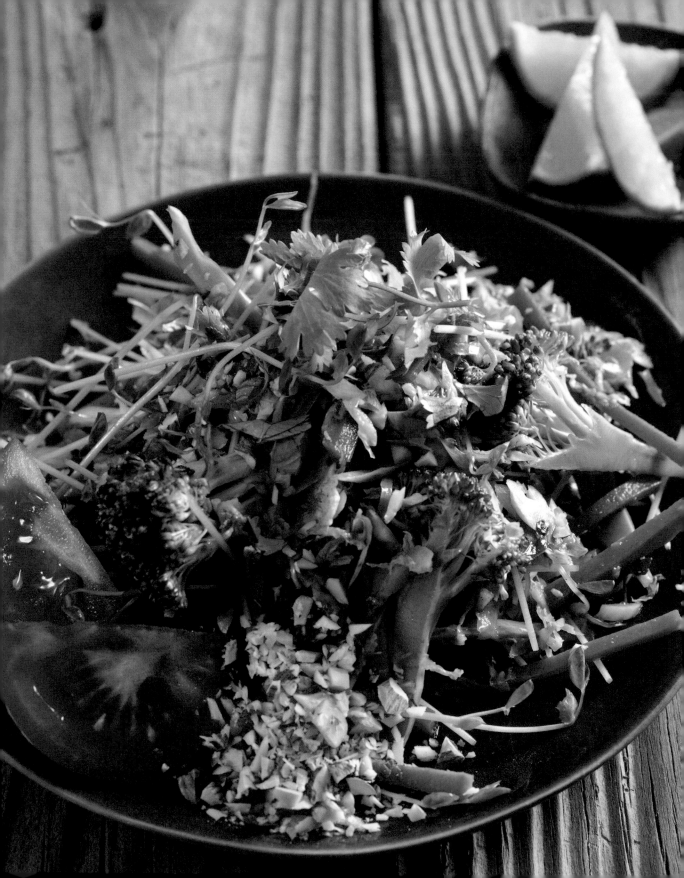

BRUSSELS SPROUTS "NOODLE" PAD THAI

Yield: 3–4 servings

Pad thai has been a favorite dish of mine ever since I started traveling to Thailand and buying it from street vendors for less than fifty cents a dish. It's also a favorite with clients, who tell me they love to order it for take-home delivery for quick dinners.

I decided to try a totally different way of making it, one that is veggie based. I replaced the traditional rice noodles with heart-supporting, mineral- and nutrient-rich brussels sprouts, which have a somewhat similar texture. Adding the carrots right at the beginning draws out their savory, earthy flavor, and this flavor emulates the fish sauce in traditional pad thai.

INGREDIENTS:

1 tablespoon coconut oil

¼ cup diced carrots

¼ cup diced tomatoes

¼ cup diced white onions

1 large clove garlic, peeled and minced

1 pound brussels sprouts, cored and shredded

¼ cup filtered water, plus more as needed to keep the veggies from sticking

1½ cups mung bean sprouts

3 tablespoons organic tamari (preferably low sodium)

1½ tablespoons coconut nectar or maple syrup

2 tablespoons freshly squeezed lime juice

1 teaspoon chili flakes (or to taste, depending on your spice quotient!)

TOPPINGS:

3 or 4 tomato wedges

3 or 4 lime wedges

⅓ cup minced scallions (green part only)

⅓ cup minced fresh cilantro

⅓ cup crushed almonds

DIRECTIONS:

▶ Heat a wok or a large saucepan over high heat. Add the coconut oil and allow it to get hot. Add the carrots, tomatoes, onions and garlic, and sauté, stirring well, for 1 minute.

▶ Add the brussels sprouts and water, and cook, stirring, for 4 to 5 minutes, or until the brussels sprouts start to soften. Add the mung bean sprouts, tamari and coconut nectar, and cook for an additional 2 minutes, adding a little more water, if necessary, to keep the veggies from sticking. Turn off the heat. Stir in the lime juice and the chili flakes.

▶ Arrange the pad thai on individual plates and top each with a tomato wedge, a lime wedge, scallions, cilantro and crushed almonds. Express your creativity by arranging the toppings according to *your* style to make the plates uniquely beautiful. Enjoy at once!

SHIVA'S KALE SALAD WITH ALMOND-GINGER DRESSING

Yield: 4 servings, or ²/₃ cup dressing

I've been making and promoting the popular Dharma's Kale Salad recipe in *The Beauty Detox Solution* for years. Here is another favorite kale salad of mine. In Hinduism, Lord Shiva represents the "Supreme Self," the formless, infinite soul seated within the innermost chamber of each of our hearts, a soul that is already perfect, as it is one with the whole. Shiva Rea is also the name of an inspiring yogini who is in touch with her true power.

Kale, ginger, almond butter from pressed almonds—all these foods are amid the bounty of nature that is provided for us. All we have to do is partake of these natural, perfect foods to feel more connected to our oneness with nature.

SALAD INGREDIENTS:

½ pound curly or lacinato kale (1 large bunch or 2 smaller bunches), torn into bite-size pieces

½ cup thinly sliced red onions

DRESSING INGREDIENTS:

⅓ cup filtered water

3 tablespoons almond butter (preferably raw)

1½ tablespoons organic miso paste (preferably mellow white)

1½ tablespoons freshly squeezed lime juice

1 tablespoon honey (preferably raw), coconut nectar or maple syrup or ½ teaspoon stevia

2 teaspoons sesame oil

½ teaspoon minced fresh ginger

Sea salt, to taste (optional)

DIRECTIONS:

▸ Toss together the kale and the onions in a large salad bowl and set aside.

▸ Combine all the dressing ingredients in a blender and process until smooth. Pour the dressing over the reserved kale salad and toss it well to coat. Next, add in your love and good energy for those about to eat your salad. Serve the salad at once.

NOTE: Feel free to add to this salad any other veggies you like, such as a generous amount of sprouts, as I usually do.

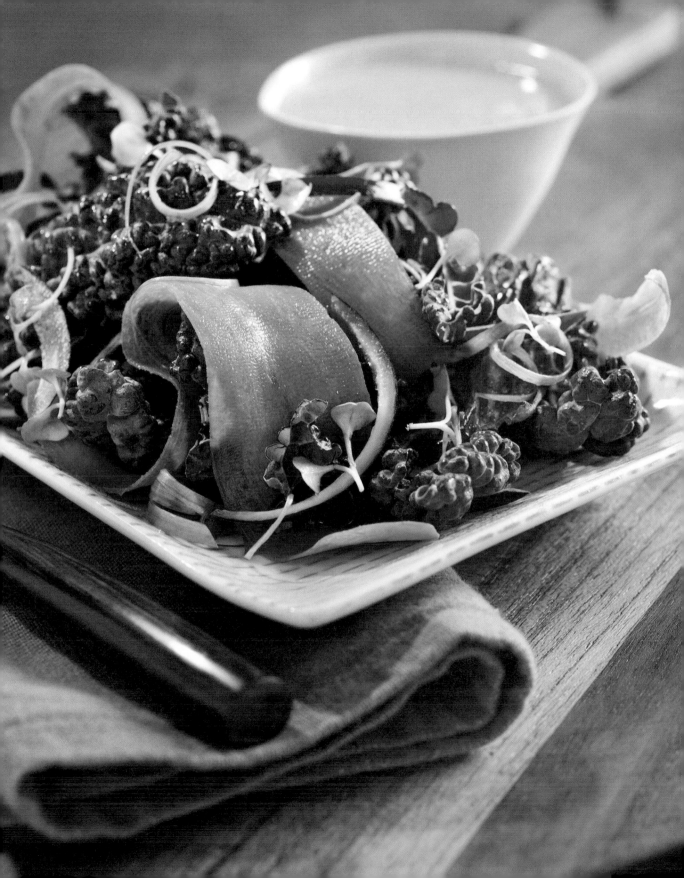

VISHUDDHA

(BLUE, ETHER/SPACE, THROAT)

....

TURKISH VEGETABLE STEW

....

Yield: 4 servings

There is something mystical about Turkey and the surrounding land. This is where one of my favorite poets, Rumi, spent a lot of time. I witnessed the Whirling Dervishes in person in that part of the world, and it was a mysterious and wondrous experience, one I'll never forget. When I was there, I also adored the fact that there were vegetarian dishes on every menu. This stew is an homage to the fabulous veggie creations from that region.

INGREDIENTS:

1½ tablespoons coconut oil

½ medium white onion, peeled and sliced thin

2 medium cloves garlic, peeled and minced

2 cups sliced carrots

2 cups sliced zucchini (I cut them into half-moons for this recipe)

2 cups baby bella (cremini) mushrooms, sliced into ½-inch thick slices

2 medium tomatoes, cut into 1-inch pieces (2 cups)

1 medium red bell pepper, seeded, deribbed and cut into 1-inch cubes

2 cups passata or tomato puree

2 cups filtered water

2 teaspoons ground cumin

½ tablespoon minced jalapeño pepper (or to taste)

1 teaspoon ground turmeric

½ teaspoon smoked paprika

High-quality sea salt, to taste

Freshly ground black pepper, to taste

DIRECTIONS:

▸ Heat the coconut oil in a large saucepan over low heat. Add the onions and sauté for 2 minutes. Do not allow them to brown. Add the garlic, and sauté for another minute.

▸ Next, fold in the carrots, zucchini, mushrooms, tomatoes and bell pepper, and sauté for about 2 minutes.

▸ Pour in the passata and the water, and mix well. Stir in the cumin, jalapeño, turmeric and paprika, and then season with sea salt and pepper to taste. Raise the heat to medium-high, bring the mixture to a boil, and then reduce the heat and simmer, covered, for 1 hour.

▸ Serve the stew with brown rice or quinoa, or, as I often do, just eat a gargantuan amount of the stew over salad.

TOMATO AND BASIL VEGAN SOUP

Yield: About 4 cups

I first started making this soup for clients while on a press tour for a film in Chicago in the middle of winter, when it was freezing. I would make it in the hotel kitchen, then bring it up to my clients' rooms during the press junkets to help warm them up. It's easy to digest and feels soothing. This soup is packed with minerals and antioxidants for many beauty benefits.

INGREDIENTS:

2 tablespoons low-sodium vegetable broth, plus 2 cups

½ cup diced white onions

1 medium clove garlic, peeled and minced

1 medium carrot, peeled and chopped

1 medium celery stalk, chopped

3 cups coarsely chopped fresh Roma tomatoes (about 2 pounds)

¼ cup tomato paste (from a glass container)

⅓ cup packed fresh basil leaves

½ teaspoon raw apple cider vinegar

1½ cups unsweetened almond milk or coconut milk

2 bay leaves

Sea salt, to taste

Freshly ground black pepper, to taste

DIRECTIONS:

▶ Heat the 2 tablespoons vegetable broth in a large heavy saucepan over medium heat. Add the onions and cook for about 3 minutes, or until they become translucent. Stir in the garlic and cook for another minute.

▶ Next, add the carrots and celery, and cook for 1 minute. Then add the tomatoes, the remaining 2 cups vegetable broth and the tomato paste. Bring the mixture to a boil, and then reduce the heat to medium-low and simmer, covered, for about 15 minutes, stirring frequently.

▶ Remove the soup from the heat and let it cool. Transfer the cooled soup to a blender, add the basil and the apple cider vinegar, and blend until fairly smooth.

▶ Pour the soup back into the saucepan, and stir in the almond milk and the bay leaves. Reheat the soup over medium heat. For a thicker consistency, allow the soup to reduce, stirring frequently, for 20 to 30 minutes. Remove the bay leaves with a slotted spoon, season the soup with sea salt and pepper, and serve at once.

AJNA

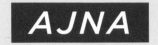

(INDIGO, THIRD EYE)

PURPLE POTATO AND ZUCCHINI BAKED FRITTERS WITH COCONUT AIOLI

Yield: 9 fritters

Purple potatoes are unusual and intensely, well, purple! They resonate with the color vibration of your *Ajna* chakra. These earthy fritters pair perfectly with the coconut-based aioli. Coconut is considered a sacred food in many cultures. The perfect inner-most white part of the coconut represents the purity of the soul, which is in tune with "seeing" with the intuition of your third eye.

FRITTER INGREDIENTS:

Coconut oil, for greasing baking sheets

1 medium zucchini, shredded (about 2 cups)

1 pound purple potatoes, shredded (about 3 cups)

1 tablespoon Ener-G Egg Replacer mixed with ¼ cup very hot filtered water

¼ cup coconut flour

½ teaspoon sea salt

½ teaspoon freshly ground black pepper

1 tablespoon minced fresh parsley, minced fresh cilantro, microgreens or sprouts, for garnishing

COCONUT AIOLI INGREDIENTS:

½ cup plain, unsweetened coconut yogurt (available at some natural-food stores; the So Delicious brand is a good choice)

2 teaspoons freshly squeezed lime juice

1 teaspoon olive oil

½ teaspoon minced fresh parsley or fresh cilantro

1 small clove garlic, peeled and finely minced

Pinch of sea salt

Freshly ground black pepper, to taste

DIRECTIONS:

▸ Preheat the oven to 375°F. Grease two baking sheets with coconut oil.

▸ Prepare the fritters. Remove as much of the moisture from the zucchini as possible by placing it on paper towels and wringing them out tightly over a bowl. Combine the zucchini, potato, Ener G Egg Replacer and water mixture, coconut flour, and salt and pepper in a large bowl, and mix well.

▸ Fill a ½-cup dry measuring cup with the vegetable mixture and unmold it on one of the prepared baking sheets. It should be loosely packed and should retain its circular shape on the baking sheet. Repeat this process until all the vegetable mixture has been used, making sure that none of the veggie shapes touch on the baking sheets.

▸ Bake the fritters for 10 minutes, and then lower the heat to 350°F and bake them for an additional 15 minutes. Remove the fritters from the oven and flip them over carefully. They are super delicate, so I use two spatulas to keep them from falling apart. Return the fritters to the oven and bake for another 20 minutes, or until they are slightly browned. (They will still be soft inside.) Remove the fritters to large plates and allow them to cool for at least 15 minutes.

▸ Meanwhile, prepare the coconut aioli. Whisk together all the aioli ingredients in a small bowl, combining well. (It's pretty delicious, but try to save the aioli for the fritters!) When the fritters are cool, spoon a small amount of the aioli on top of each and then garnish with parsley, cilantro, microgreens or sprouts.

ASIAN CUCUMBER SALAD

Yield: 4 servings

I love cucumber salad because it's so fresh tasting. We had a lot of it in my house while I was growing up, and I remember eating it out of a huge bowl when I was a child and trying to gather as much of the dressing onto each cucumber as I possibly could. I love fresh cucumbers and herbs, a combination that is an integral part of Vietnamese and Thai cooking; those cuisines were the inspiration for this recipe. I like imbuing the salad with lime flavor for extra freshness. The lime juice also helps soften the red onions—which are really purple and fall into the color vibration for your *Ajna* third eye. A little bit goes a long way with red (truly purple) onions, which are visually beautiful and stimulating.

INGREDIENTS:

1 large or 2 medium cucumbers (about 1¼ pounds)

2 medium tomatoes, cut into wedges

¼ small red onion, peeled and thinly sliced

3 tablespoons freshly squeezed lime juice

1 tablespoon raw apple cider vinegar

1 tablespoon organic tamari (preferably low sodium)

2 tablespoons coconut nectar or maple syrup (or to taste)

¼ teaspoon chili pepper flakes (or to taste)

1 small clove garlic, peeled and minced

⅓ cup minced fresh cilantro (optional)

¼ cup minced fresh basil

DIRECTIONS:

▸ If you are using nonorganic cucumbers, peel the skin off the cucumbers. (When I use organic cucumbers, I like to leave on the mineral-rich skin). Cut the cucumbers into thin slices, and combine them with the tomatoes and onions in a medium bowl. Set aside.

▸ Whisk together the lime juice, apple cider vinegar, tamari, coconut nectar, chili pepper flakes and garlic in a small bowl. Pour the dressing over the reserved vegetables and toss well so that all the vegetables are coated.

▸ Cover the salad and refrigerate it for at least 1 hour before serving. Fold in the cilantro, if using, and basil right before serving.

NOTE: I keep this cucumber salad nearby when I'm preparing dinner and I'm hungry. Instead of "tasting" the dishes I'm preparing for flavor over and over again, I just nibble on the cucumbers, and this tides me over and keeps me from spoiling my appetite.

SAHASRARA

(VIOLET, CROWN)

FIG AND OLIVE DRESSING

Yield: 1 cup

It's a great idea to pack up some of this dressing and add it to the prepared salads you get on the run if you don't have time to make a full salad yourself. While the color of figs and olives might put them in the *Ajna* chakra category, I think there is something quite mystical about these two fruits, and so I like to include them in this all-pervading *Sahasrara* chakra section. Figs and olives appear often in Greek and Roman mythology, pointing to a fascination with these fruits since ancient times. Figs have mucus-dissolving properties and can help cleanse your blood and your entire system, and olives provide a healthy dose of vitamin E, to help scavenge free radicals and keep your body full of vitality.

INGREDIENTS:

1 cup filtered water

½ cup pitted Niçoise olives

4 dried figs (unsulfured)

2 tablespoons freshly squeezed lemon juice

2 tablespoons minced fresh basil

2 small cloves garlic, peeled

1 teaspoon fresh thyme or ½ teaspoon dried thyme

½ teaspoon Dijon mustard

10 black peppercorns, crushed with a mortar and pestle, or about ¼ teaspoon freshly ground black pepper

DIRECTIONS:

▶ Combine all the ingredients in a blender and blend until smooth. The dressing will be a mauve color due to the olives. It pairs gorgeously with a kale salad tossed with some veggies in contrasting colors, such as radishes and carrots.

▶ This dressing will keep, covered, in the refrigerator for about 3 days.

STUFFED ZUCCHINI BLOSSOMS WITH PINE NUTS AND BASIL

Yield: 2–3 servings

Eating edible flowers is like eating fruit. Such flowers are a peak, ripe offering of nature's perfection, embodying the universal and divine energy flowing through the *Sahasrara* chakra. They are more often available in the summer, but in some regions of the country zucchini blossoms and other edible flowers (such as nasturtiums, lilacs, pansies, primrose or hawthorn) are available year-round. Get them from your trusty farmer at your local farmers' market. Since flowers are so delicate and perfect as they are (again, like fruit), the dressings and flavorings that go with them should be simple and simply combined so you can taste all the raw elements. I know it's popular to cook (even fry) zucchini blossoms and flowers, but here you'll enjoy them in their raw beauty and take in that beauty yourself.

INGREDIENTS:

1 cup packed fresh basil leaves

⅓ cup raw pine nuts

½ tablespoon olive oil

½ tablespoon lemon juice

1 small clove garlic, peeled and minced

¼ teaspoon dried oregano

Sea salt, to taste

10 zucchini blossoms

Edible flowers, for garnishing (optional)

DIRECTIONS:

▸ Combine the basil, pine nuts, olive oil, lemon juice, garlic, oregano and sea salt in a food processor or blender (or use a mortar and pestle, my favorite way) and process until chunky but fully mixed.

▸ With dry hands, carefully open the zucchini blossoms on a clean surface, such as a cutting board. Using a small spoon, gently stuff each blossom with the basil–pine nut mixture. Arrange the stuffed zucchini blossoms on a large plate in a beautiful way and garnish with the edible flowers, if you choose. Serve your blossoms right away!

CARBS

BEAUTY FOOD–PAIRED, VEGAN AND GLUTEN-FREE MAC 'N' CHEESE

Yield: 4 servings

Mac and cheese is among the leading carb cravings that people tell me they have. It's not just the carbs they crave; it's also all the fatty dairy. So many vegan dishes get their creamy, cheesy quality from cashews, but I wanted to avoid those here. Nuts are a protein, and combining them with pasta, even when it is gluten-free, results in a dense protein-starch combination that should be avoided for easier digestion. In this recipe, the fatty richness is derived from a blend of butternut squash and coconut milk. This recipe is a variation of the one that caterer Hope Bailey created as an appetizer and served in elegant little espresso cups at our wedding. I hope you, too, enjoy this properly combined, much healthier version of mac and cheese!

INGREDIENTS:

2 cups cubed butternut squash
(½-inch cubes)

1 cup diced white onions

2 medium cloves garlic, peeled and smashed

1 tablespoon coconut oil, plus 1 tablespoon for the bread crumbs

½ teaspoon sea salt, plus ½ teaspoon for the sauce, plus ½ teaspoon for the bread crumbs

¼ teaspoon freshly ground black pepper, plus ¼ teaspoon for the sauce, plus ¼ teaspoon for the bread crumbs

2 cups full-fat, unsweetened coconut milk

4 sprigs fresh thyme

2 bay leaves

2 tablespoons nutritional yeast, plus 2 tablespoons for the bread crumbs

½ teaspoon dry mustard

½ teaspoon ground turmeric

Few drops Tabasco sauce or other similar hot sauce (optional)

¾ cup gluten-free bread crumbs (made from about 3 pieces of toasted gluten-free bread)

1½ teaspoons paprika

8 ounces gluten-free pasta elbows or shells, cooked according to the package directions

DIRECTIONS:

▸ Preheat the oven to 375°F.

▸ Toss the butternut squash cubes, onions and garlic with 1 tablespoon of the coconut oil, ½ teaspoon of the sea salt and ¼ teaspoon of the pepper in a large bowl. Spread the squash mixture on a baking sheet and roast in the oven until the squash cubes are soft and golden brown, around 40 minutes.

▸ Meanwhile, combine the coconut milk, thyme and bay leaves in a medium saucepan, and bring to a rolling boil over medium heat. Turn off the heat and let the coconut milk steep for 15 to 20 minutes. Remove the bay leaves and thyme sprigs with a slotted spoon.

▸ Combine the cooked coconut milk, the squash mixture, ½ teaspoon of the sea salt, ¼ teaspoon of the pepper, 2 tablespoons of the nutritional yeast, the dry mustard, turmeric and Tabasco sauce in a blender and process until smooth. Set the butternut squash sauce aside.

▸ Toss the bread crumbs with the remaining 1 tablespoon coconut oil, the remaining 2 tablespoons nutritional yeast, the remaining ½ teaspoon sea salt, the remaining ¼ teaspoon pepper and the paprika. Set the bread crumb mixture aside.

▸ Arrange the cooked pasta in a large bowl. Pour the reserved butternut squash sauce over the pasta and combine well. Spoon the pasta into a 9 x 13-inch casserole dish. Sprinkle the reserved bread crumb mixture over the pasta and bake for 20 minutes, or until top is golden. Spoon out, serve at once and enjoy each bite!

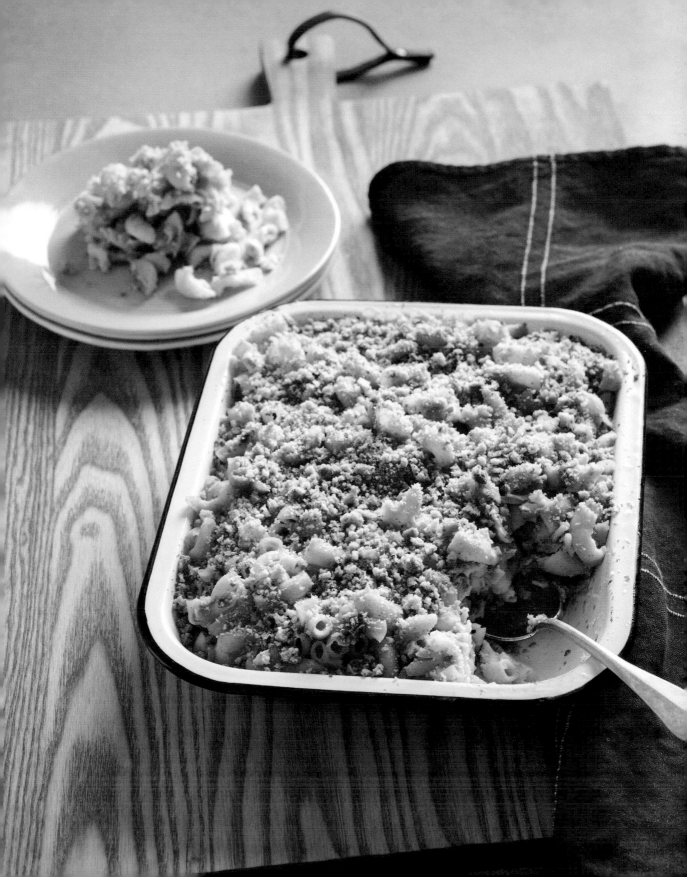

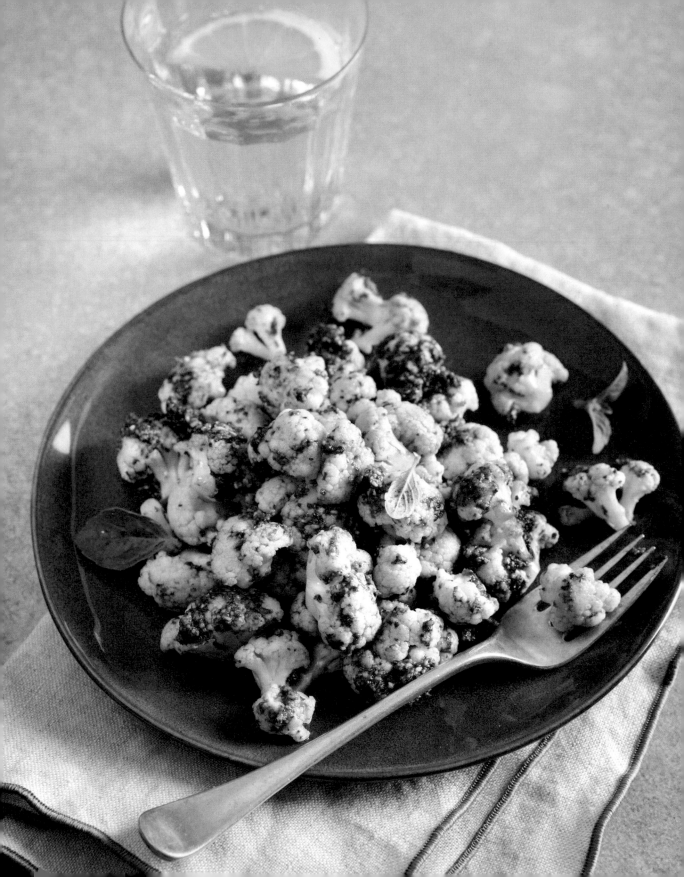

CAULIFLOWER GNOCCHI WITH WALNUT PESTO

Yield: 2–4 servings

Cauliflower, especially when steamed, has a fairly mild flavor and, much like rice and pasta, acts like a carrier for the sauce you put on it. However, pesto, which contains nuts, doesn't Beauty Food Pair with pasta. (Try to simplify meals by not combining dense proteins and starches, as this makes for easier digestion.) This veggie replacement is a perfect pasta alternative. I've been making this dish for clients for years to help abate heavy, traditional gnocchi cravings, and I sincerely hope you love and enjoy it, as well!

INGREDIENTS:

1 medium head cauliflower, cored, green leaves removed and cut into small stemless florets the size of traditional gnocchi

2 cups packed fresh basil leaves, plus more for garnishing

$^2/_3$ cup raw walnuts

2 tablespoons olive oil

2 teaspoons freshly squeezed lemon juice

2 small cloves garlic, peeled and minced

Sea salt, to taste

DIRECTIONS:

▸ Bring a medium pot of water fitted with a steamer basket to a boil over medium-high heat. Add the cauliflower, and steam, covered, for about 9 minutes, or until tender but not too crumbly. With a slotted spoon, carefully transfer the steamed cauliflower to a medium serving bowl, shaking off any water droplets in the process. Set aside.

▸ Combine the basil, walnuts, olive oil, lemon juice, garlic and sea salt in a food processor or blender (or do this by hand with a mortar and pestle), and pulse until you achieve a pesto with your preferred consistency. I do suggest breaking down the walnuts pretty finely, though, for easier digestion!

▸ Mix together the pesto and the reserved cauliflower, garnish with basil leaves for a fabulous presentation and serve at once.

ANGEL HAIR SPAGHETTI SQUASH PUTTANESCA

Yield: 6 servings

I bow down to the wonder of nature and how she created natural noodles for us to enjoy in spaghetti squash! No flour-based pasta is needed to satisfy your pasta craving. Traditional puttanesca involves anchovies, but instead I added some portobello here for a little bit of earthy flavor and texture. This is one of the few recipes you'll see me using olive oil in, though there is a pretty small amount spread out over the servings. Please be sure to follow the recipe and cook at a lower heat, as olive oil is not as heat resistant for cooking as coconut oil. Make a batch of this and reheat it for yourself over the next day or two.

INGREDIENTS:

1 medium or 2 small spaghetti squash, cut in half and seeds removed

2½ tablespoons olive oil

1 cup minced white onions

4 small cloves garlic, peeled and minced

1 medium portobello mushroom cap, diced

1 cup diced tomatoes (about 2 vine-ripened Roma tomatoes or 1 large beefsteak)

¾ cup pitted and halved Kalamata olives

2 tablespoons capers, drained

⅓ cup torn fresh basil leaves, plus more for garnishing

½ teaspoon red pepper flakes

Sea salt, to taste

Freshly ground black pepper, to taste

DIRECTIONS:

▶ Preheat the oven to 375°F. Arrange the spaghetti squash halves cut side down on a baking sheet, and bake for 45 minutes, or until softened.

▶ Meanwhile, heat the olive oil in a large pot over medium-low heat. Add the onions and sauté for about 3 minutes, or until they become translucent. Add the garlic and sauté for another minute.

▶ Next, add the mushrooms and tomatoes, and cook for about 5 minutes, or until both have softened. The tomatoes will release some liquid. Stir in the olives, capers, basil and red pepper flakes, and cook for 3 or 4 minutes.

▶ Scrape the flesh from the inside of the baked spaghetti squash halves and fold it into the sauce. Alternatively, you can scrape the flesh from the inside of the baked spaghetti squash halves onto a plate, and top with some of the sauce. Season with salt and pepper and garnish with basil leaves. Serve at once.

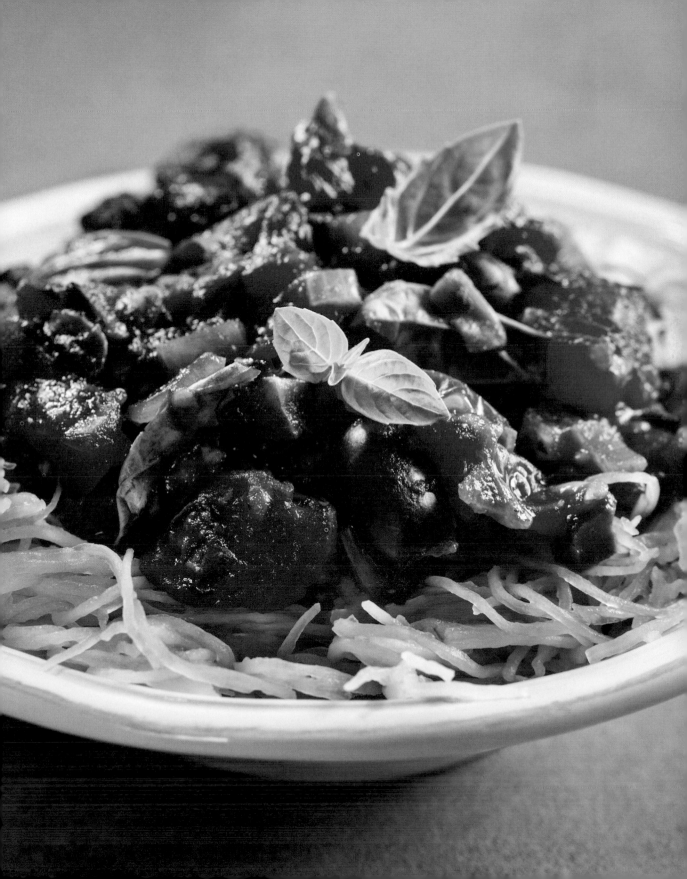

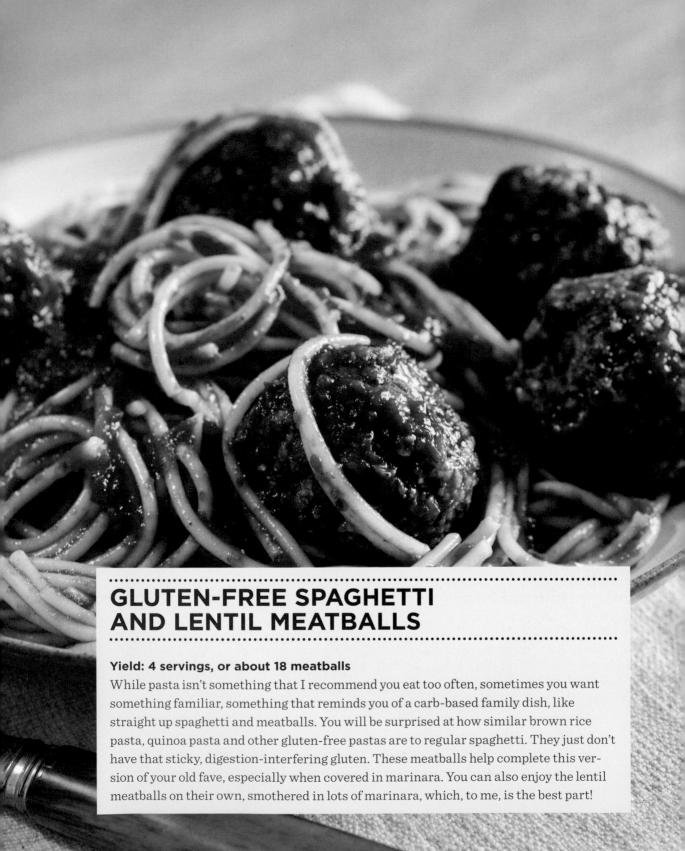

GLUTEN-FREE SPAGHETTI AND LENTIL MEATBALLS

Yield: 4 servings, or about 18 meatballs

While pasta isn't something that I recommend you eat too often, sometimes you want something familiar, something that reminds you of a carb-based family dish, like straight up spaghetti and meatballs. You will be surprised at how similar brown rice pasta, quinoa pasta and other gluten-free pastas are to regular spaghetti. They just don't have that sticky, digestion-interfering gluten. These meatballs help complete this version of your old fave, especially when covered in marinara. You can also enjoy the lentil meatballs on their own, smothered in lots of marinara, which, to me, is the best part!

INGREDIENTS:

2 cups filtered water

½ cup lentils, soaked overnight

¼ cup low-sodium vegetable broth

⅓ cup diced red onions

1 medium clove garlic, peeled and minced

½ cup diced celery

1 tablespoon minced fresh thyme

2 teaspoons minced fresh oregano

Pinch of cayenne pepper

1 cup gluten-free bread crumbs
(made from about 4 pieces of toasted

millet, brown rice or other gluten-
free bread)

1 tablespoon olive oil

2 teaspoons Ener-G Egg Replacer mixed
with ¼ cup very hot water

Sea salt, to taste

Freshly ground black pepper, to taste

Coconut oil, for greasing the baking sheet

8 ounces gluten-free spaghetti, cooked
according to the package directions

Marinara sauce, such as Homemade Bella
Marinara (page 288)

DIRECTIONS:

▸ Bring the water to a boil in a large pot over medium-high heat, and then reduce
the heat to medium and add the lentils. Cook the lentils for about 30 minutes,
or until they are tender.

▸ Meanwhile, heat the vegetable broth over medium heat in a medium saucepan.
Add the onions and garlic, and cook for about 4 minutes, or until the onions are
translucent. Add the celery, thyme, oregano and cayenne pepper, and cook for
4 more minutes, or until the onions have softened. Set the onion mixture aside.

▸ Preheat the oven to 375°F. Mash the cooked lentils with a fork in a medium bowl
to break them down a bit. Stir in the reserved onion mixture, bread crumbs, olive
oil, and the Ener-G Egg Replacer and water mixture, mixing well. Season with salt
and pepper.

▸ Grease a baking sheet with coconut oil. Form the lentil mixture in balls about the size
of Ping-Pong balls, and line the balls up on the prepared baking sheet, leaving equal
space in between them. Bake the meatballs for 10 minutes, and then turn them and
bake for another 10 minutes.

▸ Place the cooked spaghetti in a large serving bowl and toss with a generous amount
of marinara sauce. Gently fold the lentil meatballs into the spaghetti, being careful
not to break them apart. Serve at once.

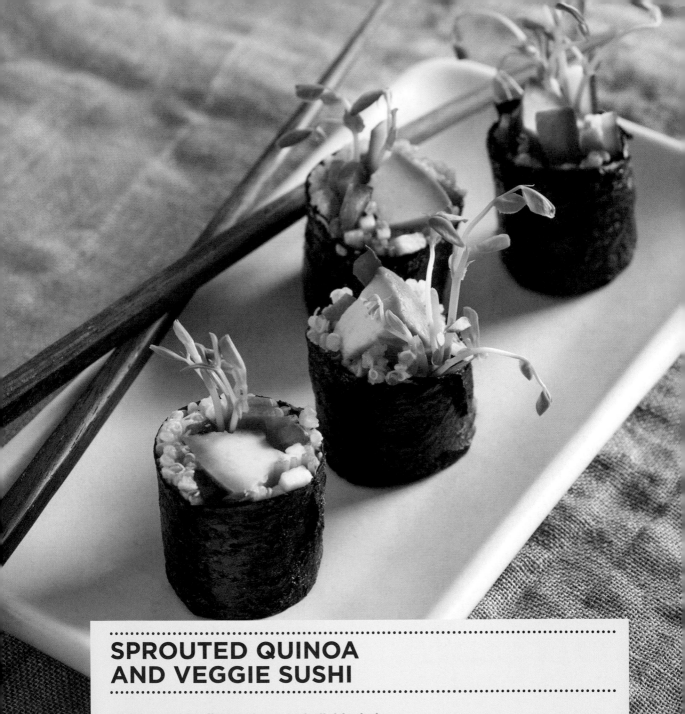

SPROUTED QUINOA AND VEGGIE SUSHI

Yield: 4 sushi rolls, or about 24 individual pieces

Making sushi at home is fun and satisfying! With a little practice, you'll love the feeling of hand rolling sushi. The "secret sauce" in this recipe helps make your sushi rolls moist without the use of mayonnaise. And as a twist on a classic sushi roll, this recipe uses quinoa, a mineral-rich, fiber-filled whole carbohydrate.

INGREDIENTS:

1¼ cups filtered water

½ cup quinoa, soaked overnight and rinsed well

¼ teaspoon ground turmeric

Pinch of sea salt

2 tablespoons coconut nectar or maple syrup

1 tablespoon Dijon mustard

1 tablespoon minced red onions

2 teaspoons organic tamari (preferably low sodium)

4 nori sheets

Bamboo mat or a cutting board, for rolling the sushi

⅓ cup julienned red bell peppers

⅓ cup julienned carrots

⅓ cup julienned cucumbers

2 tablespoons freshly squeezed lemon juice

1 medium ripe Hass avocado, peeled, pit removed, cut into ¼-inch strips lengthwise and sprinkled liberally with lemon juice

DIRECTIONS:

▸ Bring the water to a boil in a medium saucepan over medium-high heat. Reduce the heat, add the quinoa and cook for 12 to 14 minutes, or until the quinoa is tender and no water remains. Stir in the turmeric and the sea salt, and then set the quinoa aside to cool.

▸ To make the sauce, whisk together the coconut nectar, Dijon mustard, onions and tamari in a medium bowl. Set the sauce aside.

▸ Place the shinier side of a nori sheet on a bamboo mat or cutting board. (If you can't tell which side is shinier, no worries. This will just make the sushi slightly prettier, but it's not a huge deal! It won't change the taste.) With a spoon, spread ⅓ cup to ½ cup of the reserved quinoa over about half of the nori sheet (no more than that, or it will be too thick to roll, and you'll just have a jumbo sushi burrito). Leave 1 inch free of quinoa at the top and the bottom of the nori sheet. Push down firmly with the back of a spoon to compact the quinoa.

▸ Next, spoon a quarter of the reserved sauce evenly over the compacted quinoa. Arrange a quarter of the julienned peppers, carrots, cucumbers and avocado strips near (and parallel to) the bottom edge of the nori sheet, that is, the end closest to you. (This makes it easier to roll the nori.) Roll the nori up tightly and seal the top edge. (You can rub a little bit of water on the top edge to help seal the roll.)

▸ Set the finished roll on a large plate and repeat this process with the remaining nori sheets. Then, using a very sharp knife, cut each roll into 6 pieces. I find that making a slit first and then cutting all the way through the roll ensures a cleaner cut and makes cutting easier. It can also be helpful to wet your knife a bit. Try this if your veggies are slipping out too much (and if that happens, just push them back in!).

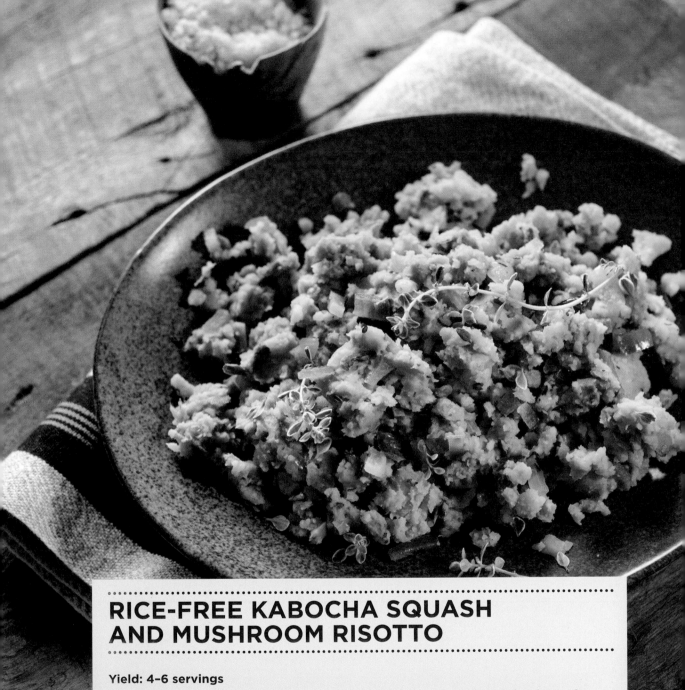

RICE-FREE KABOCHA SQUASH AND MUSHROOM RISOTTO

Yield: 4–6 servings

I love the texture of risotto, which is somewhere between smooth and chunky. In the past, I ordered some vegan versions of risotto, but they often contained processed vegan cheese, and I never felt good after eating that. In contrast, this risotto is made of pure veggies and no processed foods. Kabocha squash is an Asian variety of winter squash and hands down one of my favorite nongreen vegetables. Oh, and yes, it will definitely help "squash" your carb craving!

INGREDIENTS:

1 large or 2 medium kabocha squashes (acorn squash could work too, but cook about 20 minutes less to keep from getting too soft)

1 tablespoon coconut oil

1 cup diced red onions

2 medium cloves garlic, peeled and minced

1 pound baby bella (cremini) mushrooms, stems trimmed and thinly sliced

1 ounce porcini mushrooms (dried are okay; just rehydrate for 30 minutes in warm filtered water before using)

½ cup low-sodium vegetable broth, plus ¼ cup

2 tablespoons raw apple cider vinegar

2 teaspoons chopped fresh thyme

1 cup unsweetened coconut milk

¼ cup nutritional yeast

Sea salt, to taste

Freshly ground black pepper, to taste

DIRECTIONS:

▸ Adjust the racks in the oven so that the middle rack will accommodate the whole kabocha squashes. Preheat the oven to 375°F.

▸ Carefully make several 2-inch slits in the squashes with a sharp knife. Place the squashes on a baking sheet and roast them for 1 hour, or until they have softened. Through roasting, the squashes retain the perfect texture for this dish. Remove the squashes to a large plate or a cutting board to cool.

▸ Once cool, cut each squash in half and scoop out and discard the seeds and the stringy parts of the flesh. Cut the skin off. (If you like the taste, you can save the skin for snacking, as I do!) Working with batches that your food processor can handle—such as a quarter of a squash at a time—process the squash until the texture is chunky and resembles grains of rice. (It's better to work with smaller batches so that the squash doesn't end up with too fine a texture or even pureed.) Process all the batches and then set the squash aside. (If you don't have a food processor, you can instead dice the squash by hand.)

▸ Heat the coconut oil in a large saucepan over medium-high heat. Add the onions and sauté them for about 3 minutes, or until they become translucent. Add the garlic and sauté for another minute. Add the baby bella and porcini mushrooms, the ½ cup of vegetable broth, apple cider vinegar and thyme, and cook for about 5 minutes, stirring well.

▸ Fold in the reserved squash, stirring well. Next, stir in the remaining ¼ cup vegetable broth, the coconut milk and the yeast, and cook for a few more minutes until every-thing melds together. Don't overcook, to retain the texture. Season the risotto with salt and pepper as desired and serve at once.

HOMEMADE BELLA MARINARA

Yield: About 8 cups

It's a great idea to assemble this sauce ahead of time. Then, while it's simmering, you can make the other components of your meal. And because we're cooking with olive oil (which is not as heat-resistant as coconut oil), be sure to keep the heat on lower temperatures. Besides, you don't want to rush the sauce!

INGREDIENTS:

1½ tablespoons olive oil

⅓ cup finely diced white onions

2 medium cloves garlic, peeled and minced

14 Roma tomatoes, puréed in a blender or food processor

⅓ cup tomato paste (from a glass container)

⅓ cup coarsely minced fresh basil

¼ teaspoon dried oregano or ½ tablespoon fresh oregano

Sea salt, to taste

Freshly ground black pepper, to taste

DIRECTIONS:

▸ Heat the oil in a medium saucepan over medium-low heat. Gently sauté the onions for 2 minutes, or until they become translucent. Add the garlic and sauté for about 1 more minute.

▸ Add the puréed Roma tomatoes and the tomato paste. Increase the heat to medium and cook until the mixture is just about to boil. Immediately reduce heat to low and add the basil, oregano, sea salt and black pepper. Cook the sauce, covered, over low heat for 30 minutes, or until it has reduced and the flavors have condensed.

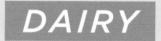

VEGAN BEAUTY RANCH DRESSING

Yield: About 1 cup

I grew up eating vinegar-based dressings, so it wasn't until later in life that I came to realize how popular ranch dressing is. I was inspired to come up with a healthier option for friends and clients who craved it. Luckily, this version is super tasty (former ranch eaters all around me love it) and delivers beauty benefits, including B vitamins, amino acids, probiotics and minerals, such as potassium. Be sure to use plain, unsweetened coconut yogurt, the purer the better.

INGREDIENTS:

$2/3$ cup plain, unsweetened coconut or almond yogurt

$1/3$ cup pine nuts

$1/4$ cup nutritional yeast

2 tablespoons minced yellow onions

2 teaspoons raw apple cider vinegar

1 small clove garlic, peeled

$1/2$ teaspoon sea salt (or to taste)

1 tablespoon minced fresh parsley

1 tablespoon minced fresh dill

DIRECTIONS:

▸ Combine the coconut yogurt, pine nuts, nutritional yeast, onions, apple cider vinegar, garlic and sea salt in a blender or food processor and process until smooth. Stir in the parsley and dill. You can "ranch it up" for about 2 days.

RAW RED PEPPER CREAM CHEESE ENDIVE BITES

Yield: 4 servings, or ⅔ cup nut cheese

I don't consume or recommend consuming cashews on a daily basis, as they are rarely truly raw and I think there are far better beauty nuts out there. Still, cashews can be transformed into an undeniably delicious plant-based cheese alternative. This nut cream cheese pairs beautifully with endive. Serve this dish as an appetizer or enjoy it as a snack.

INGREDIENTS:

1 cup non-roasted, non-salted cashews

½ cup diced red bell peppers

1 ½ tablespoon freshly squeezed lemon juice

2 tablespoons filtered water

1 small clove garlic, peeled

½ teaspoon sea salt (or to taste)

1 thick head endive, root end trimmed and separated into leaves (or 2 romaine leaves, cut into 6-inch-long and 1½-inch-wide strips)

¼ cup walnut halves, for garnishing

¼ cup microgreens, for garnishing

DIRECTIONS:

▸ Combine the cashews, red peppers, lemon juice, water, garlic and sea salt in a food processor or blender, and process until smooth. If you are using a blender, you might have to add a little bit more water to keep it going. Simply turn off the blender, add a little more water, scrape down the sides, pushing the contents into the middle, and then resume blending as needed.

▸ Next, arrange the endive leaves on a large plate. With a small spoon, spread a small amount of the nut cream cheese on each endive leaf. Garnish each with a walnut half and some microgreens, and serve at once. Enjoy each blissful bite!

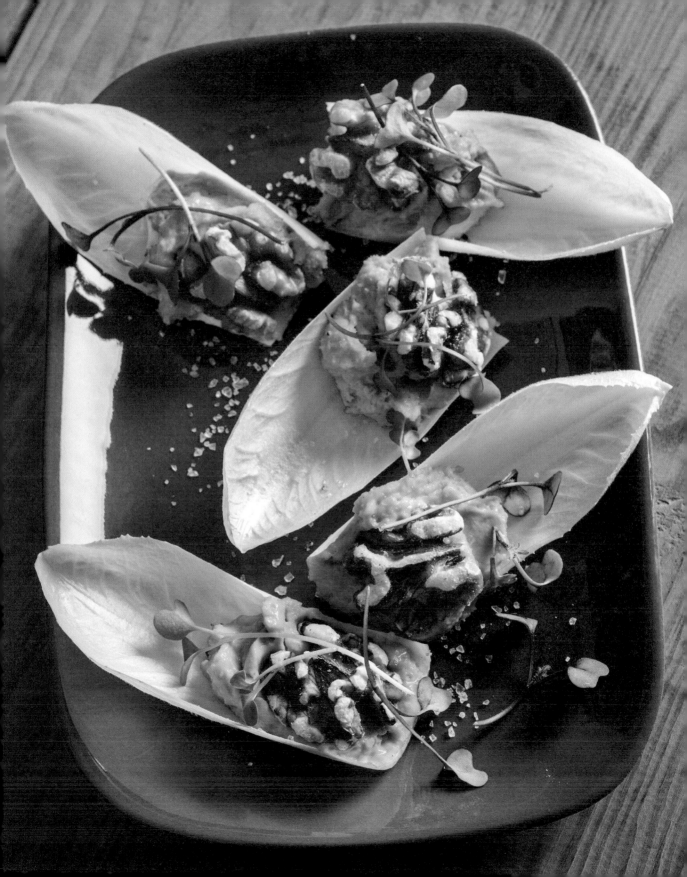

ITALIAN WALNUT PARMESAN CHEESE

Yield: ½ cup

This cheese is a variation of one that I made at a raw food café and education center that used to be in New York's East Village. I interned and hung out there a lot. It's fantastic sprinkled on salads, veggie soups and steamed or roasted vegetables. If you once loved Parmesan cheese, this one is for you!

INGREDIENTS:

½ cup raw walnuts

3 tablespoons coarsely chopped fresh parsley

2 tablespoons nutritional yeast

1 tablespoon minced fresh oregano or 1 teaspoon dried oregano

1 small clove garlic, peeled

¼ teaspoon sea salt
(or to taste)

DIRECTIONS:

▸ Place all the ingredients in a food processor or blender and pulse until well blended. During this process, you may have to turn off the food processor or blender and scrape down the sides, pushing the contents into the middle.

▸ This cheese keeps, covered, in the refrigerator for up to 5 days.

NOTE: I'd love to hear from you (on my blog) about your favorite way to use this cheese, since it's one of my personal faves!

RAW VEGGIE ROMESCO SAUCE AND STEAMED VEGGIES

Yield: 2 servings, or 1½ cups

I have noticed that for a lot of my clients, it's the sauce they are after in pasta dishes. In this dish the pasta is entirely replaced with fiber-filled veggies. The combination of the almonds, the nutritional yeast and the blended veggies in the red sauce makes for a supernutritious, satisfying, creamy sauce.

BASE INGREDIENTS:

1 cup thinly sliced zucchini

¾ cup thinly sliced carrots

3 cups small broccoli florets

SAUCE INGREDIENTS:

2 cups diced tomatoes

¾ cup coarsely chopped red bell peppers

¼ cup raw almonds, soaked overnight and rinsed well

¼ cup packed fresh basil leaves

2 tablespoons nutritional yeast

1 tablespoon freshly squeezed lemon juice

½ tablespoon olive oil

1 medium clove garlic, peeled

½ teaspoon dried oregano

½ teaspoon paprika

½ teaspoon sea salt (or to taste)

DIRECTIONS:

▸ Bring a medium pot of water fitted with a steamer basket to a boil over medium-high heat. Add the zucchini and the carrots, and steam for about 3 minutes. Then add the broccoli and steam the vegetables for another 5 to 6 minutes, or until they have softened to the desired degree. Remove the steamed vegetables to a large serving bowl and set aside.

▸ Next, combine all the sauce ingredients in a blender and blend until smooth. Transfer the sauce to a small saucepan and cook, stirring frequently, over medium heat for 3 or 4 minutes, or just until it is warm. Stir the sauce with care and love, and be sure not to overheat it. Once the sauce is warm, pour it over the reserved vegetables and toss to coat them. Serve at once.

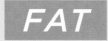

BAKED BROCCOLI AND YAM TERRINE

Yield: 4–6 servings

A terrine is a vegetable or meat mixture that has been cooked and allowed to cool or set in a tureen and then is cut into slices and served. Here's my all-veggie version, folks! It has a cheesy taste, without any dairy or faux vegan cheese. It can be sliced into nice squares—be sure to let it set and to lift the squares using two spatulas.

INGREDIENTS:

1½ pounds small yams
(or sweet potatoes or
red-skinned potatoes)

Coconut oil, for greasing
the casserole dish

1 cup plain, unsweetened
coconut yogurt

2 tablespoons Ener-G Egg
Replacer mixed with ½ cup
very hot filtered water

½ cup unsweetened
coconut milk (the So
Delicious brand is
a good choice)

6 cups small broccoli florets

Sea salt, to taste

¼ teaspoon freshly ground
black pepper (or to taste)

DIRECTIONS:

▸ Arrange the yams in a medium saucepan and cover with 2 inches of cold water. Bring the yams to a boil over medium-high heat, and then reduce the heat to medium-low and cook the yams, uncovered, for 30 minutes, or until they are tender. (If you use red-skinned potatoes, the cooking time may be shorter.)

▸ Meanwhile, preheat the oven to 350°F. Grease a 9 x 13-inch casserole dish with the coconut oil.

▸ When the yams are done, drain them in a colander, allow them to cool enough to be handled and then peel off their skins (the skins should come off easily). Transfer the peeled yams to a large bowl and then mash them with a potato masher or a fork.

▸ Next, stir in the coconut yogurt, Ener-G Egg Replacer and water mixture, and the coconut milk. Add the broccoli, salt and pepper and stir, mixing well so that all the ingredients are incorporated. Adjust the seasoning to taste.

▸ Spoon the yam mixture into the prepared casserole dish. Cover the casserole dish with aluminum foil, being careful not to touch the casserole, and bake for 45 minutes. Uncover and bake for another 15 minutes. Allow the terrine to set for about 15 minutes before slicing it into squares. Serve at once.

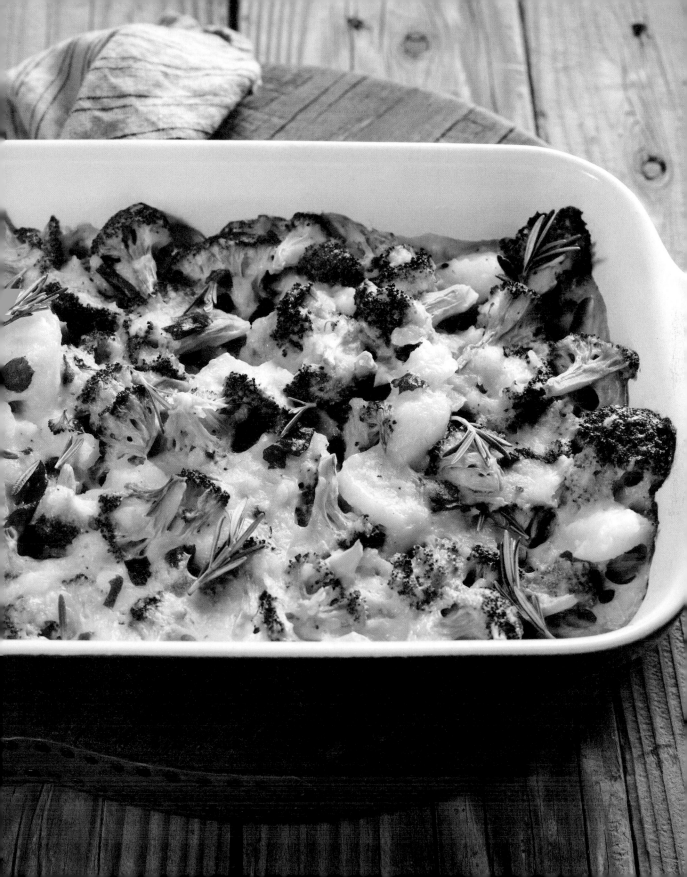

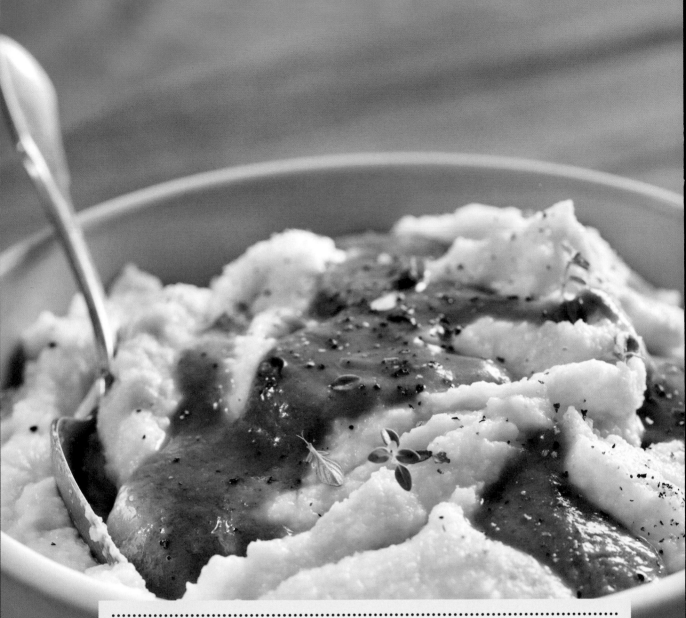

MASHED CAULIFLOWER WITH GRATIFYING GRAVY

Yield: 4–6 servings

The mushroom gravy in this dish is out of this world. It tastes decadent and richly fulfills a fat craving. The mashed cauliflower is a great conduit for the sauce and an excellent veggie replacement, and it pairs well with most of the entrées in this book. But to be completely honest, with or without the cauliflower, I could drink this gravy and be happy. Try it for yourself!

CAULIFLOWER INGREDIENTS:

One 2-pound head cauliflower, cored, green leaves removed and cut into florets

¾ cup unsweetened coconut milk

2 tablespoons nutritional yeast

1½ tablespoons olive oil

1 medium clove garlic, peeled and roasted

Sea salt, to taste

Freshly ground black pepper, to taste

MUSHROOM GRAVY INGREDIENTS:

2 tablespoons coconut oil

1 cup diced yellow onions

2 medium cloves garlic, peeled and minced

1 pound baby bella (cremini) mushrooms, thinly sliced

2 cups low-sodium vegetable broth or filtered water

3 tablespoons organic tamari (preferably low sodium)

¾ teaspoon minced fresh thyme

2 tablespoons arrowroot starch or tapioca starch

Sea salt, to taste

Freshly ground black pepper, to taste

DIRECTIONS:

▸ Prepare the cauliflower. Bring a medium pot of water fitted with a steamer basket to a boil over medium-high heat. Add the cauliflower and steam, covered, for about 9 minutes, or until tender.

▸ Place half of the steamed cauliflower in the bowl of a food processor. Add the coconut milk, nutritional yeast, oil and garlic, and process until the cauliflower is broken up. Add the remaining cauliflower and process until it reaches the consistency you prefer. Season with sea salt and pepper. Transfer the cauliflower to a medium serving bowl and set aside.

▸ Prepare the gravy. Heat the coconut oil in a medium saucepan over medium-high heat. Add the onions and garlic and sauté, stirring frequently, for about 4 minutes, or until the onions are lightly brown. Stir in the mushrooms and sauté for 5 minutes more, or until the mushrooms are tender.

▸ Next, add the vegetable broth, tamari and thyme to the mushroom-onion mixture. Bring the mixture to a boil over medium heat. Then lower the heat to medium-low and simmer, covered, stirring occasionally, until it thickens, about 25 minutes. Stir in the arrowroot starch and cook the sauce, stirring frequently, for another 5 minutes. Transfer the sauce to a blender and puree for a smooth consistency.

▸ Season the sauce with sea salt and pepper. Pour the sauce over the reserved cauliflower and serve at once.

KIK ALICHA ETHIOPIAN YELLOW SPLIT PEA STEW

Yield: 4 servings

The desire to feel "full" is often a root cause of fat cravings, and this dish creates that full feeling while being oil free and low fat. I love the food I eat when I go to Africa, and I especially love Ethiopian food. This dish is inspired by my travels there. The yellow split peas make this a satisfying and hearty stew.

INGREDIENTS:

¼ cup filtered water, plus 3 cups

½ cup diced white onions

1 medium clove garlic, minced

⅔ cup diced zucchini

½ cup diced carrots

1 cup dried yellow split peas, soaked overnight and rinsed well

¼ cup thickly sliced fresh ginger

½ teaspoon ground turmeric

Sea salt, to taste

Freshly ground black pepper, to taste

DIRECTIONS:

▸ Heat ¼ cup of the water in a medium saucepan over medium-high heat. Add the onions and cook for about 1 minute, or until they are translucent. Add the garlic and cook just until it becomes fragrant, about 1 minute. Add the zucchini and carrots, and cook for another 2 minutes.

▸ Add the remaining 3 cups water, the split peas, ginger and turmeric, and bring the mixture to a boil. Then reduce heat to medium-low and simmer, covered, stirring occasionally, for about 1 hour, or until the split peas have softened nicely.

▸ Using a slotted spoon, carefully remove the ginger slices. Season the stew with sea salt and pepper. If you like, pulse the stew in a food processor to break down the split peas even more and give the stew a less chunky texture. Serve at once.

NOTE: Be sure to soak the split peas overnight. This will help you digest them better.

GUACAMOLE PIZZA

Yield: 1–2 servings

Giving up dairy doesn't mean you have to give up all forms of pizza forever! This is a gluten-free avocado version that is satisfying—in terms of both the taste and the fun when picking it up traditional pizza-style. It's also a reliable and quick-to-make snack for when you are hungry and want something pronto that is healthy and satisfying.

INGREDIENTS:

1 gluten-free wrap (brown rice, teff or any other kind)

½ medium ripe Hass avocado

1 tablespoon freshly squeezed lemon juice

1 teaspoon minced red onions

1 small clove garlic, peeled and minced

Dash of cayenne pepper

Pinch of sea salt

1 Roma tomato, thinly sliced

DIRECTIONS:

▶ Heat a large skillet over medium-high heat. Lay the wrap flat in the skillet and heat it for about 1½ minutes before flipping it over. Heat the other side for another minute, or until it is slightly toasted. Keep a close eye on the wrap, as it will toast quickly.

▶ Next, spoon the avocado flesh into a small bowl and mash it until it has a chunky consistency. Add the lemon juice, onions, garlic, cayenne pepper and sea salt, and mix thoroughly.

▶ Spread the guacamole on top of the wrap and garnish it with tomato slices. Cut the pizza into slices with a pizza cutter or a knife. (It's so much more fun when you cut this into wedges!) Serve at once.

ZUCCHINI BEAUTY SAUCE

Yield: ²⁄₃ cup

This creamy sauce is jam-packed with vitamins C and E, potassium and enzymes. There's a reason I call it Beauty Sauce. You can use this sauce as a dip for veggies or as a thicker salad dressing.

INGREDIENTS:

1 cup thickly sliced zucchini

¼ cup coarsely chopped Hass avocado

¼ cup filtered water

3 tablespoons freshly squeezed lemon juice

2 tablespoons diced yellow onions

2 tablespoons organic tamari (preferably low sodium)

1 tablespoon coconut nectar or maple syrup

2 teaspoons sesame oil

1 small clove garlic, peeled

Pinch of cayenne pepper

DIRECTIONS:

▸ Combine all the ingredients in a blender and blend until smooth. Time to get your beauty on! Covered, this sauce will keep in the refrigerator for about 3 days.

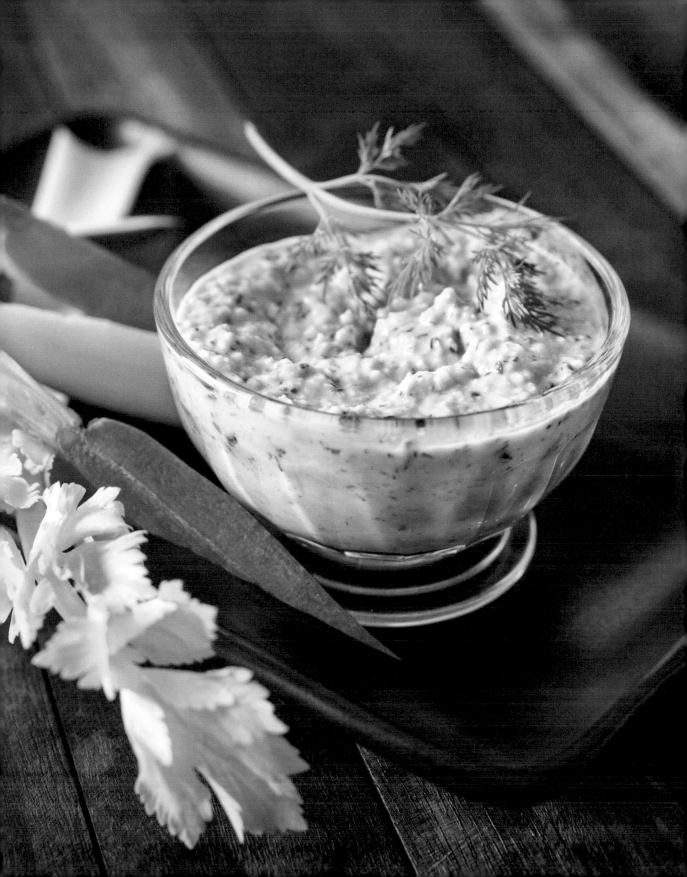

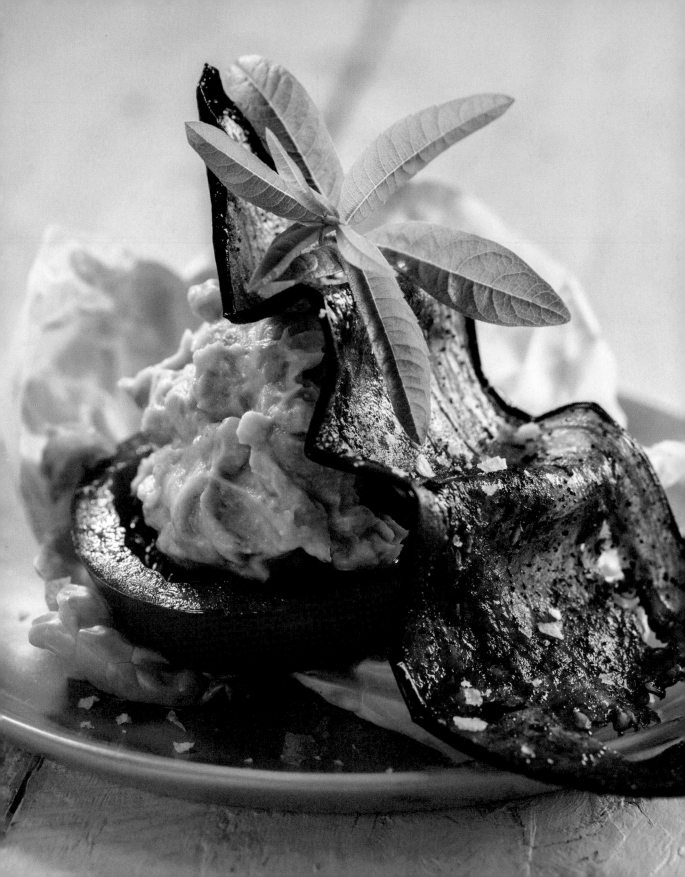

BLT STACK WITH AVOCADO-MISO SPREAD

Yield: 4 servings

This is my version of the classic BLT with a Beauty Food makeover. The fattiness of the avocado and the richness of the Wild West Eggplant Bacon will satisfy your fat craving. No bread needed! And you can have fun with the fresh tomatoes, mixing it up with colorful, funky-shaped, imperfectly perfect heirloom varieties when available.

INGREDIENTS:

1 medium ripe Hass avocado

1 tablespoon organic miso paste (preferably mellow white)

1 tablespoon freshly squeezed lemon juice

2 romaine lettuce leaves, cut in half, or 4 butter lettuce leaves

1 large tomato, cut into thick slices

4 strips Wild West Eggplant Bacon (page 315)

¼ cup minced fresh herbs or microgreens, for garnishing

DIRECTIONS:

▶ Cut the avocado in half and remove the pit. Spoon the flesh into a small bowl and fold in the miso paste and lemon juice. Set aside.

▶ Next, arrange a romaine leaf half on an individual serving plate. Top with a tomato slice, then spoon a generous dollop of the Avocado-Miso Spread atop the tomato. Top with a folded (or wavy) strip of Wild West Eggplant Bacon. Repeat this process with the remaining lettuce leaves.

▶ Garnish each with fresh herbs or microgreens for a perfect stack of ingestible beauty. Serve at once.

CRUNCHY

BACKYARD BROWN RICE PAPER WRAPS

Yield: 8 full wraps, or 16 halves

These wraps contain some of the veggies that might be growing in your or your local farmer's "backyard." My dream is to grow all these veggies and more myself one day! Till then, I'm happy with all the local farmers' markets I check out wherever I happen to be. Brown rice paper wrappers are gluten-free and are a bit stickier than the traditional ones. (Star Anise Foods is one good brand, and you can find it at health-food stores or online.) The crunchy veggies in this wrap paired with the tasty dip will keep your jaw busy for a while.... Be sure to chew well!

INGREDIENTS:

8 brown rice paper wrappers

1 cup julienned carrots (about 2 medium carrots)

1 cup julienned jicama

1 cup thinly sliced purple cabbage

1 cup fresh cilantro (no stems)

Zucchini Beauty Sauce (page 300)

DIRECTIONS:

▶ Dip a rice paper wrapper in a shallow bowl of warm water (wide enough to accommodate it), and soak it until each part is moistened, about 1 to 2 minutes. Quickly remove the wrapper and lay it on a cutting board.

▶ Place a layer of each of the veggies (½ cup of each) across the middle of the wrapper. Roll the wrapper up tightly, burrito-style, tucking the ends in first. If the wrapper gets too sticky to deal with, just wet your fingers a bit.

▶ Arrange the wrap on a plate and cut it in half crosswise. Repeat this process until all the wrappers are filled and rolled. You will need to replenish the warm water for wrapper dipping once or twice.

▶ Serve the wraps at once with Zucchini Beauty Sauce on the side.

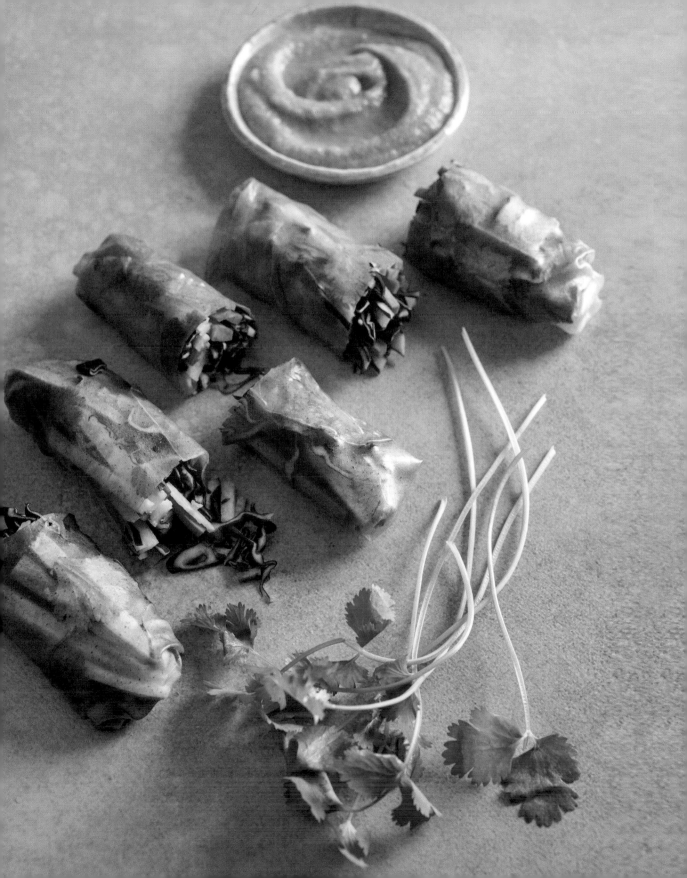

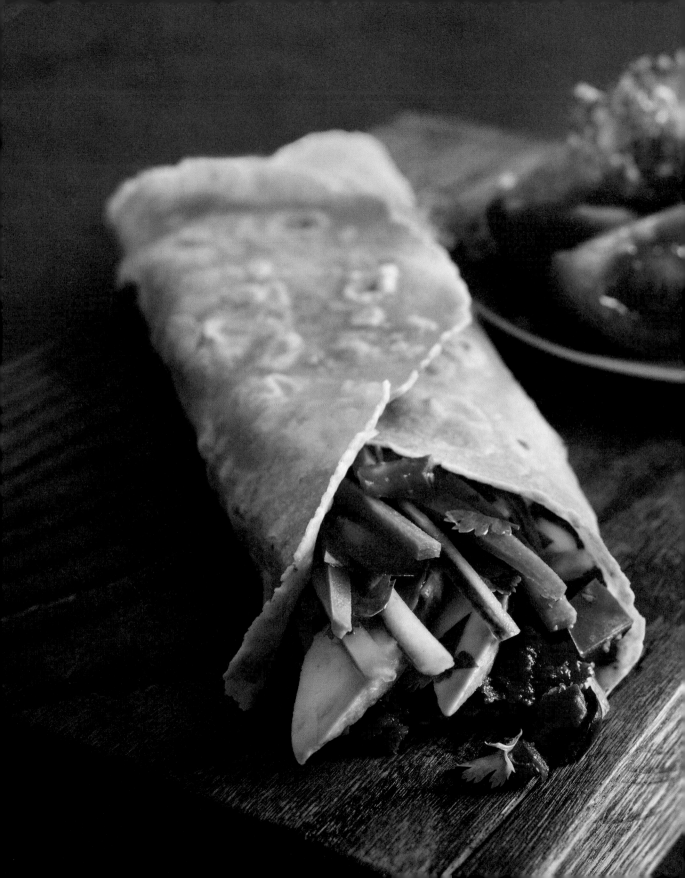

MIDDLE EASTERN GLUTEN-FREE WRAPS WITH SUN-DRIED TOMATO PÂTÉ

Yield: 4 wraps, or about 1 cup pâté

The spices and veggies that are popular in the Middle East can be unexpected to your taste buds, especially if you are new to cumin and smoked paprika or rarely eat them. Spices, a salty-sweet combo from the Kalamata olives and sun-dried tomatoes, crunchy veggies...these wraps have it all.

WRAP INGREDIENTS:

½ cup diced tomatoes

½ cup julienned cucumbers

½ cup julienned carrots

¼ cup diced white onions

2 tablespoons minced fresh parsley

1 tablespoon freshly squeezed lemon juice

1 medium clove garlic, peeled and minced

½ teaspoon ground cumin

¼ teaspoon sea salt (or to taste)

4 gluten-free tortillas (I prefer brown rice or teff, a gluten-free grain that is grown in Africa)

1 medium ripe Hass avocado, peeled, pit removed and cut into 12 slices

SUN-DRIED TOMATO PÂTÉ INGREDIENTS:

1 cup sun-dried tomatoes (use dried, rehydrating them in warm water for 30 minutes; avoid those packed in oil)

½ cup filtered water (or a bit more)

¼ cup diced Kalamata olives

1 tablespoon freshly squeezed lemon juice

2 teaspoons olive oil

½ teaspoon smoked paprika

DIRECTIONS:

▸ Prepare the veggie mixture for the wraps. Toss together the tomatoes, cucumbers, carrots, onions, parsley, lemon juice, garlic, cumin and sea salt in a medium bowl. Set aside.

▸ Prepare the pâté. Combine all the pâté ingredients in a food processor and blend well. Add a bit more water during the process to keep the mixture going, if necessary. Set aside.

▸ Assemble the wraps. Arrange a tortilla on an individual plate and spread ¼ cup of the reserved pâté on it, leaving at least 2 inches uncovered at the edges. Top with a quarter of the reserved veggie mixture and 3 avocado slices. Roll the tortilla up carefully burrito-style. Repeat this process until all the tortillas are filled and rolled.

▸ Serve the wraps at once with a large green salad.

CRUNCHY VEGGIE PURSES

Yield: 9 purses

The jicama in this recipe is blanched to make it easier to work with, but it is still pleasingly crunchy. If you're having trouble cutting the jicama thin enough to roll in these purses, you may end up with little jicama wraps, which are just as delicious! Or you can also lay the veggie mixture on the jicama strips so that they resemble tostadas or toast. Whether you end up with purses, wraps or tostadas, enjoy the crunchy combo.

INGREDIENTS:

1 medium jicama, peeled

1 medium ripe Hass avocado

1 tablespoon freshly squeezed lime juice

1 tablespoon finely diced red onions

1 small clove garlic, peeled and minced

¼ teaspoon chili powder

Cayenne pepper, to taste

Sea salt, to taste

⅓ cup finely diced red bell pepper

½ cup finely diced tomatoes

DIRECTIONS:

▸ Prepare the jicama. Bring a medium saucepan of water to a boil over medium-high heat. Prepare an ice water bath.

▸ Using a mandoline or a very sharp knife, cut the jicama into whole round slices that are as thin as you can get them. You should end up with at least 9 slices. Blanch the jicama slices in the boiling water for 1 minute, and then plunge them into the ice water bath. This makes them pliable, so they won't crack when you bunch them up. Remove the jicama slices to a plate and set aside.

▸ Prepare the avocado filling. Cut the avocado in half, remove the pit and spoon the avocado flesh into a small bowl. Mash the avocado with a fork, and then mix in the lime juice, onions, garlic, chili powder, cayenne pepper and sea salt, combining well. Next, fold in the bell peppers and the tomatoes.

▸ Assemble the purses. Arrange a reserved jicama slice on a plate. Place 1 tablespoon of the avocado mixture in the middle of the slice and then bunch up the slice to form a purse, twisting the top and dabbing a bit of water on the top to help seal it. It will look like an adorable little coin purse. Repeat this process with the remaining jicama slices. (If your jicama slices aren't thin enough and they crack when you try to bunch them up, just roll them up like a wrap. Think of it as a clutch purse variation, with the same crunchy effect.)

▸ Serve the purses at once.

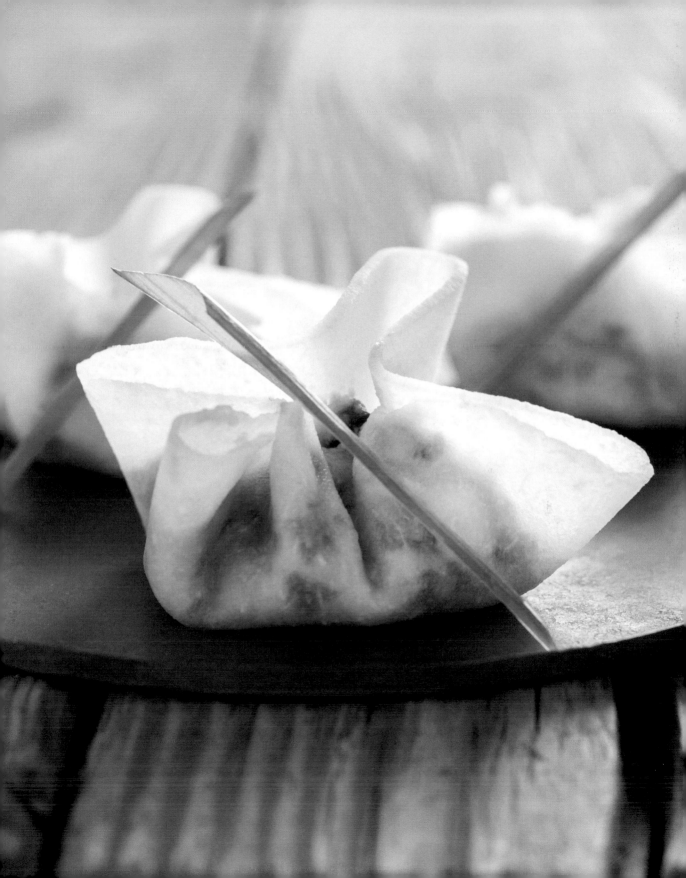

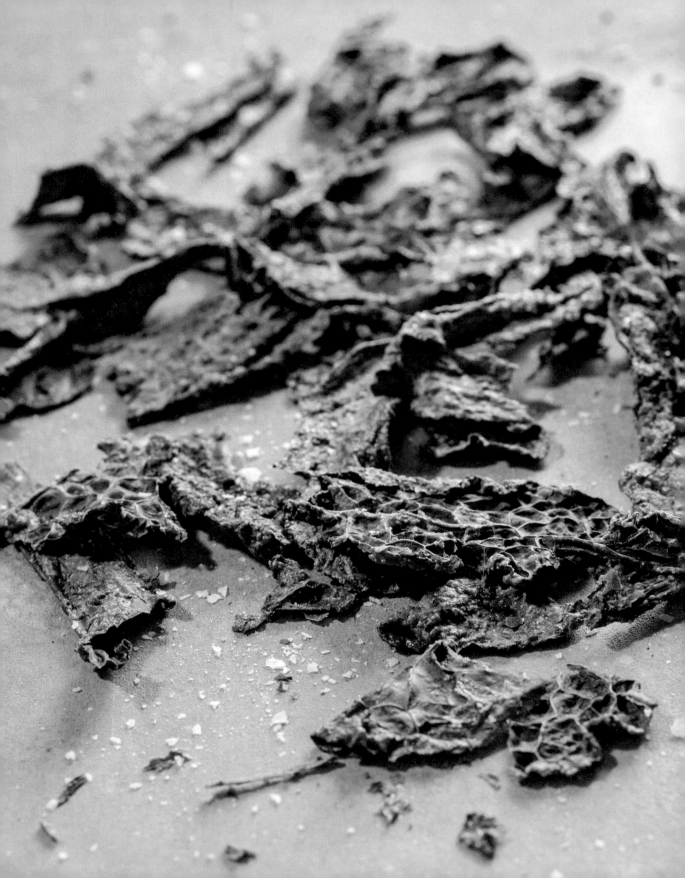

CHEESY CALCUTTA KALE CHIPS

Yield: About 6 cups

I have made many varieties of kale chips over the years, but because of my love of turmeric, which reminds me of my travels to India, and particularly to Calcutta, where I often saw it being sold by street vendors, this is one of my favorite versions. The nutritional yeast and cashews give these kale chips a cheesy flavor.

INGREDIENTS:

¾ pound curly kale (1 very large bunch or 2 medium bunches), stems and ribs removed

¾ cup non-roasted, non-salted cashews

1 medium red bell pepper, seeded, deribbed and coarsely chopped

¼ cup raw sunflower seeds, soaked overnight and rinsed

3 tablespoons freshly squeezed lemon juice

3 tablespoons nutritional yeast

2 tablespoons diced yellow onions

1 tablespoon coconut nectar or maple syrup

¼ teaspoon ground turmeric

½ teaspoon sea salt

DIRECTIONS:

▸ Rinse the kale and remove as much of the moisture as possible using a salad spinner or paper towels. Tear the kale into bite-size pieces. Let the kale air out on a clean surface while you do the next step, so that it will be saturated with the dressing and won't get weighed down by any water.

▸ Prepare the dressing. Combine the remaining ingredients in a food processor or blender and process until smooth.

▸ Place the kale and the dressing in a large bowl and mix well with your hands to ensure the leaves are well coated.

▸ If you are using a dehydrator, place the kale on the dehydrator trays, and dehydrate at 110°F overnight, or until crispy. Flip the kale about 12 hours into the dehydration process to ensure that all parts are crispy.

▸ If you are using an oven, arrange the kale on 2 baking sheets in a single layer, and bake at the lowest temperature, with the oven door cracked open. Stir the kale chips halfway through the baking process to ensure all parts are crispy. When I tested this method at my parents' house, it took about 3 hours, and the lowest setting on their oven is 170°F. Everyone's oven is different, though, so set timers and check along the way!

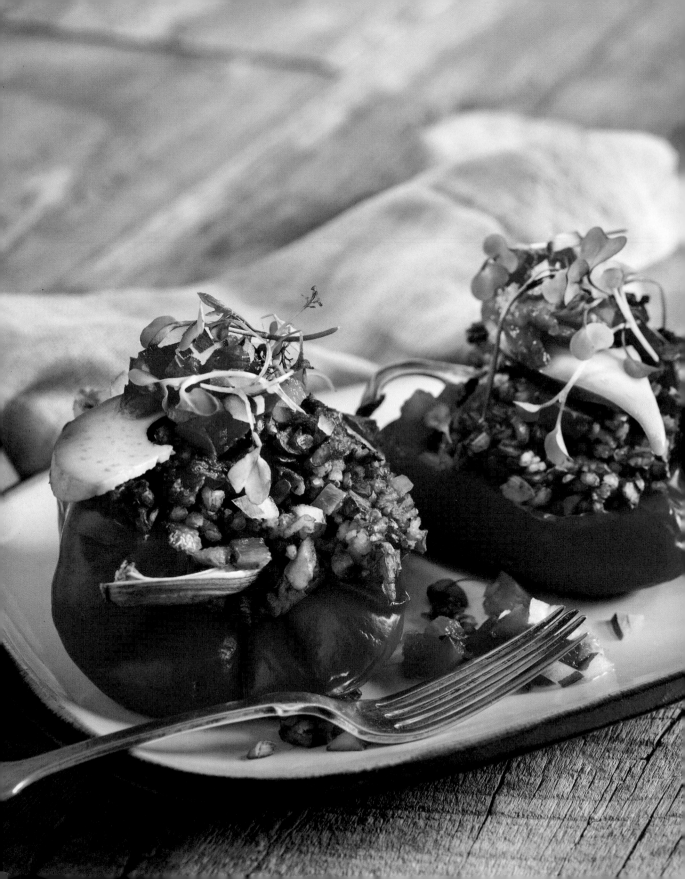

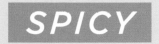

MEXICAN RED RICE AND MUSHROOM STUFFED PEPPERS

Yield: 6 full-size stuffed peppers, or 12 halves

I recently consulted with the kitchen at a beautiful Mexican resort called Esperanza, helping to add some new healthier and gluten-free ideas to their menus and giving some health classes. I have the best memories of working with all the warmhearted chefs and staff. One dish they often made for me for a late lunch was rice and mushrooms over salad. It was hearty, full of protein from the mushrooms, and filling, and it helped carry me through the dinner service, when I would walk around and chat with guests about their Beauty Detox dinner. My Mexican friends knew how I liked it—with salsa, made with very little oil, and hold the sour cream! This recipe was inspired by my experience, and I hope that you love it, too, as it satisfies your spicy cravings with its whole foods.

INGREDIENTS:

1½ cups filtered water

¾ cup dry red rice, soaked overnight and rinsed well

6 medium red bell peppers, sliced in half lengthwise, stems removed, seeded and deribbed

1 tablespoon coconut oil, plus more for greasing the baking dishes

1 cup diced red onions

2 medium cloves garlic, peeled and minced

¾ tablespoon minced jalapeño peppers

2 large portobello mushroom caps, diced (about 8 ounces)

2 cups diced tomatoes

2 tablespoons ground cumin

1 tablespoon chili powder

1 tablespoon coriander powder

1 teaspoon sea salt, to taste

TOPPINGS:

1 cup fresh salsa or *pico de gallo*

12 Hass avocado slices

12 fresh cilantro sprigs or 1 cup microgreens

DIRECTIONS:

▸ Bring the filtered water to a boil in a medium saucepan over medium-high heat. Add the red rice, reduce the heat to medium-low and cook for 45 minutes, or until the rice is tender. You can also use a rice cooker for this step. Set aside.

▸ Bring a large pot of water to a boil over medium-high heat. Prepare an ice water bath. Blanch the red pepper halves by immersing them in the boiling water, and then plunge them into the ice water bath. Remove the red pepper halves to a large plate and set aside.

▸ Preheat the oven to 350°F. Grease two 9 x 13-inch baking dishes with coconut oil.

▸ Prepare the stuffing. Heat the 1 tablespoon coconut oil in a medium saucepan over medium-high heat. Add the onions and sauté for 3 minutes, or until they become translucent. Add the garlic and the jalapeño, and sauté for another minute. Stir in the mushrooms and sauté for 3 more minutes. Next, add the tomatoes, cumin, chili powder, coriander powder and sea salt. Fold in the reserved rice and adjust seasonings to taste.

▸ Assemble the peppers. Spoon the stuffing into each of the red pepper halves and then arrange the halves in the prepared baking dish. (Depending on the size of your peppers, you may have some stuffing left over. Save it and serve it atop a salad for lunch.)

▸ Cover the baking dishes with aluminum foil, being careful not to touch the peppers, and bake for 45 minutes. Uncover and bake for another 10 minutes, or until the tops look lightly browned and a bit crispy. Top each pepper half with some fresh salsa, an avocado slice and a sprig of cilantro, and serve at once.

WILD WEST EGGPLANT BACON

Yield: About 15 strips

This spicy all-veggie bacon replacement is featured in my BLT Stack with Avocado-Miso Spread recipe (page 303). Once you try smoked paprika, you won't know how you lived without it! An essential in a plant-based kitchen, its name doesn't lie—it delivers a smoky flavor and a fiery spice. This recipe will inspire you to throw on some cowboy boots and go wrestle in some veggies from the garden!

INGREDIENTS:

Coconut oil, for greasing the baking sheet

⅓ cup coconut nectar or maple syrup

¼ cup raw apple cider vinegar

1½ tablespoons organic tamari (preferably low sodium)

1½ teaspoons smoked paprika

1½ teaspoons chili powder

1 large eggplant, thinly sliced lengthwise into long slices with a mandoline, if possible, or by hand

DIRECTIONS:

▸ Preheat the oven to 425°F. Grease two baking sheets with coconut oil (see Note).

▸ Make a marinade by mix together the coconut nectar, apple cider vinegar, tamari, smoked paprika and chili powder in a medium bowl. Set aside.

▸ Arrange the eggplant slices on the prepared baking sheets. You should have about 15 slices. Bake for 8 to 10 minutes, or until lightly browned. Remove the eggplant slices to a large plate and allow them to cool enough to be handled. Reserve the baking sheets.

▸ Dip the baked eggplant slices in the marinade, coating both sides fully. Arrange the eggplant slices on the reserved baking sheets and bake for 4 to 5 minutes, keeping a close eye on them. Do not let them burn or get too hard. The tamari will help the strips darken.

▸ Transfer the eggplant bacon to a large plate and allow it to cool and bend naturally with complete freedom. If you want to get fancy, roll up some parchment paper and bend it into wavy shapes, then lay the eggplant on top to cool, which will cause the strips to bend and create wavy shapes. Serve the eggplant bacon at once or refrigerate, covered, for up to 2 days.

NOTE: You can also line the baking sheet with a Silpat baking mat and omit the coconut oil.

SPICY TEMPEH AND VEGGIE CABBAGE ROLLS

Yield: 12–15 rolls

This is another client favorite. I love to use veggies as natural wraps and edible food containers whenever possible, and cabbage is a natural for this. In this dish it's stuffed, baked and embellished with a sauce based on fresh tomatoes, and each bite will be spicy and zesty.

CABBAGE ROLL INGREDIENTS:

1 tablespoon coconut oil, plus more for greasing the baking dishes

1 large head green cabbage

½ cup diced red onions

2 medium cloves garlic, peeled and minced

16 ounces tempeh, diced

1 cup diced zucchini

½ cup diced carrots

Sea salt, to taste

Freshly ground black pepper, to taste

SAUCE INGREDIENTS:

5 cups diced tomatoes

⅓ cup tomato paste (from a glass container)

1½ teaspoons chili powder (or to taste)

1¼ teaspoons paprika (or to taste)

¾ teaspoon sea salt (or to taste)

¼ teaspoon cayenne pepper (or to taste)

¼ teaspoon ground cinnamon (or to taste)

DIRECTIONS:

▸ Preheat the oven to 350°F. Grease two 9 x 13-inch baking dishes with coconut oil.

▸ Prepare the cabbage. Bring a large pot of water to a boil over medium-high heat. Meanwhile, carefully core the cabbage by cutting a deep triangle shape, at least 2 inches deep, into the base of the cabbage and then removing the tough stem.

▸ Immerse the cored cabbage in the boiling water, reduce the heat to medium and cook for 10 to 12 minutes, or until the cabbage starts to soften. As the outer cabbage leaves start to separate from the head, use tongs to separate them completely. (They should separate pretty easily since you made your deep triangle cut.) Once the separated leaves have softened, remove them with the tongs to a large plate to cool. Continue until all the large leaves have been removed. You can compost the small cabbage leaves at the center of the head.

▸ Prepare the tempeh mixture. Heat the 1 tablespoon coconut oil in a large saucepan over medium heat. Add the onions and sauté for 3 minutes, or until they are translucent. Add the garlic and sauté for 2 more minutes. Next, add the tempeh and sauté for about 3 minutes. If it starts to stick, add a little water, as needed, to keep things moving. Stir in the zucchini and carrots, and cook until they soften, about 8 minutes. Season the tempeh mixture with sea salt and pepper, and set aside.

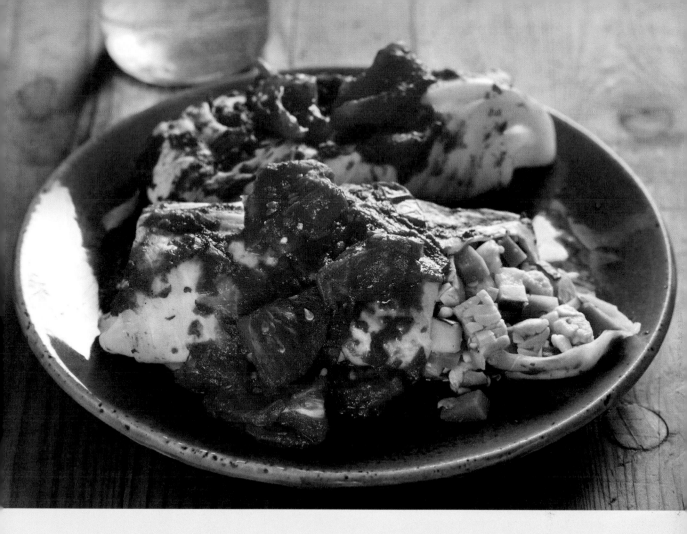

- ▶ Prepare the sauce. Add the tomatoes to a separate large saucepan, and cook over medium-high heat, stirring often, for about 2 minutes. Add the tomato paste and mix well. Reduce the heat to medium and cook the tomatoes, stirring often, for 10 to 15 minutes. Stir in the chili powder, paprika, sea salt, cayenne and cinnamon. Remove the sauce from the heat and set aside.

- ▶ Assemble the cabbage rolls. Make a deep V cut at the base of each cabbage leaf to cut out the thick stem. Arrange a cabbage leaf on a large plate or cutting board. Spoon ¼ cup to ⅓ cup of the reserved tempeh mixture down the middle. Starting with the "V cut" end, roll the cabbage leaf burrito-style, folding in the sides first. There is no need to roll too tightly. Repeat this process until you run out of the tempeh mixture. This should make 12 to 15 cabbage rolls.

- ▶ Place the cabbage rolls in the prepared baking dishes (about 7 rolls per baking dish). Spoon the tomato sauce over the cabbage rolls, covering them completely.

- ▶ Cover each baking dish with aluminum foil, being sure the foil doesn't touch your cabbage rolls, and bake for 30 minutes. Uncover and bake for another 15 minutes. Remove the cabbage rolls to individual plates and enjoy them hot!

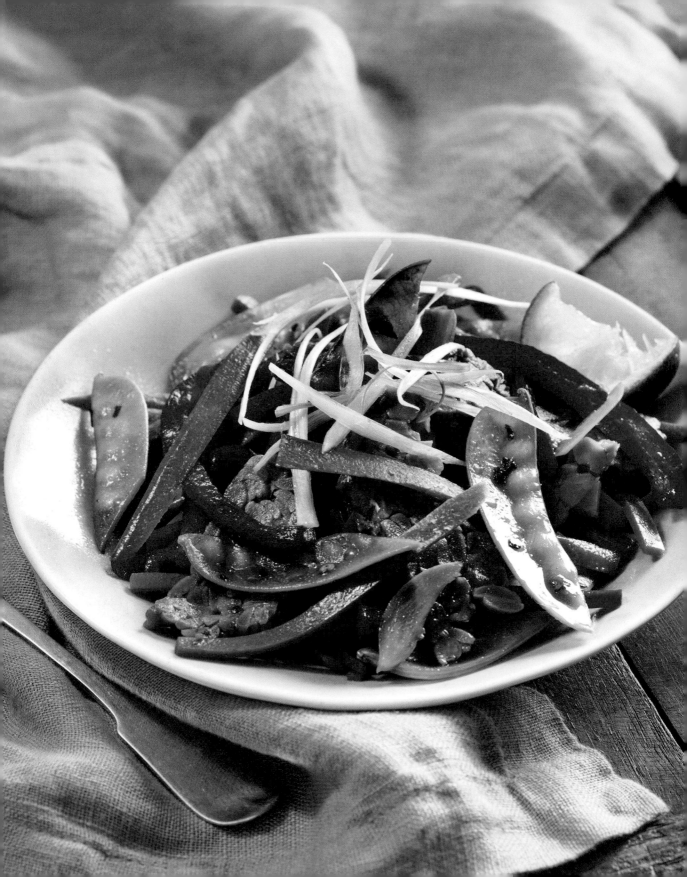

CHINESE MATCHSTICK VEGGIES AND TEMPEH

Yield: 4 servings

This is a superfun play on Asian stir-fries that have strips of beef and veggies mixed in. Who needs the beef when we have tempeh? Tempeh is not to be confused with gluten-containing seitan, which can be very difficult to digest, and which I do not recommend consuming. A fermented form of soy, tempeh is high in protein and has a nice dense texture and a nutty flavor. I like to marinate the tempeh to bring out some of the flavor of this dish. The colorful veggies and the piquant red pepper flakes make this a soul-satisfying dish.

INGREDIENTS:

4 tablespoons organic tamari (preferably low sodium)

¼ cup low-sodium vegetable broth

16 ounces tempeh, sliced into thin strips

1 tablespoon coconut oil

2 tablespoons minced scallions

1 small clove garlic, peeled and minced

2 teaspoons grated fresh ginger

3 cups julienned carrots

2 medium red bell peppers, stems removed, seeded, deribbed and sliced into matchsticks

2 cups snow peas, deveined

2 tablespoons raw apple cider vinegar or rice wine vinegar

2 tablespoons coconut nectar

¼ teaspoon red pepper flakes (or to taste)

1 tablespoon sesame oil

Pinch of sea salt (optional)

DIRECTIONS:

▸ Mix together 2 tablespoons of the tamari and the vegetable broth in a large shallow bowl or a glass pie dish. Add the tempeh, arranging it in 1 or 2 layers, and carefully spoon the marinade over it to ensure that all the slices have been coated. Cover the tempeh and refrigerate it for an hour, ideally, or at least while you prepare the other ingredients.

▸ Heat the coconut oil over medium-high heat in a large skillet or a wok. Add the scallions and garlic, and sauté for 3 minutes, stirring frequently. Next, add the ginger and sauté, stirring, for 2 or 3 more minutes, or until lightly browned. Add the carrots, and cook for 3 minutes. Keep on stirring! Toss in the bell peppers and the snow peas, and sauté for 3 or 4 minutes. Be sure not to overcook the veggies. They should stay fairly crisp.

▸ Stir in the remaining 2 tablespoons of tamari, the apple cider vinegar, coconut nectar and red pepper flakes. Next, fold in the reserved tempeh. (Be gentle so that the tempeh doesn't crumble.) Remove the skillet from the heat and add the sesame oil and sea salt, if desired, mixing well. Serve at once. Delicious!

SPICY PROBIOTIC AND ENZYME SALAD (P & E SALAD)

Yield: About 12 cups

Probiotic-rich, fermented foods are so great for your health and beauty. They help to build and maintain a clean system, one that absorbs your beauty nutrients and helps cleanse out toxins efficiently! Consuming half a cup of Probiotic and Enzyme Salad (a version of raw sauerkraut) every day is the ideal way to nourish your body. This version is spicy and flavorful. Get in the habit of making this salad regularly. There are many different ways to ferment. I have provided one easy fermentation method for you here that involves a crock (or a similar container) and not jars.

INGREDIENTS:

One 5-pound green or purple cabbage (or a combination!), outer leaves discarded, cored and shredded

3 tablespoons sea salt

1 to 2 tablespoons thinly sliced jalapeño peppers (for spicier versions, retain the seeds)

Filtered water, for the brine

DIRECTIONS:

▸ Combine the cabbage, sea salt and jalapeño in an extra-large bowl, and mix well.

▸ Sterilize *all* the equipment you use in the next steps by cleaning with hot water.

▸ Pack the cabbage mixture down into a ceramic crock, a large glass container or a food-grade plastic bucket a few inches at a time.

▸ Next, pour some filtered water into the crock so that it just covers the cabbage. (By introducing the liquid brine at the start, you help prevent spoilage.) Press down hard on the cabbage, packing it tightly, with a sturdy kitchen utensil that has a flat head. This is important, because it pushes excess air out of the crock and water out of the cabbage.

▸ Top the cabbage with a plate or a lid that fits snugly inside the crock. Place a weight on top of this plate or lid, such as a container filled with a quart or so of water or a large, clean rock. The weight helps to keep the cabbage submerged in the brine and out of the air, which will prevent spoilage. Place the crock in a cool area (65°F to 70°F).

▸ In approximately 5 to 8 days, it should have a tangy taste. Transfer the fermented cabbage to airtight containers and store them in the refrigerator. They will keep for at least a few weeks. Enjoy and then make another batch!

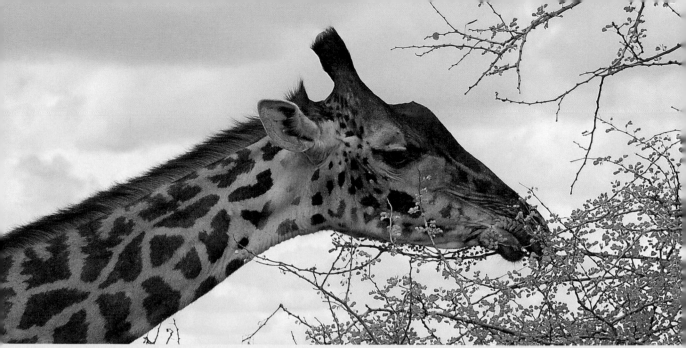

We watched this beautiful *twiga* (giraffe) enjoy his meal of acacia tree leaves during our journey to the Serengeti in Tanzania.

THE TWIGA SALAD

Yield: 4–6 servings

Twiga is the Swahili word for giraffe. While we were on safari in the Serengeti, whenever we would spot these peaceful, doe-eyed plant eaters, we would get so excited and would urge our guide, Tumaini, to stop the Jeep. He couldn't believe how long we wanted to watch the giraffes eat the leaves of the acacia trees. "Don't you want to go see more lions?" he would mutter from the front. But John and I loved watching the giraffes crunch away! Giraffes are amazing chewers, and they chew each bite so thoroughly, smacking their superthick lips. They are so adorably goofy looking, with their long eyelashes, gangly legs and all! This crunchy salad will give *you* something satisfying—as well as beauty building—to crunch on when you need it.

INGREDIENTS:

2 cups diced purple cabbage

1 cup diced carrots

1 cup diced cucumber

1 cup diced celery

Vegan Beauty Ranch Dressing (page 289)

1 cup wild arugula or mixed greens, for serving

DIRECTIONS:

▸ Combine the cabbage, carrots, cucumber and celery in a large serving bowl. Fold in the Vegan Beauty Ranch Dressing and toss well.

▸ Arrange the arugula on individual plates. Spoon the salad atop the arugula and serve at once. Chomp away, like a happy *twiga* in the Serengeti!

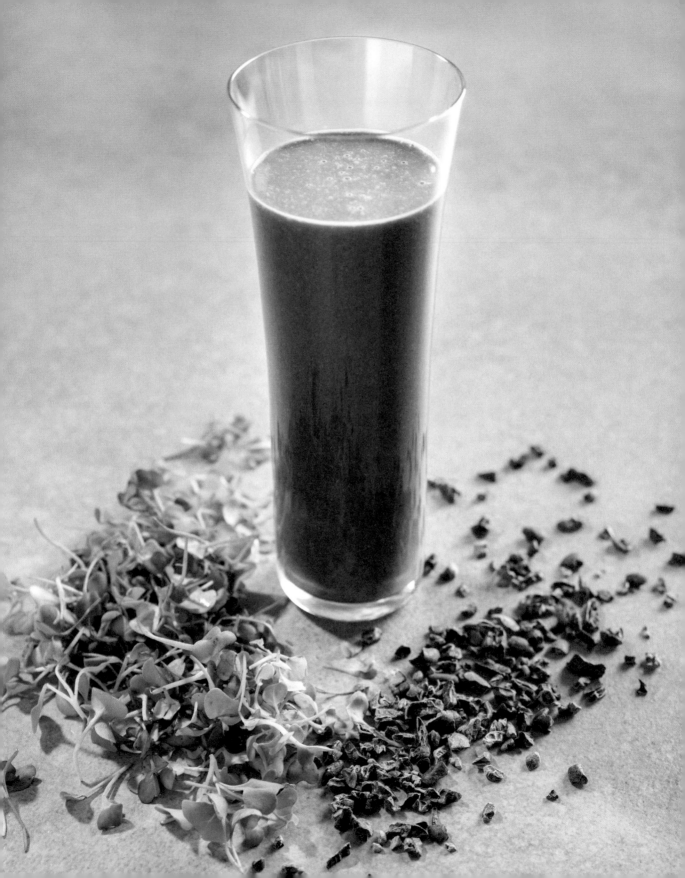

CHOCOLATE

CHOCOLATE AND SPROUT LOVE SHAKE

Yield: One 16-ounce serving

Green is the color of the heart chakra, and green sprouts are an incredibly nourishing food to consume as an act of self-love. They provide you with enzymes, antioxidants, vitamins and minerals. When a chocolate craving consistently arises, you may be seeking love at a deeper emotional level. With this recipe, you can indulge in some chocolate while simultaneously fostering more appreciation and love for yourself by including the supernourishing sprouts.

INGREDIENTS:

1 cup sliced ripe banana (frozen works best)

1 cup unsweetened almond milk

¾ cup sunflower sprouts (clover or broccoli sprouts work well, too)

1 tablespoon raw cacao powder

Stevia or coconut nectar, to taste

DIRECTIONS:

▸ Add all the ingredients to a blender and blend until smooth. Serve at once.

▸ Enjoy with gratitude for yourself, because you are awesome.

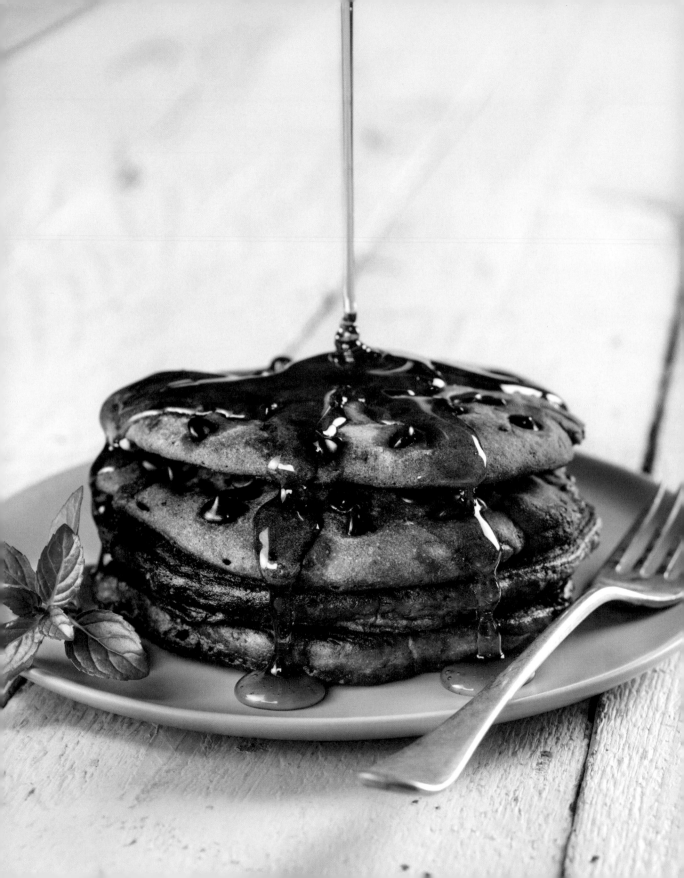

CHOCOLATE CHIP GALAXY PANCAKES

Yield: About 12 pancakes

When I was in high school, I used to go to diners with my friends after the movies, and I would always order chocolate chip pancakes. I loved them! I've devised my own gluten-free, vegan version with the help of antioxidant- and mineral-rich raw cacao, which takes these pancakes to the next level—or galaxy! Hey, I work with a lot of movie super-heroes. The batter is a bit thicker than regular pancake batter, so it holds together and the pancakes can be flipped pretty easily.

INGREDIENTS:

¾ cup brown rice flour

⅓ cup dark chocolate chips or carob chips

½ cup sorghum flour or millet flour

⅓ cup tapioca starch

¼ cup raw cacao

2 teaspoons baking powder

½ teaspoon sea salt

1½ cups unsweetened almond milk

⅓ cup coconut nectar or maple syrup

¼ cup Ener-G Egg Replacer mixed with ⅓ cup very hot filtered water

1 teaspoon vanilla extract

DIRECTIONS:

▸ Combine all the dry ingredients in a medium bowl and mix well. Stir together all the wet ingredients in a separate medium bowl. Fold the flour mixture into the almond milk mixture and whisk until smooth.

▸ Heat a large non-Teflon, nonstick skillet (such as a ceramic or "green" pan) over medium-high heat. Add just enough coconut oil to lightly coat the skillet.

▸ Cook the pancakes in batches. Flip the pancakes over once you start to see bubbles on the surface. Each side should cook for a few minutes.

▸ These pancakes are best served at once, with coconut nectar as a topping, if desired. However, if you manage to have any left over, you can save them for later or for tomorrow!

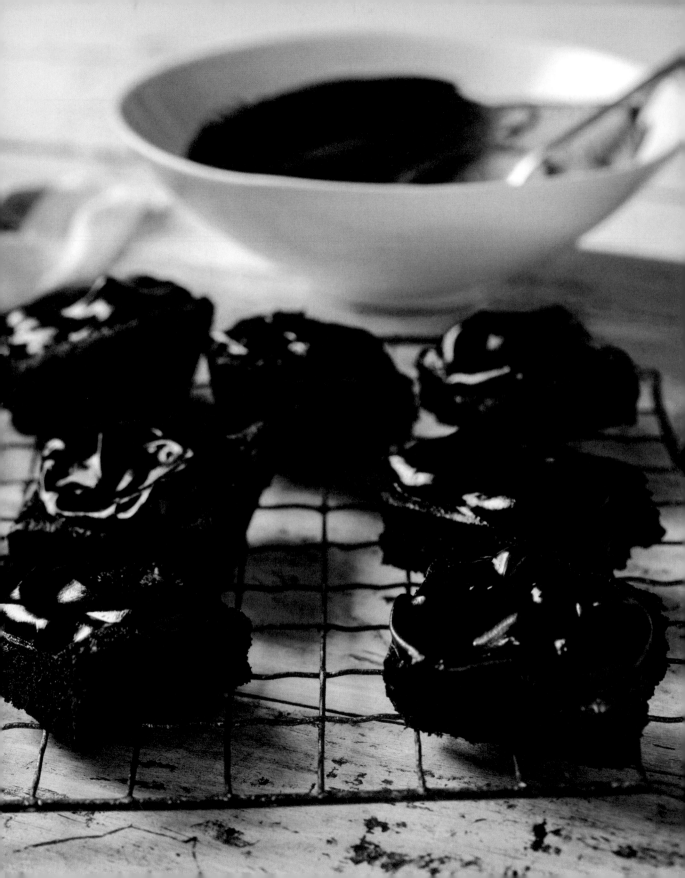

KIMBERLY'S BROWNIES WITH RAW CACAO GLAZE

Yield: About 16 brownies

It seems I end up sending these brownies all around the country, to wherever my clients might be at that moment. We all love chocolate sometimes, don't we! These brownies are treats, but they are far healthier than other varieties. I mentioned it earlier, but let me reiterate: these brownies are plant-based, gluten-free and soy-free, are well combined (no mixing of nuts/protein and starches), and don't contain any vegetable oils or vegetable oil–based products (such as vegan butters). It took making a lot of versions to perfect these brownies, and it ended up being a true labor of love to make them both simple and foolproof, so adding my name here is a way of offering my love to *you* when you make them for yourself.

BROWNIE INGREDIENTS:

¼ cup coconut oil, plus more for greasing the baking dish

½ cup brown rice flour

¼ cup sorghum flour

½ cup tapioca starch

½ cup raw cacao powder

1 teaspoon baking powder

½ teaspoon Celtic or Himalayan sea salt

½ cup coconut nectar or maple syrup

2 teaspoons vanilla extract

½ tablespoon Ener-G Egg Replacer mixed with 2 tablespoons very hot water

GLAZE INGREDIENTS:

½ cup mashed Hass avocado

¼ cup coconut nectar

¼ cup raw cacao powder

3 tablespoons coconut oil

2 tablespoons filtered water

1 teaspoon vanilla extract

1 teaspoon stevia

Pinch of sea salt

DIRECTIONS:

▸ Preheat the oven to 325°F, and grease a 9 x 9-inch baking dish with coconut oil.

▸ Mix together all the dry brownie ingredients in a large mixing bowl. Add the ¼ cup coconut oil, the coconut nectar, vanilla extract, and the Ener-G Egg Replacer and water mixture, and whisk until smooth and well combined. Transfer the batter to the prepared baking dish and bake for 12 minutes.

▸ While the brownies are baking, combine all the glaze ingredients in a small bowl and whisk until thoroughly combined. Really work out those avocado chunks! Cover the glaze and allow it to set in the fridge while the brownies continue to bake.

▸ Remember that you want your brownies to be moist. They do take a little bit of time to set, so keep that in mind instead of overbaking them. No brownie rocks here! After baking, let the brownies cool at room temperature for at least 30 minutes, or stick them in the freezer to help them set. If the middle still feels too gooey after 30 minutes at room temperature, just stick the brownies in the freezer for a few moments to harden them. (Remember, there are no eggs or dairy or anything else in them that has to be fully cooked to be safe to eat).

▸ Once the brownies are cool, spread the glaze on top. Cut the brownies into squares and enjoy!

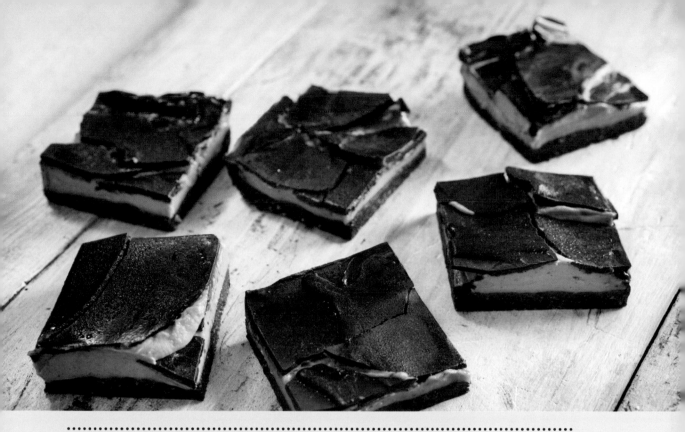

TRIPLE-LAYER RAW CHOCOLATE MINT CREAM BARS

Yield: About 12 bars

The multiple layers to this dessert add some prep time, but it is well worth it! A little piece goes a long way, and you can store these bars in your fridge for a few weeks. This recipe will always remind me of my beloved friend Tony, since I first made it as a "birthday cake" for him one year. Try it for yourself as a celebration dessert. No one will miss the cake.

BASE INGREDIENTS:

Parchment paper, for lining the loaf pan

½ cup raw almonds

½ cup raw pecans

1 cup medium Medjool dates, soaked and well drained

¼ cup cacao powder

Pinch of sea salt

MINT CREAM FILLING INGREDIENTS:

2 small ripe Hass avocados, peeled and pits removed

⅓ cup chopped fresh mint

⅓ cup coconut nectar

¼ teaspoon organic peppermint flavor

¼ cup melted coconut oil

CHOCOLATE TOPPING INGREDIENTS:

¼ cup coconut oil

¼ cup raw cacao powder

2 tablespoons coconut nectar

½ teaspoon stevia

⅓ teaspoon organic peppermint flavor

DIRECTIONS:

▸ Line the bottom of a 9 x 5-inch loaf pan with parchment paper. Be sure to leave an overhang so it's easier to remove the finished bars. Set aside.

▸ Prepare the base. Combine the almonds and pecans in a food processor, and process to form a coarse meal. Add the dates and process until the dates are broken down. Add the cacao powder and sea salt, and pulse to combine. The nut-date mixture should stick together when pressed between two fingers. Press the nut-date mixture into the bottom of the prepared loaf pan and set in the freezer to make a crust while you prepare the filling.

▸ Prepare the filling. In a high-speed blender, process the avocados, mint, coconut nectar and peppermint flavor until smooth. You may need to stop the blender and scrape down the sides a few times. Add the melted coconut oil and blend for a few seconds to combine. The mint mixture should be thick and creamy. (If your blender doesn't process the mixture very well, try blending it in batches until smooth.)

▸ Remove the loaf pan from the freezer. Pour the avocado-mint mixture on top of the nut-date crust, smoothing it out with an offset spatula or the back of a spoon. Return the loaf pan to the freezer and let the avocado-mint layer get firm, at least 1 hour.

▸ Prepare the chocolate topping. You're almost there! Last layer, here we go. Whisk together all the ingredients in a small bowl until smooth.

▸ Remove the loaf pan from the freezer once again and pour the chocolate topping on top of the avocado-mint layer, smoothing it out quickly with an offset spatula or the back of a spoon. Return the loaf pan to the freezer one last time and allow the topping to set, at least 1 to 2 hours.

▸ To cut this into bars, remove the triple-layer block from the loaf pan by pulling up on the parchment paper. Set it on a cutting board. Place a sharp serrated knife in a jar of hot water for several minutes, wipe it with a kitchen towel, and then, using a light sawing motion, cut the block into squares. It's okay if the top cracks (I think it actually looks pretty that way), but try to keep all the layers intact. Warm the knife in the water as needed to cut all the squares.

▸ Store the bars in an airtight container in the freezer for up to 3 weeks (if they last that long!).

BEVERAGES

FRESH CUCUMBER COOLER

Yield: 1 serving

I created this invigorating cocktail with my wonderful team at Glow Bio, my organic juice, smoothie and cleanse company. We have a lot of passion about putting life-changing drinks into people's bodies to make a healthier world. Never doubt that a drink can change your life. This one is a great one to sip after a long day or on the weekends, as a nice reward. Well done, for just being you and taking care of yourself!

INGREDIENTS:

1 medium cucumber (about ¼ pound)

2 tablespoons fresh mint leaves, plus a few sprigs for garnishing

¾ cup cool filtered water

2 tablespoons freshly squeezed lime juice

Stevia or coconut nectar, to taste

DIRECTIONS:

▸ Peel the cucumber if it is nonorganic. Cut a single thin slice from one end of the cucumber and reserve. Juice the cucumber and the mint together in a juicer. If no juicer is available, blend the cucumber, mint and water in a blender or food processor, and then strain the mixture through a cheesecloth. Pour the cucumber juice into a tall glass.

▸ Stir in the lime juice and filtered water (if you did not blend the water in already), and sweetener if you choose to add. You can shake this drink in a cocktail shaker with a little ice if you really want to emulate a cocktail, though digestion-wise drinking this cool but without ice is more ideal.

▸ Garnish the cooler with a beautiful sprig of fresh mint and the reserved cucumber slice.

CRANBERRY, LIME AND BASIL SPRITZER

Yield: About 3 servings of fizzy deliciousness

This is a fizzy drink that you can whip up in batches to help get over any soda addictions. The basil steeps in the drink and adds a fresh herbal flavor. Bonus: the cranberry is a great natural de-bloater!

INGREDIENTS:

1 pint sparkling water

¼ cup freshly squeezed lime juice

3 tablespoons unsweetened cranberry concentrate

1½ teaspoons stevia or 1 tablespoon coconut nectar (or more for a sweeter spritzer)

¼ cup packed fresh basil leaves

DIRECTIONS:

▸ Mix together the sparkling water, lime juice, cranberry concentrate and stevia in a carafe or pitcher until well combined. Stir in the basil leaves. Serve at once! Or you can store this spritzer in an airtight container for an hour or so to let the basil flavor seep in more, without losing the carbonation.

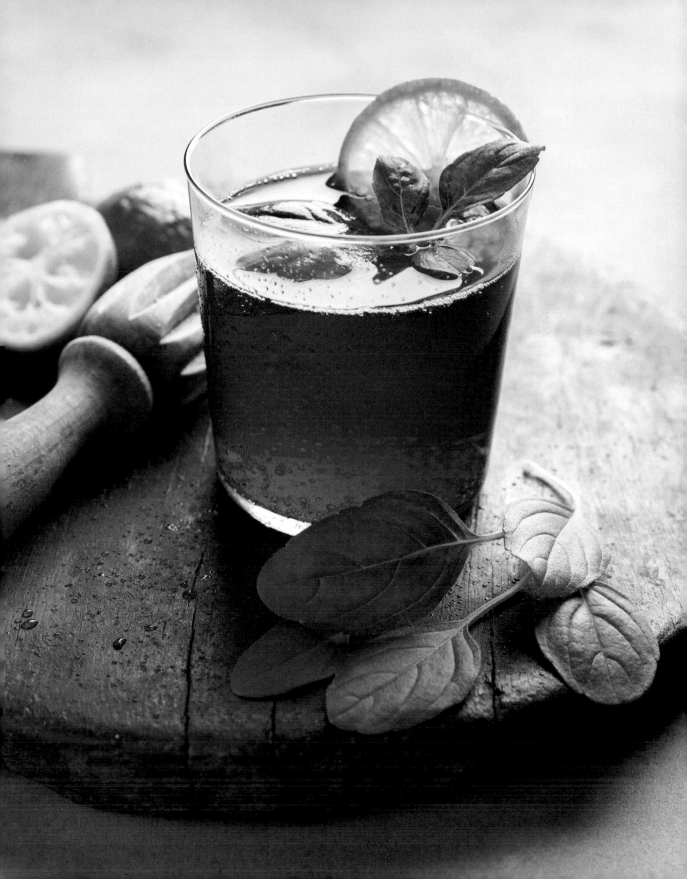

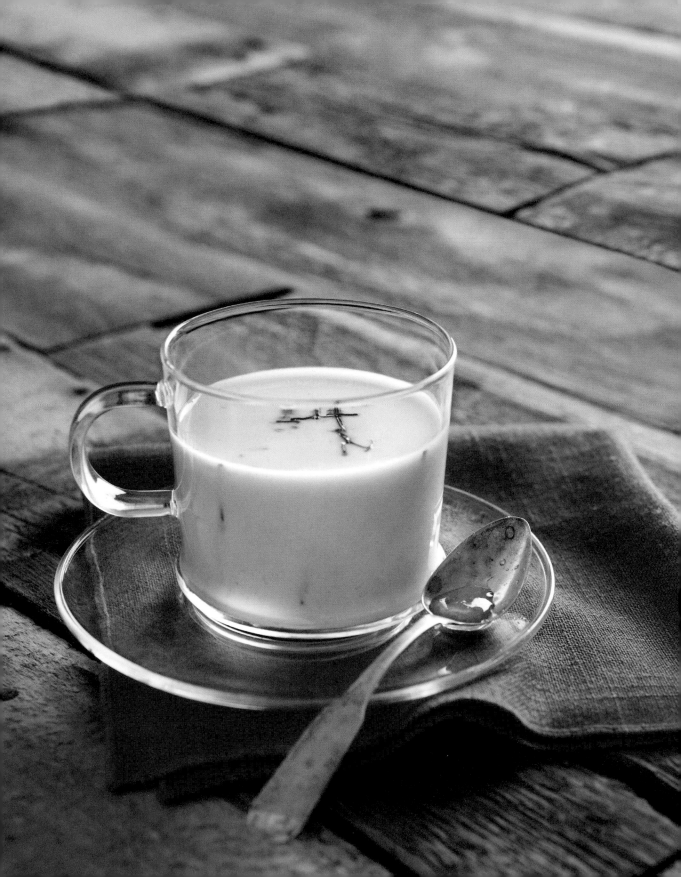

NOURISH YOUR NERVOUS SYSTEM ELIXIR

Yield: 1 serving

This elixir is based on Ayurveda principles of nourishing your nerves. Your nerves are coated in a layer of fat, called the myelin sheath, which insulates, protects and guides the electric impulses of your neurons. All the ingredients in this recipe have been chosen for their specific enriching qualities. Almonds, with their beauty fat, vitamins and minerals, feed this protective fatty barrier, which helps you handle stress without allowing it to accumulate and overstimulate you. Cardamom is related to ginger and has warming, digestive-enhancing properties. It is also a diuretic, and so it helps flush toxins out of your kidneys. Saffron improves circulation and purifies the blood. This is a great recipe to sip in the evening, as you start to wind down, to help encourage peaceful beauty rest.

INGREDIENTS:

1½ cups unsweetened almond milk

2 teaspoons honey (preferably raw) or coconut nectar

½ teaspoon ground cardamom

Pinch of saffron (or turmeric)

DIRECTIONS:

▸ Heat the almond milk in a small saucepan over medium heat to just under a boil. Stir in the honey, cardamom and saffron, and enjoy at once.

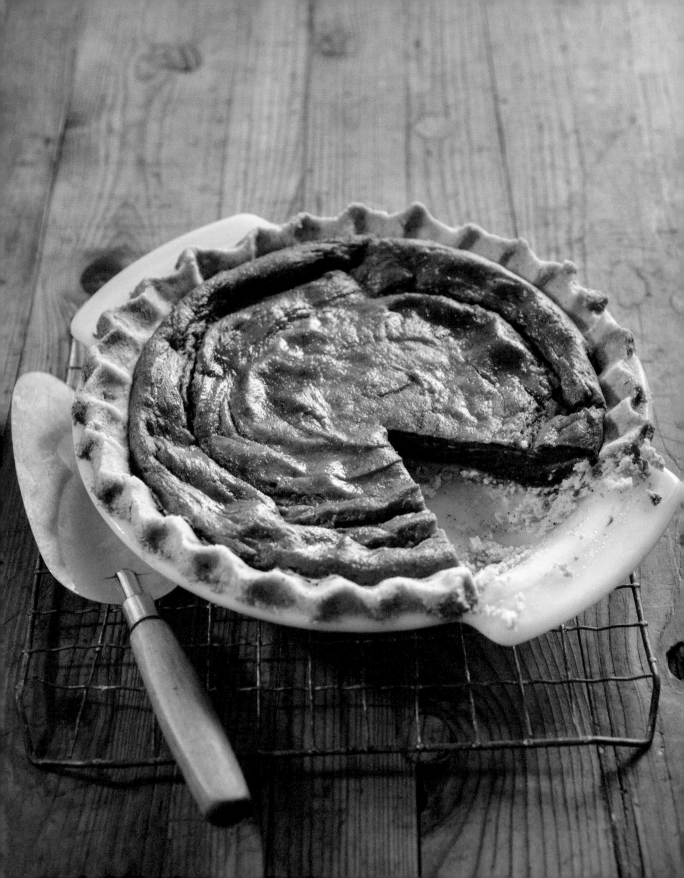

SWEETS

JOHN'S CRISPY CRUST PUMPKIN PIE

Yield: One 9-inch pie

I consider this crust to be a masterpiece, if I do say so myself! Properly Beauty Food paired, gluten-free and crispy. Woo-hoo! I love that you can get organic pumpkin puree in cartons rather than in aluminum cans, and it really makes the filling of the pie much easier to create. This is for my hubby, John, who does have a sweet tooth and loves this pie.

CRUST INGREDIENTS:

½ cup coconut oil, plus more for greasing the pie plate

1 cup brown rice flour

¼ cup tapioca flour

¼ cup filtered water

3 tablespoons arrowroot starch

¾ teaspoon xanthan gum or guar gum

½ teaspoon sea salt

PUMPKIN FILLING INGREDIENTS:

1½ cups organic pumpkin puree (from a carton)

¾ cup unsweetened coconut milk

¼ cup brown rice flour

½ cup coconut nectar or maple syrup

2 tablespoons tapioca starch

1 tablespoon Ener-G Egg Replacer mixed with ¼ cup very hot filtered water

2 teaspoons vanilla extract

2 teaspoons baking powder

1 teaspoon ground cinnamon

½ teaspoon xanthan gum

½ teaspoon sea salt

½ teaspoon ground nutmeg

DIRECTIONS:

▸ Preheat the oven to 400°F. Lightly grease a 9-inch glass pie plate with coconut oil.

▸ Combine all the crust ingredients in a food processor and process until well blended. Press the dough into the sides of the pie plate. Cover the pie plate and place it in the fridge to let it set while you work on the pumpkin filling.

▸ Combine all the pumpkin filling ingredients in a large mixing bowl. Beat with an electric mixer until smooth and creamy. Stop and scrape down the sides of the bowl, if necessary, to incorporate all the dry ingredients.

▸ Pour the pumpkin filling into the prepared crust and spread it out evenly, smoothing it with a spatula or a spoon. Pour some love in, as well, which is essential for baking.

▸ Bake the pie in the center of the oven for 10 minutes. Lower the oven temperature to 350°F and continue to bake for an additional 45 minutes, or until the pie is firm but still gives a little when lightly touched.

▸ Transfer the pie to a wire rack to cool completely. Once the pie is cool, cover and chill it in the refrigerator for at least 4 hours to achieve the best taste and texture. Chilling the pie overnight is even better.

RAW HALVAH WITH A CHOCOLATE LOVE LAYER

Yield: 12 pieces

This dessert is a little unexpected, especially if you are like me and don't eat plain sesame seeds that often. Though I eat tahini on a semiregular basis, plain sesame seeds have a different, earthier flavor. They are an excellent source of calcium, zinc, iron and other minerals, as well as protein. The chocolate atop the halvah adds an extra layer of love.

HALVAH INGREDIENTS:

Plastic wrap or parchment paper, for lining the baking pan

2 cups raw sesame seeds, soaked overnight and rinsed

⅔ cup unsweetened coconut flakes

½ cup honey (preferably raw) or coconut nectar

3 tablespoons coconut oil

½ teaspoon sea salt

CHOCOLATE LOVE LAYER INGREDIENTS:

½ cup raw cacao powder

⅓ cup coconut nectar or maple syrup

¼ cup coconut oil, softened

DIRECTIONS:

▸ Line an 8-inch square baking pan with the plastic wrap or parchment paper, leaving 2 inches hanging over the edges so it's easy to lift the halvah out of the pan.

▸ Make the halvah. Grind the sesame seeds in batches in a spice grinder or a food processor. Let those little seed babies really grind down for easier digestion of their nutrients! Next, add the coconut flakes, honey, coconut oil and sea salt and process until smooth. Press the sesame seed mixture into the bottom of the prepared baking pan, and cover and place in the refrigerator to set while you make the Chocolate Love Layer.

▸ Make the Chocolate Love Layer. Mix together all the Chocolate Love Layer ingredients in a small bowl until well blended.

▸ Remove the baking pan from the refrigerator and pour the Chocolate Love Layer mixture (with love, of course!) over the halvah, spreading it evenly with a spatula or a spoon. Cover the baking pan, place it back in the refrigerator, and allow the halvah to set for at least an hour.

▸ To serve, lift up on the plastic wrap edges and pull the entire square of halvah out of the baking pan. Transfer it to a cutting board. Cut the halvah into 12 pieces and arrange them on a serving plate. You can store the halvah, covered, in the refrigerator for about a week or in the freezer for a few weeks.

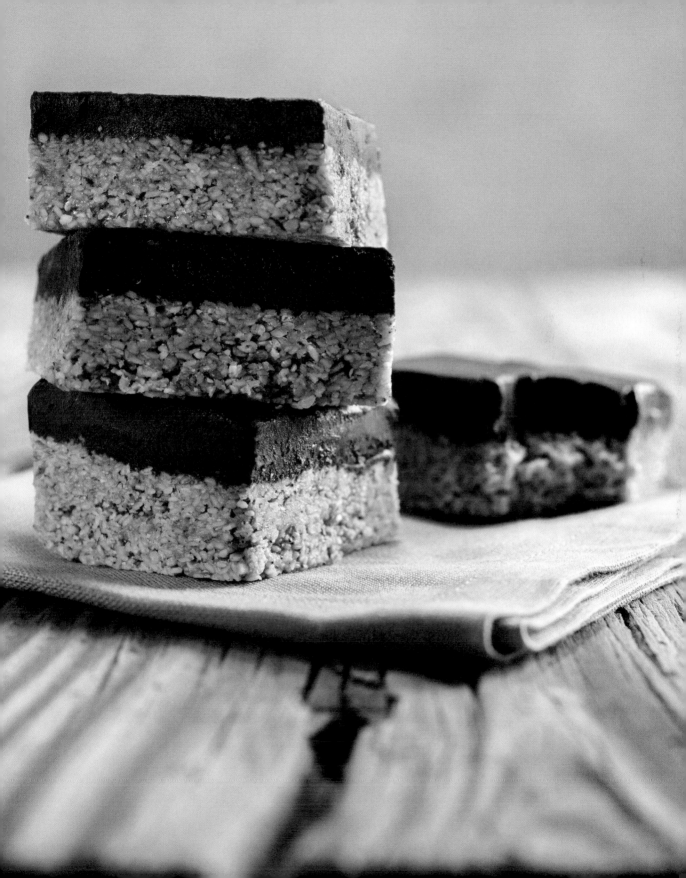

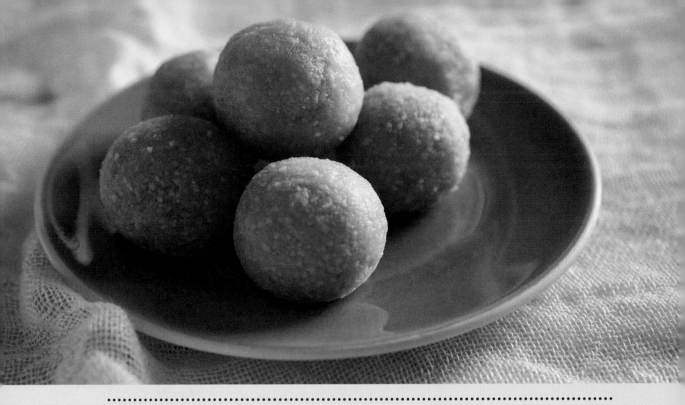

BLONDE BEAUTY TRUFFLES

Yield: About 12 truffles

The combination of these ingredients is simply decadent and incredibly satisfying. You can keep these truffles in the freezer, as I do, and just pop one out when you need a sweet indulgence. If it's hard for you to stick to just one or a few, reserve them for special occasions or make some for yourself and give the rest to your friends, who will be *very* grateful.

INGREDIENTS:

2 cups unsweetened coconut flakes

⅔ cup ground raw almonds

2 tablespoons maple syrup

2 tablespoons coconut oil

1 teaspoon vanilla extract

½ teaspoon sea salt

DIRECTIONS:

▸ Process the coconut flakes in a food processor to make a powder. Add the ground almonds and pulse to combine. Next, add the maple syrup, coconut oil, vanilla extract and sea salt, and process again to blend well. The coconut-almond mixture will be quite sticky and moist.

▸ With clean hands, roll the coconut-almond mixture into balls the size of gum balls and arrange them on a plate. Try not to eat too much! Cover and refrigerate the truffles for at least 10 minutes before serving so that they harden and chill slightly.

Endnotes

A full list of references used in the

writing of this book can be found at

WWW.KIMBERLYSNYDER.COM

Metric Conversion

WEIGHT MEASUREMENT CONVERSIONS

U.S.	METRIC
¹/₄ oz	7 g
¹/₂ oz	15 g
1 oz	30 g
2 oz	60 g
3 oz	90 g
4 oz	113 g
5 oz	150 g
6 oz	170 g
7 oz	200 g
8 oz (¹/₂ lb)	225 g
9 oz	250 g
10 oz	300 g
11 oz	325 g
12 oz	350 g
13 oz	375 g
14 oz	400 g
15 oz	425 g
16 oz (1 lb)	450 g
1¹/₂ lb	750 g
2 lb	900 g
2¹/₄ lb	1 kg
3 lb	1.4 kg

VOLUME MEASUREMENT CONVERSIONS

U.S.	METRIC	IMPERIAL
¹/₄ tsp	1.2 ml	
¹/₂ tsp	2.5 ml	
1 tsp	5.0 ml	
1 Tbsp (3 tsp)	15 ml	¹/₂ oz
¹/₄ cup (4 Tbsp)	60 ml	2 fl oz
¹/₃ cup (5 Tbsp)	80 ml	2.5 fl oz
¹/₂ cup (8 Tbsp)	120 ml	4 fl oz
²/₃ cup (10 Tbsp)	160 ml	5 fl oz
³/₄ cup (12 Tbsp)	180 ml	6 fl oz
1 cup (16 Tbsp)	250 ml	8 fl oz (¹/₂ pint)
1¹/₄ cups	300 ml	10 fl oz
1¹/₂ cups	350 ml	12 fl oz
2 cups	475 ml	16 fl oz (1 pint)
2¹/₂ cups	625 ml	20 fl oz
4 cups (1 quart)	950 ml (1 liter)	32 fl oz (2 pints)

OVEN TEMPERATURE CONVERSIONS

GAS MARK	FAHRENHEIT	CELSIUS	GAS MARK
¹/₄	225	107	¹/₄
¹/₂	250	120	¹/₂
1	275	135	1
2	300	150	2
3	325	170	3
4	350	180	4
5	375	190	5
6	400	200	6
7	425	220	7
8	450	230	8
9	475	240	9

Index

Acknowledgments

I'd like to express the greatest gratitude first and foremost to my husband, John, for being my love and best friend. I am incredibly grateful for our sacred and rare connection. Thank you also for being an incredible rock of support. It's an honor to walk the path together. I love you. Thank you to my parents, Sally and Bruce Snyder, who have been there for me, with love and support, through the many waves of the adventure of my life. I love you both. And big thanks to my amazing Mom for also helping me test all these recipes (a few times)! Deep thanks also go to my beloved Auntie, other family members, all my dear friends, my clients and my teachers, who, in many different ways, have taught me countless invaluable lessons about love, evolution and growth at every step of my life journey. The entire Beauty Detox community deserves my thanks. You are an important part of the whole, and I appreciate you deeply.

I am beyond grateful for my close Beauty Detox team, including and especially AJ Chauhan, who is highly talented in creative and analytical realms alike, and is a beloved "coach" to me, and Tony Flores, who is also brilliant in countless intellectual and intuitive ways and is the heart to help hold everything together. And for Katelyn Hughes, our amazing, tireless and fearless Community and Project Manager. I love and appreciate you all more than I can express here. You guys are the best.

Thank you so much to the whole publishing team at Harlequin for working with me on our third Beauty Detox book together, for allowing me the freedom to write what was in my heart and for supporting the message. I am sincerely thankful. I'd like to express my deepest gratitude and love for my wonderful editor, Cara Bedick, and my creative director, Margie Miller, who connected with the material in this book on a heart level. I appreciate our collaboration so much, ladies. I am so grateful for my wonderful literary agent, Hannah Brown Gordon. Thank you for being here every step of the way! And a big thanks goes to Jodi Lipper, my project manager, for helping me organize all my thoughts and streamline the material.

Thanks must also be given to my dear friend and an extraordinary photographer, Ylva Erevall, who shot the cover, as well as many of the interior shots. I also want to thank my hubby John here (again), who is also a great photographer and captured some of the great moments in this book. And I owe a huge thank-you to our beloved Maggie Kinnealy for her commitment and incredible hard work, and for leading the ship. I must express deep gratitude to Forrest, Harry and Lisa Masters, who provided me with a little writing casita in Puerto Rico, where the foundation of this book was written. And thank you to Noelle Beaugureau for helping to style me for some of the interior shots.

A big thank-you especially to Renee Bargh for being such an amazing friend and person. Thank you to Deepak Chopra for the support. I am deeply appreciative. Thank you also to all the great thought leaders who have had an influence on my work, including T. Colin Campbell, Eckhart Tolle, Louise Hay and Dr. Mehmet Oz, among others. And a deep thanks to my amazing team at Glow Bio for helping to spread the GGS and Beauty Detox message of health every day. First, last and through everything, I am eternally grateful to Guruji Paramahansa Yogananda for showing the path to truth and joy. I am a humble *celaa. Tat tvam asi.* Om.

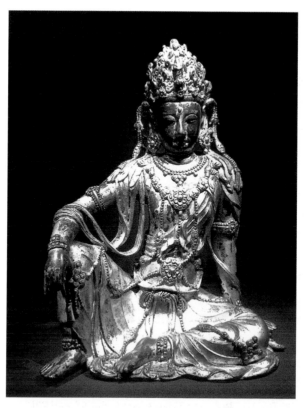

Kuan Yin or *Avalokiteshvara Bodhisattva* that inspired the cover pose.

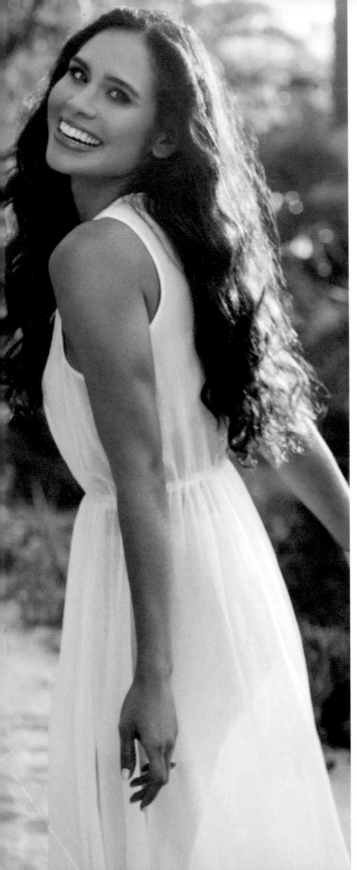

KIMBERLY SNYDER

LIFESTYLE

VISIT US AT

WWW.KIMBERLYSNYDER.COM

Health and beauty information, delicious and healthy recipes, natural weight loss tips, product recommendations and more.

FOLLOW US

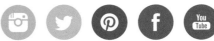

AND JOIN THE COMMUNITY :)

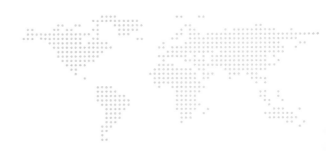

Community members in over 150 Countries